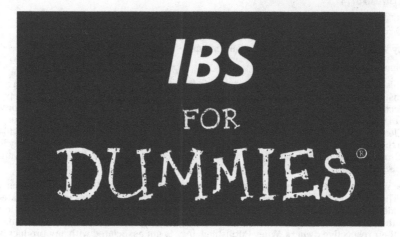

IBS
FOR
DUMMIES®

by Carolyn Dean, MD, ND and
L. Christine Wheeler, MA

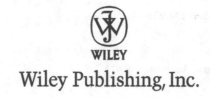
WILEY

Wiley Publishing, Inc.

IBS For Dummies®

Published by
Wiley Publishing, Inc.
111 River St.
Hoboken, NJ 07030-5774
www.wiley.com

Copyright © 2006 by Wiley Publishing, Inc., Indianapolis, Indiana

Published by Wiley Publishing, Inc., Indianapolis, Indiana

Published simultaneously in Canada

For general information on our other products and services, please contact our Customer Care Department within the U.S. at 800-762-2974, outside the U.S. at 317-572-3993, or fax 317-572-4002.

For technical support, please visit www.wiley.com/techsupport.

Wiley also publishes its books in a variety of electronic formats. Some content that appears in print may not be available in electronic books.

Library of Congress Control Number: 2005932583

ISBN-13: 978-0-7645-9814-2

ISBN-10: 0-7645-9814-7

Manufactured in the United States of America

C10003515_081318

1O/RS/RQ/QV/IN

WILEY

About the Authors

Carolyn Dean, MD, ND: Carolyn Dean is a rare breed of medical doctor. She is one of a handful of doctors who has received dual degrees in medicine and naturopathic medicine and bridges the gap between the two. Dr. Dean graduated from Dalhousie Medical School in Nova Scotia in 1978. She is also a graduate of the Ontario Naturopathic College and presently on the board of the Canadian College of Naturopathic Medicine in Toronto, Canada.

Dr. Dean is licensed to practice medicine in California, but her base is in New York, where she publishes, writes, consults, and travels frequently to present rousing lectures to eager listeners on health and wellness issues.

In her private practice, which she ran for 12 years in Toronto (from 1979 to 1992), Dr. Dean treated thousands of patients who came to her with symptoms of IBS. Having seen similar symptoms in her own family and she, herself being sensitive to wheat and dairy, Dr. Dean understands the impact of diet, exercise, and stress on the bowel.

Dr. Dean has written many books, including *Natural Prescriptions for Common Ailments, Menopause Naturally, Homeopathic Remedies for Children's Common Ailments, The Miracle of Magnesium, Death by Modern Medicine,* and *Hormone Balance*. She has also coauthored *Women's Book of Natural Health* and *The Yeast Connection and Women's Health*. She is an advisor to *Natural Health* magazine and the medical advisor for www.yeastconnection.com. Dr. Dean is a regular guest on TV and radio, appearing many times on *The View* as well as Fox, CBS, and NBC, and she has her own radio show.

Christine Wheeler, MA: Christine has been a freelance researcher and writer for 15 years. For the past seven years, she has focused mainly on health and medical topics, including extensive research on the health benefits of nutritional products. She has especially enjoyed providing writing and editorial support to Dr. Dean on various book projects.

In 1999, Christine discovered Emotional Freedom Techniques (EFT). After extensive training and preparation, she opened her private practice in 2002. She has worked with hundreds of people to help them alleviate stress, anxiety, emotional traumas, and the accompanying physical manifestations, including IBS symptoms.

Having had a brush with IBS herself, and using EFT to alleviate the condition, cowriting this book seemed to be a perfect fit and a unique opportunity to help others suffering with this condition.

Dedication

Carolyn would like to dedicate this book to the memory of our parents, Rena and Harold Wheeler. To Mum for her wry sense of humor and amazing spirit, and to Dad for his way with words. And to both of them for giving us early insight into the world of IBS.

Christine would like to dedicate this book to her sweetie, husband, partner, and spouse, Ken Lawson, a constant support and source of fun and inspiration while she worked on what was affectionately known as "the poo book."

Authors' Acknowledgments

First of all, the authors would like to acknowledge each other — this sisterly collaboration made for a sometimes riotous voyage through the research and writing on this serious yet scatological topic.

We thank our agent, Jacky Sach of Book Ends, for offering the opportunity to do this project and helping to get it underway. We have great appreciation for Stacy Kennedy, our acquisitions editor at Wiley, who felt we had what it took to get to the bottom of IBS. We thoroughly enjoyed working with Joan Friedman, our editor at Wiley. She took great care of our words while patiently guiding us through the Dummies process.

We would also like to thank Dr. Irene Grant, our professional reader, for her input and kind words about the book. And thanks to Pam Floener for her insights on the topic of mercury poisoning and mercury detoxification.

We especially appreciate our past and current patients and clients with IBS who, in their efforts to find relief from their condition, have given us the gift of learning. We hope that this book is helpful and that we can continue the dialogue as they delve into this material.

Christine would like to thank Therese Dorer for her limitless friendship, crystal clear insights, and the great rounds of laughter. And to her in-laws, Doug and Sherry Lawson, thank you for understanding when she couldn't come out to play.

Publisher's Acknowledgments

We're proud of this book; please send us your comments through our Dummies online registration form located at www.dummies.com/register/.

Some of the people who helped bring this book to market include the following:

Acquisitions, Editorial, and Media Development

Project Editor: Joan Friedman

Acquisitions Editor: Stacy Kennedy

Technical Editor: Irene H. Grant, MD, CAC

Editorial Supervisor: Carmen Krikorian

Editorial Manager: Michelle Hacker

Editorial Assistants: Hanna Scott, Nadine Bell

Cover Photos: © Max Dannenbaum/ Getty Images/The Image Bank

Cartoons: Rich Tennant (www.the5thwave.com)

Composition Services

Project Coordinators: Adrienne Martinez, Shannon Schiller

Layout and Graphics: Andrea Dahl, Lauren Goddard, Stephanie Jumper, Barbara Moore, Barry Offringa, Heather Ryan, Brent Savage

Special Art: Kathryn Born, MA

Proofreaders: Leeann Harney, Jessica Kramer, Joe Niesen, Carl Pierce, Sossity R. Smith

Indexer: TECHBOOKS Production Services

Publishing and Editorial for Consumer Dummies

Diane Graves Steele, Vice President and Publisher, Consumer Dummies

Joyce Pepple, Acquisitions Director, Consumer Dummies

Kristin A. Cocks, Product Development Director, Consumer Dummies

Michael Spring, Vice President and Publisher, Travel

Kelly Regan, Editorial Director, Travel

Publishing for Technology Dummies

Andy Cummings, Vice President and Publisher, Dummies Technology/General User

Composition Services

Gerry Fahey, Vice President of Production Services

Debbie Stailey, Director of Composition Services

Contents at a Glance

Table of Contents

Introduction

*I*rritable bowel syndrome (IBS) is a functional medical problem that's something of a well-kept secret, even though up to 20 percent of the population suffers from it. Why do we use the word *functional* to describe IBS? Because it doesn't cause structural changes in the body, and there are no laboratory tests that can diagnose it. Why do we call it a well-kept secret? Because even though up to 60 million people in the United States alone may suffer from this condition, you don't hear much about it in the media.

These days, most medical conditions and diseases have networks of fundraisers and public events to help raise money for research. But not many celebrities want to be identified with a bowel disease. (Cybill Shepherd is an exception; she has become the poster girl for IBS-constipation.)

Having IBS can be a very isolating experience, so we want you to know up front that you aren't alone. Most people with IBS don't talk about their problems — not even to their families or doctors.

Luckily, the Internet has really opened up the dialogue on IBS. More people are seeking information and help on IBS Web sites than ever before. And you can even order books like this online, which may prevent some embarrassment.

What's it like to have IBS? Chances are you know all too well! IBS is a condition of bowel disruption. Constipation, diarrhea, or alternating constipation and diarrhea are the hallmarks. Abdominal pain, gas, and bloating make people miserable and unable to function normally. If you don't have IBS (maybe you're reading this book to better understand what a loved one is going through), recall a time when you had food poisoning or a stomach flu and you couldn't stop running to the bathroom. Or think about the worst constipation you've ever experienced. Now, multiply those sensations by 100, and you have some idea what it's like to have IBS.

We dispel two persistent myths in this book:

 ✔ IBS is all in your head.
 ✔ There is no cure.

Because IBS doesn't cause structural damage, and because no lab tests can confirm it exists, some doctors have a hard time accepting it as a valid diagnosis. And some dispute the degree of disability and suffering it creates. But we're here to tell you that IBS is real, and it causes real pain and hardship. And, despite what you may have read or heard, stress does not cause IBS. Stress can certainly aggravate your symptoms, so you want to keep stress to a minimum, but you aren't to blame for bringing IBS upon yourself.

And regarding a cure for IBS, well, the myth is true to some degree: There is no *one* cure that works for everyone. However, there are many remedies, which we discuss in detail in this book. Knowledge is the first remedy, because if you can identify what triggers your IBS, you have the means to halt your symptoms. (And you may even discover that your symptoms aren't the result of IBS at all but a condition that's been hiding from you for years.)

About This Book

Our goals in writing this book are to confirm that IBS is real and to show you the many ways you can successfully deal with your symptoms. Because there is no wonder drug to cure IBS, people desperate for help try all sorts of therapies to find relief. We sort through the good, the bad, and the ugly and present you with the best of the best remedies and therapies for IBS.

While reading this book from beginning to end would make you an IBS genius, you don't really have to do that. You can read Chapter 1 and get a great overview of the book. You can check out the Part of Tens chapters at the end of the book for some great food for thought. Or you can use the table of contents or index to locate chapters and sections that interest you most.

Although there is nothing funny about having a chronic condition, we try to keep things light for one major reason — laughter really is the best medicine.

Conventions Used in This Book

The following conventions are used throughout the text to make things consistent and easy to understand:

- ✔ New terms appear in *italics* and are closely followed by an easy-to-understand definition.
- ✔ **Bold** is used to highlight key words in bulleted lists.
- ✔ All Web addresses appear in `monofont`.

What You're Not to Read

Although we're really fond of this book and obsessed over every word, we recognize that you don't need to read every word in order to benefit from it. If you're looking for just the facts you need to start managing your IBS effectively, you can skip two types of text without missing crucial information:

- ✔ Sidebars, which appear in shaded gray boxes, include information that may interest you but isn't critical to your understanding of IBS.

- ✔ Paragraphs that appear next to the icon called "Technical Stuff" may contain a bit more detail than you want, depending on how intense you want to get in your study of IBS.

Foolish Assumptions

In writing this book, we made some basic assumptions about you. We assume that

- ✔ You have IBS, think that you may have it, or have a friend or family member with IBS.

- ✔ You want information that can help you or a loved one manage IBS more effectively.

- ✔ You want to understand how your bowel works.

- ✔ You want to know if your symptoms could be caused by something other than IBS.

- ✔ You want information on the latest treatments for IBS.

- ✔ You want to work with your doctor to obtain optimal care — and yes, you want to impress him.

- ✔ You want to take charge of your body.

- ✔ You like books with black and yellow covers.

How This Book Is Organized

We have divided this book into six parts so you can skip directly to the ones that draw your interest. Following is a brief overview of each part.

Part I: Just the Facts about IBS

IBS is not something you would wish on your worst enemy, but the more you know about it, the better your quality of life can be. In this part, we first explain what IBS is, what it isn't, and how it differs from bowel conditions that have similar symptoms. Next, we give you the rundown of how your gastrointestinal tract is supposed to work and what can go awry.

Identifying what triggers your IBS symptoms is crucial to improving your health, and in this part we offer a comprehensive discussion of known IBS triggers. Finally, we explain who is most at risk for having IBS and why. (Here's a hint: We're guessing that most of the people reading this page are women!)

Part II: Getting Medical Help

We all want doctors who are knowledgeable and up-to-date on the current research, have great bedside manners, and work with us to provide the best care possible. That goes double for someone with IBS. Because this is a functional condition, your doctor first has to understand that IBS is real and know how to diagnose it. Then, she needs to be willing to help you sort through various treatment options to find the one(s) that make the most sense for your situation.

In this part, we offer advice on what to look for in a doctor, and we explain steps you can take to make your doctor's job easier. We also discuss how IBS is diagnosed so you can talk knowledgeably with your doctor about the tests he orders.

Finally, we devote a chapter to current pharmaceutical treatments for IBS that you and your doctor may consider. No wonder drug exists to alleviate IBS symptoms in everyone, so you need to think long and hard about whether medication is the right avenue for you. We provide the pros and cons so you can make the decision more easily.

Part III: Healing and Dealing with IBS

Healing is a powerful word, and in this part, we aim to give you power over your IBS symptoms.

We start by discussing dietary supplements, herbs, and homeopathic remedies that may improve your IBS symptoms. Next, we move to the all-important topic of diet; an IBS-friendly diet is the cornerstone of any IBS treatment plan. Exercise is also key to good health, especially if you suffer from IBS-constipation, gas, and/or bloating.

We round out this part by presenting information on therapies that can reduce your stress, thus eliminating a possible trigger of your IBS symptoms. We cover acupuncture, the Emotional Freedom Techniques, the relaxation response, biofeedback, transactional analysis, and hypnotherapy.

Part IV: Living and Working with IBS

Having IBS can make you feel isolated, embarrassed, and afraid. It can greatly affect how you interact with your family, your coworkers, your friends, and the world at large. In this part, we offer specific advice on how to tackle your worst fears about public embarrassment so you don't feel trapped in the house. We also discuss how to minimize IBS's impact on your work life.

Children with IBS require special care. The emotional trauma from having such a debilitating condition can potentially cause lifelong strain. In this part, we offer tips for parents so they can help a child with IBS cope.

Finally, we show you some of the most promising current research on IBS, which may translate into an improved quality of life in the near future.

Part V: The Part of Tens

This part is a standard in the *For Dummies* series. The chapters are short and chockfull of crucial information. We present ten common IBS triggers to avoid, ten things you should do when you're diagnosed with IBS, and ten things you don't want to do.

We talk about ten medical tests you should know about so you and your doctor can work together to secure a diagnosis of IBS. And finally, we offer ten resources you may want to check out for even more information on IBS.

Appendixes

The first appendix is a chart that shows you common sources of two types of fiber: soluble (which you want to eat lots of) and insoluble (which you may want to avoid). The second appendix is a handy glossary of IBS-related terms.

Icons Used in This Book

We use icons in the margins of this book to help you find specific types of information. Here's what each icon means:

We use this icon when we tell a story about a client or patient.

This string around the finger highlights information you may want to tuck into your mental filing cabinet for future reference.

The paragraphs next to this icon contain material that's a little more detailed than the rest. You don't need to read these paragraphs to effectively manage your IBS, so you can skip it if you prefer.

This icon points out practical information that you can put into use immediately.

When you see this icon, be on alert: The text next to it warns of potential problems or threats to your health.

Where to Go from Here

This book is designed to be so user-friendly that you can dive in anywhere that interests you and get valuable information. It's a reference book, so you don't have to worry about keeping up with the plot. You can even read the last chapter first if you like!

Part I
Just the Facts about IBS

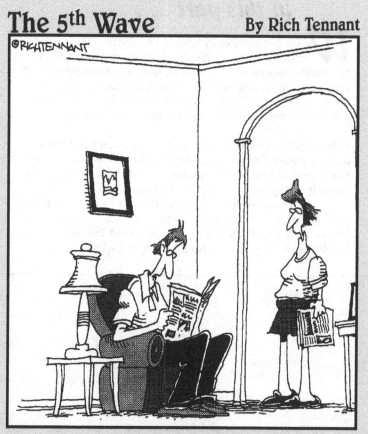

The 5th Wave   By Rich Tennant

"IBS isn't all bad. It was largely responsible for me winning 6 sprinting medals in college track."

In this part . . .

We wish it were easy to give you a list of facts about IBS and move on. But it's not an easy topic. IBS is a *functional* disease, which means it doesn't create structural symptoms in your body to help with diagnosis. Neither does it have a specific medical treatment. And IBS is sometimes mistaken for other conditions.

In this part, we classify IBS and distinguish it from inflammatory bowel disease and other bowel conditions. We give you a peek at your gastrointestinal system, show you how digestion is supposed to work, and tell you why it can go wrong. Triggers for IBS, which we discuss in detail in this part, are especially important to know about because you can avoid many of them and decrease your IBS symptoms. Finally, we let you in on who gets IBS and why.

Chapter 1

IBS Is Real

. . . .

. . . .

*I*BS is a reality for many people. Up to 20 percent of the North American population suffers IBS symptoms, and no single, definitive cure is in sight. That's quite a double whammy.

But here's the good news: We know a whole lot more about this condition today than we did even five or ten years ago. And while there is no miracle drug that can cure IBS, a lot of treatment options exist that can provide relief if you're willing to take some time to figure out what works for you.

In this chapter, we paint a picture of IBS with a broad brush. We give you an overview of what it's like to have IBS (in case you don't have first-hand knowledge). We talk briefly about possible causes and IBS *triggers* — a variety of things that can spark symptoms in someone who has IBS. We also touch on ways you can adjust your diet and take advantage of other remedies and therapies, all of which we cover in-depth in later chapters.

Hiding the Evidence

Even though up to 20 percent of the population has symptoms of IBS (that's an amazing 60 million people in the United States alone), many people won't even mention it to their doctors. Why? Partly the culprit is embarrassment, and partly it's a perception that nobody can help. A majority of people with IBS suffer in silence.

If you have been to a doctor and mentioned your symptoms, you may have been told not to worry. (That's easier said than done when you have pain and your bowels are acting like they're inhabited by alien beings.) Or maybe you were told to just increase the fiber in your diet, which made you feel even worse. Or maybe you were given medications that didn't work. These types of experiences can affect your attitude toward your condition, perhaps making you feel that your situation is hopeless and nobody can help.

As we discuss in Chapter 2, some doctors don't quite grasp the seriousness of IBS or the fact that it's a real medical condition. And even those doctors who really want to help and do understand IBS are limited in the medications that they can prescribe. Unless they spend time counseling you about diet, exercise, stress reduction, and how to handle the emotional impact of IBS, they aren't giving you the best tools available to manage your condition. Throughout this book, we give you those tools.

If you read this entire book, you may actually find yourself educating your doctor about IBS. You will know everything from how IBS is defined (see Chapter 2) to how it's diagnosed (see Chapter 7) to the key role that diet plays in your health (see Chapter 10). You'll be aware of medications that are available to help you through times of acute crisis (see Chapter 8), as well as over-the-counter herbs and homeopathic medicines that can boost your long-term health (see Chapter 9). You'll even find out about stress-reducing therapies, many of which you can do yourself (see Chapter 12).

So, you see, you are in good hands. And there is a wealth of information about IBS at your fingertips that will help change your life.

Knowing IBS Is Real

IBS is a *functional* condition. That means it doesn't cause structural damage to your body, the way a disease does. As a result, there is no laboratory test that your doctor can order to get a quick, easy diagnosis. To diagnose IBS, your doctor must rule out a whole list of other possible bowel conditions and diseases first. All this uncertainty makes IBS seem unreal to some people, who may wonder whether this condition is all in your head.

But you know that IBS couldn't be more real; you have daily symptoms that impinge on your life. Having to urgently go to the bathroom may wake you up in the morning. Or you may wake up feeling fine but be gripped by painful gas and bloating as soon as you eat your first bite of breakfast. If you have constipation, you may have incredible discomfort, and even though you always feel a certain pressure that makes you think your bowels are about to move, nothing ever seems to happen to alleviate your discomfort.

If you're looking for some solid evidence that IBS is real, skip right to Chapter 16. Look for our discussion about the new research into IBS that indicates this condition is related to a biochemical difference in people with IBS: an imbalance of serotonin in the digestive system. Even researchers who used to suspect IBS was a condition of the mind now realize it's a condition firmly rooted in the gut.

What's serotonin got to do with it? Serotonin is a mood-enhancing neuro-transmitter, which can be affected by drugs like Prozac. Amazingly, more than 90 percent of the serotonin in the body is actually produced and found in the intestines. Serotonin affects the movement of food and feces through the intestines.

Recognizing Your Symptoms

IBS is defined by the following symptoms, which most people have in some measure at some point in their lives. What distinguishes IBS from an occasional bout of stomach upset is the _degree_ of the symptoms. Having IBS doesn't mean that once a month you have a loose bowel movement after eating too much fruit. Having IBS means you're chronically affected by one or more of these symptoms:

- Diarrhea
- Constipation
- Alternating diarrhea and constipation
- Abdominal cramps and pains
- Intestinal gas
- Abdominal bloating

To make it easier for you to identify your IBS symptoms, we present a questionnaire in Chapter 7 that you can complete and take to your doctor.

We should warn you up front that if you're female, you have a much greater chance of having IBS than if you're male. As we discuss in Chapter 5, hormones may be partly to blame. Also, young people (even children, who get our full attention in Chapter 15) are more at risk for IBS than older people. After you hit the age of 40, your chances of having IBS decrease significantly. In fact, at menopause, many women with IBS see a significant drop in their IBS symptoms.

Finding a Doctor Who Knows about IBS

Unfortunately, there is no IBS specialty in medicine — and there should be. The next best thing is a doctor who believes IBS is real, listens to your symptoms, does a thorough history and physical exam, rules out all other conditions and diseases, offers you advice on diet and lifestyle, and supports you while you manage your IBS on a day-to-day basis. How do you find such a person? We give you lots of suggestions in Chapter 6.

Half the worry about IBS can be wondering if your symptoms are indicative of something worse. If your doctor does a thorough job diagnosing you (as we explain in the next section), you can be reassured that it's IBS. When you know what you're dealing with, you can focus on treating it.

Diagnosing IBS

Diagnosing IBS is tough, and many people see more than one doctor before getting an accurate diagnosis. Luckily, a group of researchers has created something called the *Rome II Diagnostic Criteria* that outlines the common symptoms of IBS, as well as the frequency and duration of their occurrence, so doctors can know just from your symptoms whether IBS is a possibility. You can find the Rome II Diagnostic Criteria in Chapter 2.

Tangled up in the difficulty of diagnosing IBS are a couple key factors: First, there is no single known cause of IBS, so your doctor can't just look for the existence of some troubling gremlin in your bloodstream or intestines. Second, IBS doesn't cause structural damage to your body, so your doctor can't just look inside you and get a clear picture of what's happening.

Instead, the diagnostic process, which we detail in Chapter 7, involves ruling out a host of other possible diseases and conditions that could be mirroring IBS. Here's a partial list of what your doctor needs to rule out:

✔ **Food intolerances:** Lactose intolerance, gluten intolerance (celiac disease), and fruit intolerance fall into this category. In plain English, these intolerances mean you can't digest dairy, you can't digest wheat, or you can't digest fruit. We discuss these conditions in Chapters 2 and 4.

✔ **Inflammatory bowel disease (IBD):** There are two IBDs: Crohn's disease and ulcerative colitis. They are more serious conditions than IBS, and they cause structural damage to the intestines, such as strictures or ulcerations. Their symptoms often mirror those of IBS but also include rectal bleeding. Crohn's can give symptoms outside the intestines, such as ulcers in the mouth and fissures and fistulas around the anus. We introduce you to both IBDs in Chapter 2.

✔ **Cancer:** Bowel cancer may take the form of a tumor that gradually blocks off the intestines and causes cramping pain that worsens over time. The symptoms of cancer differ from IBS because they can be more localized and more severe.

Considering Causes and Triggers

There is no single cause of IBS that we can pinpoint. We know that some people develop IBS after having an intestinal infection — a nasty bout of stomach flu, food poisoning, or traveler's diarrhea. But we don't know whether the germs themselves or the antibiotics used to treat these infections act as the catalyst to create IBS. And we don't know if the people who get IBS after an infection had a case of smoldering IBS all along.

Quite a few theories exist about why other people get IBS, and we present some of them in Chapter 2. Just keep in mind that these are theories, and all need further investigation before we can know for certain whether they are true causes.

Triggers for IBS are a little easier to identify. A *trigger* is something that causes you to have symptoms after you've already got IBS. We devote Chapter 4 to a discussion of known triggers. Here, we want to just alert you to some of the main culprits:

- ✔ **Antibiotics:** These medications kill off both good and bad bacteria, leaving room in your intestines for yeast to overgrow. An overgrowth of yeast can invade and irritate the intestinal lining, causing micropunctures and the absorption of yeast toxins into the bloodstream. Gas and bloating can also result, triggering additional IBS symptoms.

- ✔ **Yeast:** The overuse of antibiotics, a high sugar diet, stress, cortisone, hormones, and other factors can all lead to an overgrowth of yeast in your gut, which has the nasty effects we describe in the previous bullet.

- ✔ **Food:** Spicy and fatty foods irritate the gastrointestinal tract. Coffee, alcohol, and food additives such as aspartame and MSG also do damage and trigger IBS attacks.

There is far more to the food picture than these triggers. You need to know about conditions that can masquerade as IBS, including food allergies and food intolerances. You may discover that you cannot eat dairy or wheat, or even fruit. (If the thought of giving up any of those foods seems depressing, we urge you to focus on the positive — the reduction in symptoms you'll experience if you can eliminate problematic foods from your diet.)

- ✔ **Stress:** Stress is a major trigger for IBS because many of us hold tension in our guts. That tension causes muscle cramping and can easily escalate into an episode of IBS.

Treating IBS

Just as there is no one cause of IBS, there is no one treatment. Instead, you have a smorgasbord to choose from: medications, herbs, homeopathy, diet, exercise, acupuncture, hypnotherapy, biofeedback, the Emotional Freedom Technique — the list goes on. We discuss each of these options in detail in Chapters 8 through 12.

By far, the most important aspect of treating IBS is getting a firm grip on your diet. We know what a problem that can be, so we devote Chapter 10 to that topic. We walk you through an elimination and challenge diet that allows you to find out what foods are your friends and what foods are not. We also advise you that there is no one diet that works for everyone with IBS. Each person with IBS needs to find what works for her.

We urge you not to let medication be your only treatment protocol. If your doctor insists that a pill is the only answer to your IBS symptoms, fight back with the knowledge you gain from this book. What you eat, how you move your body, and how you process stress are much more important to your long-term health and to managing this chronic condition. Medication certainly has a role to play in helping people get over their worst short-term IBS symptoms, but it simply isn't effective in treating IBS over the long haul.

The combination of IBS symptoms is different from person to person. The cause of IBS is different from person to person. The triggers are different from person to person. Our goal in this book is not to tell you exactly what will work for you. Instead, it's to give you the most complete information possible about what treatments are available, so you can develop your own treatment plan that tackles your particular symptoms.

Coping with IBS

Coping means successfully dealing with a difficult situation. And we have no doubt that if you have IBS, you've got a difficult situation to deal with. But we're here to help you do even more than cope; if you apply the information in this book, you should be able to reduce or even reverse the symptoms that may be plaguing you on a daily basis.

At home, at work, at school — IBS symptoms can strike anywhere. But if you improve your health in the long-term, and if you have plans in place for dealing with even your worst symptoms in the short-term (and even in public), you can break the boundaries that IBS may be placing on your life right now. (If you've been stuck in the house because of IBS and want tips for getting your life back, run — don't walk — to Chapter 13.)

Chapter 2

Classifying the Condition

● ●

● ●

The cause of IBS is difficult to figure out. In fact, the cause seems *impossible* to figure out. When you define a disease like the flu, you imagine that a virus is the cause, and you end up with symptoms of fever, chills, nausea, vomiting, and the like. But in the IBS community, the only thing that everybody seems to agree upon is that there's no agreement about what causes IBS.

The symptoms of IBS, however, are easy to name: Does abdominal pain, diarrhea, or constipation sound familiar?

In this chapter, we help you become more familiar with IBS by discussing possible causes and symptoms, as well as diseases that are often misdiagnosed as IBS. The medical community doesn't yet have all the answers about this condition, but here we provide an overview of what we know so far.

Defining Our Terms

Before we go any further, we want to clarify how we're using several key terms in this chapter and the rest of the book, such as *cause, trigger,* and *associated condition*. Here's how we're describing and distinguishing among them:

✔ **Cause:** An accepted physical reason that your body develops the symptoms of IBS.

✔ **Possible cause:** A possible reason that your body develops the symptoms of IBS; something still up for debate.

✔ **Mistaken identity:** A disease or condition that has the same symptoms as IBS but requires a whole different treatment protocol; it is very important to distinguish between the two.

✔ **Trigger:** A stimulus that sets off an action, process, or series of events. (The event in this case is an episode of IBS, and the action may involve running to the bathroom!) We discuss IBS triggers in detail in Chapter 4.

✔ **Associated condition:** One of several conditions that seem to occur frequently in people with IBS.

So what are the causes, possible causes, mistaken identities, triggers, and associated conditions revolving around IBS? Fair question. It took us months of research to compile the information you find in this book. Here, in a nutshell, is what you can expect to read about:

✔ **Cause:** As we explain in this chapter, many theories exist about the cause of IBS. However, only one cause of IBS is currently accepted by doctors and researchers: IBS can occur after a bowel infection, involving either bacteria or parasites. We discuss this cause in detail in the section "Blaming bowel infections" later in this chapter. However, to be clear, not all people with IBS have had a previous bowel infection. So this is not the *only* cause of IBS — it's just the only one we know for certain at this time.

✔ **Possible causes:** Several possible causes of IBS are being considered:

- *Use of analgesics:* In survey studies, researchers have found that acetaminophen, the ingredient in Tylenol, has been frequently used by people who develop IBS-diarrhea. This drug is known to cause elevated levels of serotonin, and research indicates that serotonin may become elevated in patients with IBS-diarrhea after eating. In Chapter 16, where we talk about current research on IBS, we discuss serotonin-blocking drugs that are being used to treat IBS-diarrhea.

- *Brain-bowel chemical imbalance:* The brain and the gut are intimately connected by both the nervous system and by neurotransmitter chemicals, such as serotonin and norepinephrine. Both chemicals may be involved with the production of IBS symptoms.

  So far, we know that diarrhea can occur when high amounts of serotonin inhibit norepinephrine and cause levels of acetylcholine to increase. On the other hand, when norepinephrine levels increase, the result is constipation, as well as a lowering of serotonin levels and blockage of acetylcholine.

  For IBS patients, this chemical dance may lead to the fluctuating bowel symptoms of constipation and diarrhea. But we must ask what the cause of the imbalance is in the first place. We talk more about the brain-bowel connection in Chapter 12, where we discuss stress and how to manage it.

- *Female hormones:* Considering that men don't have high amounts of female hormone, and men do suffer from IBS, female hormones are not *the* cause of IBS. However, women have twice the incidence of IBS as men. In Chapter 5, we pay particular attention to that discrepancy and discuss how female hormones may play a role.

✔ **Mistaken identity:** The four most common conditions that are mistaken for IBS are covered in this chapter:

  - Gluten enteropathy (celiac disease)

  - Wheat allergy

  - Lactose intolerance

  - Dairy allergy

✔ **Triggers:** In Chapter 4, we address possible triggers of IBS, which come under the following headings:

  - Food allergy or sensitivity

  - Antibiotics

  - Stress

  - Candida albicans

✔ **Associated conditions:** In Chapter 5, we outline a number of conditions that seem to occur in higher numbers in IBS sufferers:

  - PMS

  - Fibromyalgia

  - Insomnia

  - Painful periods

  - Urinary frequency

  - Chronic pelvic pain

These conditions are experienced mostly by women (especially the painful periods!). Fortunately, most experts agree that IBS is *not* associated with inflammatory bowel disease (Crohn's disease or ulcerative colitis, which we discuss in this chapter) or cancer.

Trading Theories about Causes

Often, discussion of the cause of IBS overlaps with discussion of its triggers, which can get confusing. We don't know for certain whether a trigger may be enough to cause IBS in some people — or, if not, whether multiple triggers may do the trick. Is there a recipe for IBS where you have to have a certain amount of triggers to create the symptoms? And if all the triggers are eliminated, will IBS stop?

Whenever this type of uncertainty exists regarding a medical condition, many theories are thrown about to fill in the vacuum. In this section, we share some theories about the cause of IBS that you may be wondering about.

Moving past the stress test

Karen had been to several general practitioners regarding her symptoms of chronic diarrhea, pain, and bloating. She became increasingly dissatisfied with the treatment she was getting from doctors who were unable to make a diagnosis. As she was waiting for one doctor to come into the office, Karen took a peek at her chart and was alarmed by what she read. She saw the word *hypochondriac* in the notes. She realized she was never going to be diagnosed by doctors who simply didn't believe her.

Doctors originally thought that IBS was caused by stress and emotional reactions. There was a *yes, but* approach to anyone with IBS: *Yes*, it's a real condition, *but* people with IBS are really just anxious, depressed, and upset. The condition was equated with an overzealous nervous stomach, and it didn't get much respect.

We do know that bouts of IBS may be *triggered* by stress — we discuss this fact in Chapter 4. However, if stress is *the* cause of IBS, why wouldn't 100 percent of the population have IBS instead of 20 percent?

Quite frankly, IBS still doesn't always get the respect it deserves. We found one 2004 survey of family doctors that indicates the majority of them believe people with IBS and chronic fatigue syndrome are simply slacking off and not pulling their weight in society. That bias can have serious consequences for people trying to obtain a diagnosis and treatment for IBS. (We discuss this topic in detail in Chapter 7.)

But the bias isn't universal; most gastroenterologists (especially those who stay current with IBS research) now know that IBS is a very real condition. However, because IBS doesn't have a single trademark sign or symptom to call its own, just knowing that it's real doesn't mean a doctor can easily diagnose it.

Blaming bowel infections

Sheila had a horrible stomach flu. She was laid up with vomiting, diarrhea, and fever for a week. After she recovered, she dragged herself to work but couldn't seem to get her energy back. She was still having bouts of diarrhea four weeks later that didn't seem to be improving. Her doctor told her not to worry because the problems would eventually go away. But *eventually* began to seem like *forever* to Sheila, and three months after the flu she was diagnosed with IBS.

Frank and his wife, Sally, went to Mexico for a much-needed vacation. Within three days they were both getting the runs and fighting for time in the bathroom. They took an antibiotic that the hotel doctor recommended, which seemed to sort things out for Frank. But Sally didn't get much better. When they got home, Sally's doctor (after several false starts with antidiarrhea medication) finally diagnosed parasites. The antiparasite medications were harsh, but after several weeks Sally was feeling somewhat better. However, she never completely recovered and was finally diagnosed with IBS.

For some people with IBS, like Sheila and Sally, the cause can be identified definitively as a bowel infection. The infection may be due to either bacteria or parasites, and the IBS that results from it is called *post-infectious IBS*. (Something to keep in mind: Women seem to suffer more bowel symptoms for a longer period of time after a gastroenteritis attack than men. We compare IBS in women and men in Chapter 5.)

According to a paper published in the journal *Gut* in 2003, chronic bowel turmoil resembling IBS develops in approximately 25 percent of patients after an episode of infectious diarrhea. The researchers admitted that the research community had previously shown that psychosocial factors operating at the time of, or prior to, the acute illness appeared to predict the development of post-infectious IBS. (As we explain in the previous section, many people have incorrectly placed the blame for IBS on stress.) The new research, however, showed an increased number of inflammatory cells in the rectum persisting for at least three months after the acute infection. The researchers concluded that there is definitely an organic component involved in the development of post-infectious IBS.

How infection can cause IBS

IBS research on why and how infection causes IBS focuses on two areas:

✔ How the inflammation that accompanies a bowel infection damages nerves in the gut lining and alters the way the gut nervous system works

✔ How a low-grade inflammation remains in the gut following the infection

In general, acute GI infections cause inflammation of the mucus membrane lining the intestines. They initiate a cascade of events that don't stop when they're supposed to. The inflammatory process seems to have a life of its own where immune cells infiltrate the intestinal lining and become a local irritant to the nervous system.

Consuming *probiotics* (good bacteria) either in yogurt or in capsule form is a worthwhile preventive measure when you have an episode of infectious diarrhea. Replacing your good bacteria that may be lost with continuous diarrhea may help to avoid the future development of IBS. The best types of probiotics are those that guarantee that each capsule contains one billion live organisms. See Chapter 9 for much more on probiotics.

Bacteria in the small intestine

Doctors have been looking for the cause of IBS in all the wrong places, according to researchers in California. IBS affects the large intestine; however, no studies have shown inflammation or signs of abnormal bacterial overgrowth or bacterial infection in the large intestine. Going a little further up the food digestion chain, researchers have found an abnormal overgrowth of bacteria in the small intestine.

It seems that bacteria that are supposed to reside in the large intestine are immigrating to the small intestine where the grass is greener. Away from their normal confines, these bacteria begin to feed on the rich smorgasbord of partially digested food in the small intestine.

Let this serve as a warning to those of you who chew once and gulp: If not properly digested, that mouthful of food becomes someone else's dinner.

Feeding, growing, and reproducing, these bacteria release enough bacterial waste to make you feel gassy and bloated. Some of that waste is absorbed into the walls of the small intestine and even into the bloodstream. The immune system is prepared for just such an event and mounts an immune response that leads to flu-like symptoms that are so common in IBS.

With the small intestine under attack, symptoms of joint and muscle pain, headaches, arthritis, chest pain, fibromyalgia, difficult urination, and chronic fatigue are easier to explain. The immune system responds to all these waste products by creating *antigen antibody complexes* — combinations of a toxic protein and an immune system protein — that sometimes, instead of neutralizing the toxic protein, just add to the amount of foreign substances in the bloodstream and body tissues.

It's pretty impossible to get into the small intestine to count bacteria, so researchers use what's called a *hydrogen breath test*. The patient takes a strong drink of milk sugar, and as the bacteria in the small intestine feed on this sugar, they excrete gas that can be measured in the breath over the next several hours. A 2003 study found that 84 percent of patients with IBS had abnormal breath test results suggesting small intestinal bacterial overgrowth. When given either a placebo or antibiotic therapy, breath tests showed that patients who were given antibiotics eliminated their bacterial overgrowth and reported a 75 percent improvement in their symptoms.

But despite these findings, the treatment for IBS is not as simple as taking antibiotics. In fact, antibiotics are also a possible trigger of IBS, as we explain in Chapter 4. They wipe out good and bad bacteria and allow yeast to set up housekeeping in your colon. So before you run out and take antibiotics to wipe out the bacteria in your small intestine, be sure to read Chapter 4 and consider whether you're trading one problem for another.

One doctor's experience with parasites

Dr. Marcelle Pick, an obstetrician and gynecologist, says that when she started her practice in the early 1980s, she was shocked at the number of women who came to her clinic suffering from symptoms of intestinal pain and distress including constipation, diarrhea, gas, bloating after eating, and fatigue.

Dr. Pick would refer these women to gastroenterologists who often diagnosed IBS and simply recommended increased fiber in the diet, which brought minimal relief. Referrals to psychiatrists brought little relief as well. Dr. Pick came to the conclusion that IBS was being used as a catch-all diagnosis for a complexity of symptoms that needed deeper exploration.

Tapping into her own experience of traveling in developing nations where she experienced GI distress due to parasites, Dr. Pick began testing every woman with bowel symptoms for parasites. She says that other doctors are shocked when she tells them that 40 percent of her female IBS patients, even some who have never traveled, test positive for parasites.

Dr. Pick also believes that an overgrowth of Candida due to overuse of antibiotics creates a yeast infection in the intestines that leads to symptoms of IBS. We also believe that Candida infection can cause IBS, but we don't find consensus in the medical community to include it under causes. Instead, we refer to Candida as a trigger and include it in Chapter 4. In Chapter 7, we discuss state-of-the-art tests for Candida overgrowth that will eventually bring Candida into the list of causes of IBS.

Travelers' precautions: We are not alone

It may come as a shock to realize that most of the cells in our bodies are not our own. We carry around about two pounds of hitchhikers wherever we go. There are fungi on our toes, viruses in our nose, and about 100 trillion bacteria and yeast in between. (The cells of our body only number about 10 trillion!) Quite a lot of diarrhea can happen when these bugs get out of control.

You would be hard pressed to find someone whose bowels stayed completely on schedule while traveling. The U.S. Food and Drug Administration says that traveler's diarrhea ruins about 40 percent of vacations for Americans. Water, germs, and a change in diet are bound to either speed up or slow down intestinal movement. You may be used to the bugs in your own environment but not the foreign ones in another country.

Montezuma II was the great chief of the Aztec nation in Mexico at the time of the Spanish conquest leading to the decimation of the Aztec population. The revenge of Montezuma comes in the form of debilitating traveler's diarrhea that almost half the visitors to Mexico take home with them. Water and food may contain bugs that the natives are perfectly comfortable with but that can cause IBS-like symptoms in unsuspecting visitors.

Preparing for air travel

If you have IBS with diarrhea, you may hesitate to travel at all. However, if you plan ahead, you can board a plane without having to fear the worst:

✔ Book your flight in advance and choose a seat that is near the washrooms.

✔ Bring a small roll of toilet paper with you on a flight. Sometimes the sheets provided in an airplane washroom just don't provide the coverage you need.

✔ Pack your own food and water. Take a selection of tried-and-true foods with you on the plane (see Chapter 10 for help figuring out what they may be). Don't rely on airline foods, which could trigger diarrhea.

✔ Consider wearing an adult diaper during the flight if you're concerned about having an accident. (See Chapter 13, where we discuss this option in detail.)

✔ Consider whether you may benefit from taking Pepto-Bismol or Imodium before your flight, which some doctors recommend. But be careful with these medications, which are said to bind together the toxins produced by bacteria in your bowel. You don't want those toxins staying around too long!

When you are traveling, practice safe eating and drinking habits. Quite simply, that means *no tap water*.

✔ Do not drink tap water. That means drinking fountains too.

✔ Do not brush your teeth with tap water.

✔ Do not use ice cubes made with tap water.

✔ Do not eat watermelon, which may be injected with local water to increase weight.

✔ Eat raw fruits and vegetables only if you have peeled them yourself. (That's right; otherwise they may be washed with tap water.)

✔ Do not purchase food from street vendors, because they may not wash their hands (even with tap water).

If tap water, harboring bugs and germs, makes its way into your food, you may be able to avoid a calamity by taking grapefruit seed capsules with every meal. The seeds of grapefruit are very bitter and poisonous to bugs. Another name for these capsules is *citricidal,* and they can be bought in health food stores and some pharmacies.

Considering possible effects of vaccines

We now know that many children with autism suffer symptoms of IBS. Several prominent researchers indicate that they have true intestinal inflammation, which is caused by the live measles, mumps, and rubella vaccine (MMR). Because most of the U.S. population has received MMR shots, the implications of this research are vast. The possibility that some vaccines may trigger bowel inflammation is being heavily researched.

Dr. Andrew Wakefield in the United Kingdom initiated this research at the request of parents of children with autism. These children almost always suffer from symptoms of IBS and also seem to be allergic to wheat, dairy, and other foods. While a child is under anesthetic, Dr. Wakefield inserts a small scope through the nose, down the throat, and into the intestines to find live measles virus in the lymphatic tissue of almost every child he studies.

The immune system of a child who has a cold or some other infection when he is given a vaccine often cannot identify the vaccine virus and fight against it. There is just too much going on in a child's little body. Therefore, the measles virus from the vaccine can stay in the gut and start causing mild inflammation that is barely recognized but that starts to cause food digestion and absorption problems.

Pointing the finger at pent-up gas

In 2004, a group of Italian doctors pulled together all existing data on IBS in an effort to define it clearly. Here's what they concluded:

> *IBS is a functional, multifactorial condition characterized by abdominal pain and irregular bowel habit.*

We talk about what *functional* means in the upcoming section "Faulty Functioning." A *multifactorial* disease or condition is one that has several different causes or contributing factors, such as genetics and environmental influences.

This group of doctors also determined that IBS happens when the muscles of the intestines act erratically. They explain that IBS is more likely to assault people who seem to have an unconscious internal overreaction to bowel gas and bloating and who also pick up more than their share of stress from their environment.

The Italian group added a twist to the mystery of IBS — a new finding of their own. The researchers were excited to find that people with IBS are not able to expel intestinal gas. (You're probably not as excited as they are.) This brilliant new discovery — which some researchers are saying may be a cause of IBS — may come as a shock to you, because people with IBS often feel that they are nature's own gas producers. But apparently people with IBS have a special attachment to gas and don't like to let it go. Most people produce about one to three pints of gas a day, although some people can produce as much as a gallon. Obviously, if even a portion of that amount gets stuck in your system, you're going to be uncomfortable.

Gas with no way out will cause you to bloat and cause your bowel to stretch, creating abdominal pain (the most frequent symptom of IBS). The Italian researchers say that when gas stretches the rectal area of the bowel, the pain activates certain areas of the brain, which makes people feel more symptoms. What they don't say, however, is *why* this problem occurs — what is causing this inability to expel gas in the first place?

Here's our two cents about this theory: People with IBS are fully aware of the phenomenon of *sharting*. (If you haven't heard the word before, it's a colorful combination of our two favorite IBS words: *shitting* and *farting*.) When you experience both at the same time, what's your natural reaction whenever you feel the need to pass gas? Right, you do your best to hold everything in until you know you're safe! And who wouldn't?

In Western culture, passing gas in public is simply not polite. So from a very young age we are conditioned to refrain from farting in public and are often shamed if we happen to let one rip. Another observation is that boys are more likely to be free with their farts than girls. Young ladies are not young ladies if they pass gas in public. Young men, however, have been known to even have farting competitions, which can include shooting *blue angels* — the term for farts that have been lit on fire!

Does this theory fully explain the male/female discrepancy in IBS sufferers? Probably not, but we'd love to see some further research on this topic!

Faulty Functioning

In the previous section, we mention that IBS is defined as a functional condition. We tackle the definition of *functional* here.

We know that the symptoms of IBS are real. Some people with IBS-diarrhea have 10 to 15 bowel movements a day and all the associated painful cramps, gas, bloating, and social discomfort. But IBS does not damage the colon; there is no bleeding, no ulcer, and no tumor. Therefore, it's not a diagnosable *structural* disease. Perhaps, in the future, a blood test or a tissue sample of an

IBS colon will help to identify the ailment, but until then, the condition is labeled a *functional disorder*.

Functional is another way of saying, "Sorry, pal, we really don't know what's happening, but we grudgingly admit that something is wrong, mainly because you keep bugging us about it and running to the bathroom and using up all the toilet paper." Don't quote us on this definition, but many people with IBS spend an average of three years trying to get a doctor to believe that something is really wrong. If that's been your experience, the definition probably rings true.

Science is based on observation, x-rays, laboratory blood tests, and solid evidence of disease. But the sum total of your intestines' daily output is not what doctors and researchers are looking for. Because no structural damage can be observed in an IBS colon, the only explanation available for your symptoms is that your colon isn't functioning properly. This functional impairment results in very real twisting, spasming, gripping, and swelling of the colon, but it does not bleed or ulcerate like other colon diseases, such as ulcerative colitis and Crohn's disease. (We discuss these inflammatory bowel diseases later in the chapter.)

Because of the lack of structural evidence of disease, a diagnostic cloud hangs over IBS. In our experience, most people would rather have a real diagnosis than be in limbo, even though a diagnosis of an inflammatory bowel disease is more serious than IBS. We discuss the diagnostic process in detail in Chapter 7.

Roaming the Criteria

As we explain in Chapter 7, you can be *officially* diagnosed with IBS only when all other infections and related conditions are ruled out. Therefore, most doctors depend on symptoms to define the disease.

Rome seems to have a special place in its heart for IBS. (Maybe it's all that pasta and cheese; we discuss the symptoms of wheat allergy and lactose intolerance later in the chapter.) In 1988, the 13th International Congress of Gastroenterology was held in Rome. That congress developed the Rome II Diagnostic Criteria for IBS, which is the current model followed worldwide.

If you think it's hard to figure out whether or not you have IBS, you're in good company. It took ten multinational working teams collaborating for more than four years to arrive at a consensus for the following symptom-based diagnostic standards.

Note that the Rome II Diagnostic Criteria presumes "the absence of a structural or biochemical explanation for the symptoms."

The Rome II Diagnostic Criteria for IBS state that IBS can be diagnosed based on "At least 12 weeks, which need not be consecutive, in the preceding 12 months of abdominal discomfort or pain that has two out of three features:

1. Relieved with defecation; and/or
2. Onset associated with a change in frequency of stool; and/or
3. Onset associated with a change in form (appearance) of stool."

Rome II also identifies the following symptoms "that cumulatively support the diagnosis of irritable bowel syndrome:

✔ Abnormal stool frequency (may be defined as greater than 3 bowel movements per day and less than 3 bowel movements per week);

✔ Abnormal stool form (lumpy/hard or loose/watery stool);

✔ Abnormal stool passage (straining, urgency, or feeling of incomplete evacuation);

✔ Passage of mucus;

✔ Bloating or feeling of abdominal distension."

For many people, this last item is an ongoing source of discomfort. Bloating can occur to such an extent that a woman with IBS actually appears to be pregnant.

Living the Symptoms

IBS has a way of interfering with your quality of life. By that we mean your home life, your work, sleep, social life, travel, diet, and sex. Did we miss anything? Oh yes, IBS also creates a financial burden, costing you directly for medical expenses and indirectly for time off work or school and lost productivity. The costs of decreased quality of life are immeasurable. (We discuss all these issues in Part IV of this book.)

In the following sections, we discuss various symptoms of IBS, as well as the spectrum of severity that people with IBS can experience.

Listing primary symptoms

IBS has several major symptoms, and not everyone has all of them. Some people have a predominant symptom, such as

✔ Diarrhea

✔ Constipation

✔ Pain 30 minutes to 2 hours after eating

In one survey of almost 9,000 people, 25.4 percent mostly suffered diarrhea, 24.1 percent had a predominance of constipation, and 46.7 percent had alternating symptoms.

The symptoms of IBS that most people experience are

✔ **Abdominal cramps:** These cramps can be achy or colicky and tend to occur in the lower abdomen. They are sometimes relieved by a bowel movement or passing gas. If they start up in a public place, you probably automatically try to put a clamp on them for fear of passing gas or having a messy accident. That reaction only adds to the pain.

✔ **Bloating:** Ninety-two percent of IBS patients regularly let their belts out to accommodate bloat. Bloating comes and goes so fast that you have long since learned that you can't wear anything tight around your waist. Low rider jeans were made for people with IBS. And maybe that's why the pants you see on so many men and women these days are dangling around their hips!

TIP

If you are short-waisted, which means you have very little space between the top of your hip and your last rib, you have very little room for bloat and may experience more discomfort. Are you in this category? Feel for the space at your sides between your hipbone and the bottom of your ribs. If that space is more than 5 inches, you're high-waisted and you have more room for the 20 feet of intestine that go into that space. If you've got less than 5 inches (possibly even as little as 1 inch!), you're short-waisted.

✔ **Diarrhea:** Diarrhea may be the most distressing symptom of IBS. Running to the bathroom, especially at work or in public, can be embarrassing. The anxiety of worrying about finding a bathroom and getting there in time only adds to the problem. Everyone has had an anxious moment when the trigger from the brain makes the bowels churn. For people with IBS, that moment may occur many times a day.

✔ **Constipation:** Chronic constipation is often characterized by straining and pain and a feeling of not fully evacuating the bowel. Although you may have a bowel movement only three or fewer times per week, we know you probably spend much of your time contemplating the relief it will bring. When the evasive bowel movement comes, the stool is often hard and lumpy, and your relief is rarely absolute.

✔ **Alternating constipation and diarrhea:** Having alternating diarrhea and constipation may not seem so bad in theory. But when your days of running to the bathroom constantly are replaced by broken promises of a bowel movement, you end up with another kind of misery. Whereas a bowel movement can relieve the pain and cramping of gas buildup, constipation makes you feel like an uncomfortable beached whale.

Some doctors say that the manner in which stool exits the body can distinguish IBS from infective or inflammation bowel movements. The IBS stool leaves in very brief squirts, whereas the infectious or inflammatory bowel movement vacates with a gush lasting several seconds. This appears to make sense because people with IBS tend to have rectal spasms, which means the rectal contents can be released only in brief squirts. In other conditions such as infection or inflammatory bowel disease (IBD), the rectum is not in spasm, and the contents can flood out.

Recognizing other common symptoms

Aside from the primary symptoms of IBS, some people also experience the following:

- **Excessive gas:** According to the fine folks at the University of Maryland, having gas and burping or passing gas is not life-threatening. (Whew!) Most gas is odorless, consisting of oxygen (from swallowing air), nitrogen, hydrogen, and sometimes methane (which is what gets lit at frat parties). The noxious odor we associate with flatulence is produced by sulfur.

- **Nausea:** Feeling queasy is pretty easy when your stomach and intestines are bloated and pressing up into your diaphragm. Fullness in your digestive system can make you want to gag. When you are constipated, toxins with descriptive names like cadaverine and putrescine can be absorbed into the bloodstream and make you feel sick to your stomach. (The names alone can make you ill!) Other toxic byproducts from infectious bacteria, parasites, and yeast can also be absorbed through the intestinal lining and make you feel unwell. Chapter 4, where we discuss Candida albicans, explains this aspect of IBS.

- **Incomplete bowel movements:** When you have an incomplete bowel movement, you have the sensation that there's more to come. When you experience that sensation, you may or may not actually have more stool to pass. The feeling is strange and makes you *too* aware of your bowels. It's difficult to know what causes the sensation; it may be due to mucus in the intestines.

A severe form of the sensation of an incomplete bowel movement is called *tenesmus,* where the constant feeling of the need to go is painful and involves cramping and involuntary straining efforts. Tenesmus is not associated with IBS but with inflammatory bowel disease.

Another cause of incomplete evacuation is a *fecalith,* which is a hard intestinal mass formed from feces. If it partially blocks the rectum, it can cause symptoms of alternating constipation, diarrhea, pain, and an obvious feeling of incomplete evacuation.

- ✔ **Mucus in the stool:** Don't be alarmed when you see mucus in the toilet. Mucus that coats the stool comes from an irritated intestinal lining from all the cramping, gas, and bloat. The mucus is actually trying to coat the intestines and protect them from the irritation. It also may be partly responsible for the sensation of not quite finishing a bowel movement.

- ✔ **Diarrhea after eating or after waking in the morning:** It is a harsh condition when the mere act of eating causes your symptoms. But, for most people with IBS, the stomach and intestinal juices, sphincters, and muscles can go into overdrive when they simply chew and swallow. And yes, the very act of opening your eyes stimulates your metabolism and can trigger the urge. Standing up adds to the process as gravity drops your intestinal contents to their inevitable end.

Many people with IBS, both with constipation and diarrhea, have reported abdominal cramping and pain that was comparable to child birth and relieved only after several bouts of diarrhea. While seemingly unbearable pain is rare, it is very frightening and can result in trips to the emergency room.

Considering less frequent symptoms

There are even more IBS symptoms, some of which occur in the colon and others that occur in the stomach and esophagus. These symptoms can be rare, but for the sake of being thorough, we want to discuss them here.

The following symptoms occur in the large intestine:

- ✔ Pain under the left ribs that is not relieved by a bowel movement
- ✔ Bloating that subsides at night but comes back the next day
- ✔ Stabbing pains in the rectum, called *proctalgia fugax*

Here's a fun fact: The gurgling in your gut that can be heard across the room actually has a name; it's called *borborygmi*.

The following symptoms occur in the stomach:

- ✔ Stomach pain that can be confused with ulcers
- ✔ An inability to eat a large meal due to pressure from bloating

The following symptoms occur in the esophagus:

- ✔ A sensation like having a golf ball in your throat, which does not interfere with swallowing (called *globus hystericus*)
- ✔ Heartburn, which is burning pain often felt behind the breastbone
- ✔ Painful swallowing, which is called *odynophagia*

IBS does not cause food to become lodged in the esophagus. This problem is called *dysphagia*. If you experience it, talk to your doctor.

Dealing with mild cases

IBS symptoms come in various shades of mild, moderate, or severe. Some fortunate people with IBS have only mild symptoms and maybe an occasional flare-up when the triggers turn into explosions. (See Chapter 4 to find out what your triggers may be.) The majority of people with IBS are lucky enough to be in this group. If you are, you probably have never even seen a doctor about your symptoms. That's why you secretly picked up this book and told the cashier, "It's for a friend." You wanted to see if having three bowel movements a day was abnormal. Rather than make you read the whole book to find out, we'll tell you right now — you're just fine.

Morning movements

Many people have two or three bowel movements in the morning, which is perfectly normal. The excitement of getting up, having breakfast, and maybe drinking one too many cups of coffee may be enough to give you an extra bowel movement or two.

But, as we mention in the previous section, the rise and shine time can trigger IBS in some people. The stress of getting ready for your work day can increase your urgency to visit the bathroom. And if you add a few extra trips to the bathroom in the morning, that can make you run late and further increase your stress, thus increasing your symptoms.

If we've just described your morning, here's a simple solution: Set the alarm 30 minutes earlier, and allow your bowels to get moving. You will have a more relaxed preparation time and perhaps reduced bowel stress. If you have more time before running out the door, you may spend less time running to the bathroom.

Three a day

Having three bowel movements a day, especially if they come shortly after meals, is not a symptom of IBS. In fact, it's just what the doctor ordered. (Well, some doctors believe that a single bowel movement a day is normal, but others of us — especially those who practice traditional medicine dealing with dietary supplements and natural remedies — think otherwise.)

Think of your body this way: What goes in must come out. So when you eat a meal, it makes perfect sense that you need to make room for it. It's only natural. Perhaps you're wondering why we don't absorb more of our food, so that there isn't so much waste. But, as we discuss in Chapter 5, there are billions of bacteria in the intestines that add bulk to your stool.

Even though having more than three bowel movements a day is one criterion for IBS, it's only *part* of the whole picture. If you don't have pain and bloating as well, you probably don't have IBS — your symptoms may be entirely due to what you eat.

Linking other problems to IBS

There are a whole host of problems that may be related to your IBS. In other words, if you have IBS, you have a greater chance of having these other conditions. We talk more about them in Chapter 5, but here is a list of possibilities:

- ✔ Back and groin pain
- ✔ Fatigue
- ✔ Depression
- ✔ Frequent urination
- ✔ Insomnia
- ✔ Painful periods
- ✔ Pain during intercourse

If you're experiencing one or more of these problems, your doctor may be treating them as if they are not associated with IBS. We encourage you to ask your doctor about the possible connection so that you won't be treated for symptoms rather than addressing IBS.

Mistaking Identity

Several conditions have symptoms that are similar to IBS: gluten enteropathy (celiac disease), wheat allergy, lactose intolerance, and dairy allergy. Your intolerance for certain foods can slip by unnoticed for decades, and then one day you hear an item on TV, read an article in a magazine, go online, or read this book, and *wham!* — you just know that wheat or dairy is no longer your friend. You know that eating bread and bagels and pizza and toasted cheese sandwiches is doing you in. Identifying a food allergy can be exciting, because if you stop eating certain foods you have a chance of getting your IBS-like symptoms off your back.

In the following sections, we explain how these four conditions that look like IBS actually work.

Gluten enteropathy (celiac disease)

Gluten is a protein that is mainly found in four grains: wheat, rye, oats, and barley. (Yes, that's toast, rye crackers, oatmeal, and barley soup!) *Enteropathy* is quite simply defined as a disease of the gastrointestinal tract. In this case, the disease is caused by gluten. Some people are extremely allergic to gluten, and some of the symptoms are identical to IBS.

This disease is also called *celiac disease* and used to be called *tropical sprue* (don't ask us why!). It's a genetic disease, but most people don't know they have it. Many families who share the condition just think all that farting and running to the bathroom is normal.

The classic symptoms for celiac disease include diarrhea, short stature, anemia, and weight loss. Doctors are now finding that liver problems, thyroid problems, gas and bloating, skin lesions, and chronic fatigue may also be related to celiac disease.

Gluten enteropathy occurs because the immune system gets the idea that gluten is bad and attacks it using IgA and IgG antibodies. The lining of the small intestine suffers major collateral damage during the assault. As you find out in Chapter 3, the small intestine is the absorption site for vitamins and minerals. When it is damaged, malabsorption and malnutrition are the results.

This disease is more common than people think. Researchers consider it one of the most common lifelong genetic diseases in the West. It is widespread in Scotland and Ireland, with an incidence of 1 in 122 people of Scottish and Irish descent. It occurs in 1 in 200 people in Sweden, but only in 1 in 10,000 in Denmark. There is some speculation that celiac disease is so common in Scotland and Ireland because of the heavy grain diet in those countries.

Beatrice Trum Hunter, in her book called *Gluten Intolerance* (Keats Publishing), says that there may be an inherited susceptibility to multiple sclerosis from lesions in the small intestine caused by gluten. Such lesions may lead to the classic demyelination of nerves in MS. (*Demyelination* means that the myelin sheath covering nerves is broken down.) Other researchers have supported this theory by noting the high incidence of MS in Canada, Scotland, and western Ireland, where the most popular wheat is very high in gluten. In contrast, in African nations, MS is rare and people mostly eat nongluten grains such as millet.

Starting young

If you have the gene that says gluten is bad, you can start getting symptoms when you first begin eating cereal, as early as 6 months of age. Children with this disease have abnormal stools, gas, bloating, failure to thrive, and poor appetite — they're miserable.

Getting gluten enteropathy later in life

Not everyone with gluten enteropathy had the disease as a child; some people develop it as they get older. Why does the disease develop later in life?

Gluten enteropathy is a genetic condition, but sometimes genes can turn on and off. The field of medicine called *epigenetics* studies this very fact. Researchers are mostly focusing on animal research at this stage, but they have already found that in mice who have a gene for a certain condition — obesity — particular behaviors can trigger that gene to turn on and off.

Specifically, mice with the obesity gene will all develop obesity if they're fed a normal diet of mice chow. But if they are given extra B vitamins, they don't get fat. And if they are given a diet that's very low in B vitamins, they get even fatter!

We may find out in the future that because of a deficiency in certain nutrients, the gluten allergy gene can get turned on during a person's life. That's one of the reasons why we tell you about vitamins and minerals and other nutrients in Chapter 9.

Adults who get past their childhood without a proper diagnosis can continue to experience diarrhea with bowel movements that are bulky and highly odoriferous. They also may have abdominal cramps, bloating, gas, and even constipation. This is where the rubber meets the road and gluten enteropathy meets IBS.

Diagnosing gluten enteropathy

It used to be that a surgical biopsy of the small intestine was needed to diagnose gluten enteropathy. "No, thank you" was the response of many parents when offered this very uncomfortable test for their children. Now, there are several blood tests that can show antibodies to various grains that can make the diagnosis.

Avoiding gluten foods and watching your life come back clinches the diagnosis. However, some researchers still say that they have to get a look at a biopsy of the intestine to really tell. Trouble is, if you have been on a haphazard gluten-free diet — meaning that you cheat a lot — then the bowel will partly heal, and a biopsy will no longer show as much gluten damage. We talk more about the tests for gluten enteropathy in Chapter 7.

Treating gluten enteropathy

Surprise, surprise! The way to treat gluten enteropathy and gluten allergy is to stop eating gluten. Period. If you suffer from gluten enteropathy or suspect you may, in Chapter 10 we enlighten you about a host of nongluten grains that may fill in that gap in your diet. Because grains supply vitamins and minerals necessary to the body, diet is important, as are dietary supplements (which we address in Chapter 9).

Wheat allergy

If you have gluten enteropathy, you're allergic to the protein found in many grains. But some people have an allergy only to wheat, which makes the task of changing your diet a bit less daunting. Wheat allergy can happen to anyone, unlike gluten enteropathy, which is inherited.

When people react badly to foods, they think they have allergies. But medically-defined true food allergies aren't really that common. Only about 1 percent of adults and 5 percent of children actually have a true food allergy, which is defined as an adverse reaction to a food that is triggered by the immune system. Most people have food *intolerance,* which is an unpleasant reaction to food without the immune system being involved. A true food allergy is also called a *hypersensitivity,* and it can cause serious problems and even death. Think of peanut and shellfish allergies, which can cause anaphylactic shock.

Removing wheat from your diet is a surefire (and inexpensive) way to determine whether it's the culprit behind your IBS-like symptoms. Blood tests for antibodies to wheat are available. We list reference labs in Chapter 21.

One of the common side effects of wheat in susceptible people, believe it or not, is depression. There are numerous other symptoms that you may find surprising:

- ✔ Arthritis
- ✔ Bloating
- ✔ Chest pains
- ✔ Chronic cough
- ✔ Diarrhea
- ✔ Faint feeling
- ✔ Fatigue
- ✔ Gas
- ✔ Headache
- ✔ Muscle and joint aches and pains
- ✔ Nausea or vomiting
- ✔ Palpitations
- ✔ Psoriasis
- ✔ Sinus blockage, post nasal drip
- ✔ Skin rash, eczema

You can replace wheat in your diet with rice pasta, spelt bread, and kamut cereal.

Lactose intolerance

Lactose (milk sugar) intolerance occurs when your body doesn't produce enough lactase enzymes to digest dairy products. You may be one of the more than 50 million Americans who are lactose intolerant or lactose sensitive — yes, *50 million.* The symptoms of lactose intolerance are just like the symptoms for IBS:

- Abdominal pain and bloating
- Constipation
- Diarrhea (usually very runny)
- Alternating constipation and diarrhea
- Cramps
- Gas
- Vomiting

Here's what happens when you don't digest milk and cheese: Dairy that is not broken down properly by enzyme action travels through your intestines, attracting a considerable amount of fluid in order to dilute it. This mass of fluid alone is enough to cause an episode of watery diarrhea. If that isn't bad enough, the unabsorbed lactose (which is, after all, a sugar) becomes food for the *trillions* of bacteria and yeast in your intestines. Through a process of digestion and fermentation, these sugar-loving organisms create what amounts to a gas-producing factory in your gut.

A certain group of people with lactose intolerance develops chronic constipation. We've heard horrible stories of people going from doctor to doctor for decades because they can only have a bowel movement every two or three weeks. When it finally comes out it is hard as a rock and can cause bleeding and tearing of the rectum. They're told to eat more fiber, drink more water, and exercise, but doing so makes no dent in this type of constipation. The cure is to stop consuming dairy products.

Some people can be allergic to even just a few molecules of lactose and develop symptoms that can encompass the sinuses, lungs, skin, and intestines.

There are many stages in lactose intolerance. Some people are able to tolerate milk that contains added lactase enzymes, but for many people with lactose intolerance, any amount is too much. Another group can eat dairy up to a point, and when they reach that point they head for the bathroom. Unfortunately for them, their lactose limit comes as a surprise every time.

Hold the pizza

An interesting study published in the *Italian Journal of Gastroenterology* spells disaster for many pizza lovers. Researchers indicated that the inability to digest and absorb lactose could induce gut symptoms that could pass for IBS. Of 230 patients with possible IBS, 157 were diagnosed with lactose intolerance. Only 110 patients could be talked into giving up their pizza and cream sauce. But for the ones that were brave enough to bite into soy cheese, the results were pretty impressive. In 48 of the 110 patients who complied with the diet, their symptoms subsided; in 43 the symptoms were somewhat reduced; and in 17 they remained unchanged.

Yogurt and *kefir* (a fermented milk product popular in Europe) seem to be much less of a problem because the fermentation process digests much of the lactose in these products. Plain yogurt and kefir are the best kinds to eat — organic is even better. They contain good bacteria called *probiotics* and don't have the high amounts of sugar that are in the sweetened varieties.

Dairy allergy

You can also be allergic to some dairy products even if you have enough lactase enzymes to do their work of digesting. (We say *some* because yogurt is off the hook; the previous section explains why.) Even if your lactose tolerance test is negative, you may still be allergic to a protein in dairy called *casein*.

Being allergic to casein adds more symptoms to the pain, gas, bloating, and bowel changes that make us think of IBS. You may also have the following if you have a casein allergy:

- Allergic "shiners" (black circles under the eyes)
- Coughing
- Eczema
- Hives
- Itchy, red rash
- A runny nose, which you are always rubbing
- Shortness of breath
- Sneezing
- Swelling of the lips, mouth, tongue, face, or throat
- Watery and/or itchy eyes

Although this seems like a horrible load of symptoms to have, the good news is that if you do have them you can read Chapter 10, where we guide you through an elimination diet to get rid of the offending white stuff.

Also, dairy products like milk and cheese have nondairy substitutes made of soy. (Remember to consume only organic soy, as other types of soy may be genetically modified and more difficult to digest.) You can replace dairy with soy cheese, almond milk, and rice milk. See, it's not so bad after all!

Letting Genes Off the Hook

Now that scientists have finished the Genome Project, which defines every gene in the body, people with IBS want to know if their condition is genetic. The thinking usually goes something like this: "If I can blame my IBS on my genes, then maybe there's a chance that gene therapy can just snip out the bad gene and replace it."

Even though we now know the whole genetic sequence of the human body, we are no further ahead in replacing bad genes with good ones. Eventually, we may be able to perform these types of procedures, but we are probably looking at 100 years from now, not 10. Also, the gene would have to be entirely responsible for the condition to have any effect. That does not seem to be the case with IBS.

People with IBS often report that members of their family also suffer from the condition, so researchers recently conducted a study of IBS in families. Relatives and in-laws of IBS patients were asked some delicate questions about their bowels. (In-laws were chosen because they are not genetically related to the patients.) The in-laws' incidence of IBS was compared to incidence in relatives of IBS patients, and the results were not that conclusive. The in-laws experienced a 7 percent incidence of IBS. The relatives of IBS patients had a higher incidence at 17 percent, which suggests that IBS runs in families but is not high enough to be conclusive of a genetic link.

In the hallowed halls of science, the ultimate study to prove that genes cause a disease is the twin study. If you can prove that identical twins have the same incidence of IBS whereas non-identical twins do not have the same incidence, you know you have a disease that is caused by some genetic malfunction. One study involved about 12,000 pairs of twins who completed detailed questionnaires concerning 80 health problems. In identical twins, 17.2 percent of people whose sibling had IBS also had the condition. The rate of incidence with non-identical twins was 8.4 percent. Again, the findings indicate that genes may somehow play a role, but if IBS were purely a genetic condition, the rate of incidence among identical twins with IBS would be much higher.

Separating IBS from IBD

As we explain in Chapter 7, IBS is a diagnosis of exclusion. That means your doctor has to rule out the really bad guys before settling on a diagnosis of IBS. The really bad guys in this story are Crohn's disease and ulcerative colitis. Together, they are called *inflammatory bowel disease* (IBD). An IBD causes damage to the gastrointestinal tract that shows up on an x-ray, through a diagnostic scope, or even on blood tests.

The symptoms of IBS can mirror a mild case of an IBD. For that reason, diagnosing abdominal pain and diarrhea based on symptoms alone can be difficult. With moderate to severe IBD, there are many associated symptoms and a great probability of bloody discharge or actual bleeding from the bowels.

In general, Crohn's disease and ulcerative colitis affect two different areas of the bowel. Crohn's mostly attacks the small intestine, and ulcerative colitis attacks the large intestine.

If you are experiencing bleeding from the bowel, put down this book and call your doctor immediately.

Crohn's disease

Crohn's disease is a bowel disease that seems to run in some families and affects men and woman equally. It typically settles into the lower part of the small intestine, but it can also cause troublesome signs and symptoms in any part of the GI tract, from the mouth to the anus. The inflammatory process that occurs affects layers of intestinal tissue, causing chronic pain and diarrhea.

Like IBS, Crohn's disease does not have an identified, definitive cause. The current theory about the origin of Crohn's is that the immune system overreacts to a viral or bacterial invasion, which initiates a chronic inflammatory reaction. Immune system abnormalities show up on blood tests, but even then it's a chicken-and-egg situation. Does the disease cause the abnormalities, or do the immune system abnormalities cause the disease? Scientists don't yet know.

Crohn's disease abdominal pain tends to be focused on the lower right side. Rectal bleeding, weight loss, and fever, which occur in moderate to severe cases, distinguish Crohn's from IBS. We talk more about differentiating Crohn's from IBS using special diagnostic tests in Chapter 7.

Because Crohn's attacks the small intestine, which is the site of nutrient absorption, many people with this disease become nutritionally deficient. Protein, caloric, vitamin, and mineral deficiencies are all common in Crohn's. People may also just feel too sick with abdominal pain and fever to eat regular meals, so they develop malnutrition. The result is stunting of growth in children and weight loss in adults.

Unlike IBS, Crohn's patients are susceptible to bowel complications with their disease. In a Crohn's patient, the intestinal wall can become thick with inflammation and scarring and cause narrowing of the *lumen* (the cylindrical area inside the bowel) and even blockage. In severe cases, the inflammation can cause ulcerations that penetrate through the intestinal wall to the skin or into the bladder or vagina. Ulcerations around the anus can be particularly nasty, causing *fistulas* (tunnels) that can become infected.

The list doesn't end there. Other complications associated with Crohn's include skin rashes, arthritis, kidney stones, gall stones, liver and gall bladder diseases, and inflammation of the mouth and eyes. When the bowel symptoms are treated and resolve, some (but not all) of the complications improve. Others have a life of their own and must be treated separately.

Ulcerative colitis

Ulcerative colitis, like Crohn's disease, also may run in some families and affects men and woman equally. It is most often diagnosed in people 15 to 30 years old.

In ulcerative colitis, the large intestine and the rectum are the focus of not only inflammation but also *ulcers* — shallow depressions in the lining of the gut wall. It rarely affects the small intestine, except at the site where the large and small intestines are joined. Abdominal pain and diarrhea are common symptoms caused by the inflammatory process in the intestine, but as with Crohn's and IBS, nobody knows for sure what causes the inflammation in the first place.

As with Crohn's, the cause of ulcerative colitis is thought to be the immune system overreacting to a viral or bacterial infection in the intestines. Either because the large intestine is much wider or because the ulcerations are not as deep, ulcerative colitis does not tend to cause blockage or scarring like Crohn's disease. The ulcers in ulcerative colitis can, however, cause bleeding and produce pus.

The symptoms of ulcerative colitis are abdominal pain, bloody diarrhea, weight loss, fatigue, lack of appetite, fluid loss, and nutrient loss. Fifty percent of patients have mild symptoms. The other fifty percent aren't so fortunate, and they go on to experience fever, nausea, and severe abdominal cramps.

Associated conditions in ulcerative colitis include arthritis, eye inflammation, liver disease, skin rash, anemia, and osteoporosis. These conditions are likely caused by the immune system triggering inflammatory processes in sites far removed from the bowels.

Chapter 3

How Your Digestive System Works

*T*he gastrointestinal track (GIT) can act just like a *git* sometimes, which is defined as an annoying, troublesome, unpleasant, and thoughtless person. But problems with the GIT usually happen when we eat or drink something that upsets it.

The GIT is an independent system that travels inside the body in a long cylinder from mouth to anus. Some researchers even say that the GIT is a *complete* system within the body. However, it does need help from two major organs — the pancreas and the liver. Its main function is to process food and liquids. Everything we eat or drink goes through that long hollow tube and is worked upon by dozens of different chemicals.

Don't take your digestive system for granted. It is constantly working on its own, digesting and processing your food without you having to think about it. But even though you don't have to think about the work it is doing, you still have to think about what work you are making it do — especially if you have a gastrointestinal disorder like IBS.

When we eat or drink something that our GIT doesn't like or can't process, the whole body seems to suffer. You only have to go to Chapter 2 and see the long list of symptoms that can be attributed to IBS to know how true that is.

Unfortunately, there is no guard at your mouth making you stay away from things that are bad for you. You have to be the guard for your GIT, because you want to avoid those stages of digestion where the GIT can react harshly to the things you eat.

In this chapter, we take you on a journey through the GIT. By the end of the chapter, you will know what it's like to live in your gut, as well as what happens in a GIT gone awry.

Getting to Know Your Gut

We go into much more detail later in the chapter, but for now, here are the basic facts about the structure of the GIT, which you can see in Figure 3-1: The GIT is an enclosed system within the body that travels from mouth to anus with about 20 feet of small intestine and 6 feet of large intestine in between.

If you've ever eaten a lot of corn on the cob, you may have witnessed things going in one end and out the other undisturbed. The point of the GIT, however, is to transform those corn niblets into something that helps build or repair the body. That's what digestion is all about.

Don't be confused if, during a meal, you have to run to the bathroom. It's not your present meal that you are eliminating but the one you ate a few hours earlier. We give you some clues on how to determine the transit time of food entering and leaving your body later in the chapter.

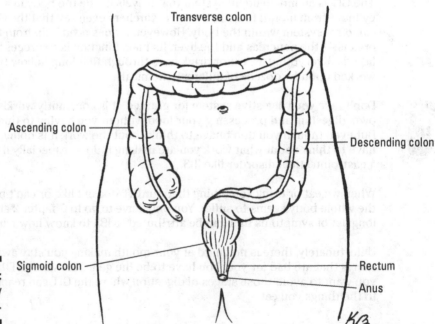

Transverse colon

Ascending colon

Descending colon

Sigmoid colon

Rectum

Anus

Figure 3-1:
A healthy colon.

Getting to Know the Food You Eat

Carol and Pat had busy lives and felt like they were always on the run — often to the bathroom with IBS symptoms. They had been trying for a year to get pregnant, but so far their attempts were unsuccessful. They decided to make some changes in their lives.

The first change they made was to clean out the oven and actually use it for cooking instead of storage. They researched some recipes and, using fresh and organic foods, began cooking their meals instead of eating fast food or frozen dinners. Both of them felt better, and their IBS symptoms cleared, only to return when they treated themselves to their favorite fast food.

Within a year after changing their diets, they had a healthy baby girl.

Hunting and gathering

Let's talk for a minute about how food gets to your table. Our days of hunting and gathering — of living off the land and enjoying its bounty — are far behind us. Our new hunting and gathering skills consist of finding the time to walk or drive to the nearest grocery store and stock up for a few days or a week with fresh, frozen, canned, and packaged food items.

What you may not realize is that many of these food items come from thousands of miles away. Fruits are mostly picked before they ripen, and they go through the important ripening process deep inside storage vans. Many other foods are processed beyond recognition and mixed with dozens of ingredients in colorful packages.

Because we are so removed from our food supply, we may not even realize that the processing, the chemical additives, and the multiple combinations of food ingredients in a grocery product may not be good for our bodies and can easily throw our digestion out of whack. Maybe your gut does not look kindly upon chemical additives and genetically modified foods. It mainly wants living foods from natural sources — especially if you have IBS.

It's a lot of extra work for the digestive system to decide what is natural, safe, and digestible versus what is foreign, unsafe, and undigestible. Sometimes the GIT rebels and rejects foods that are too complex, too spicy, or contain too many chemicals. Doing so is part of the GIT's way of protecting the body. The GIT appears to have a wisdom of its own when it rejects a food or drink today that was acceptable yesterday.

Giving your GIT a break

Knowing what you are eating and knowing what to eat may be the most important way to protect your digestive system. For example, it's wise to know if a food contains MSG or aspartame, two of hundreds of chemicals that can irritate your intestines. Be your own scientist. Reading labels is your first clue to what's in a food. Most labels are complete, but food additives like MSG can hide in the label "hydrolyzed protein." We talk about MSG, aspartame, and other additives in Chapter 4.

Buying organic food and making it from scratch may not be what you had in mind when you picked up this book, but it may be something you can do to heal your bowels. We talk more about diet in Chapter 10 with a focus on finding safe foods that won't bother you.

In the next section, we discuss the impact that your senses have on the digestive process. Perhaps the most important sense to proper digestion is common sense. Everyone agrees that IBS can be triggered by what you eat and how you eat, so it's very important to get a handle on what goes in your mouth. See Chapters 2, 4, and 10 for much more information about how food can affect your IBS.

Eating and Digesting

Have you ever just looked at a food and noticed that your mouth started watering? Have you ever been overcome with the memory of a delicious meal and noticed that saliva burst into your mouth? Triggering the production of saliva is the start of the digestive process, and any of your senses may be involved in that work. Right now, if you think about the taste of fresh raspberries bursting into your mouth, you may start salivating on the spot.

Smell is often the first sense that triggers the digestive process. The aroma of a home-cooked meal filling the kitchen can certainly get the digestive juices flowing. (People who don't have a sense of smell don't enjoy their food nearly as much as those who do.)

Digestive juices consist of digestive enzymes in your saliva and in your stomach that start pouring out to help break down a meal. If these juices are triggered by the smell or sight of delicious food and you don't start eating soon, you begin to drool.

But if you're like us, you probably don't wait too long before diving into that delicious food. The following sections explain exactly what happens when you do.

Chewing your way to health

Your teeth are designed for ripping, grinding, and chewing. They chop up food into smaller pieces that are more manageable in the mouth. While your teeth are doing their work, your salivary glands pump out saliva that is loaded with enzymes for digesting food.

We produce an average of one quart of saliva every day and barely even notice. Only when you get a sore throat do you become aware of how many times a day you swallow.

Saliva is sticky with mucus, and mucus is important because it helps coat your food so that digestive enzymes can remain attached to their work. The enzymes are mainly *amylase* enzymes that digest carbohydrates, especially grains.

Kick-starting good digestion

Why are we talking about something as mundane as chewing? What does chewing have to do with IBS? A lot. Here's some food for thought: If you chew your food properly, which means at least 30 times per bite, you can accomplish almost one-third of your digestion in your mouth.

Over a century ago, French psychotherapist Emile Coue had people visiting his clinic from all over the world to find out about his famous cure for digestive disorders. He would tell patients that his treatment was highly confidential and not to repeat his recommendations to anyone. But he told everyone the same thing — to chew their food 50 times per bite and repeat this optimistic phrase, "Day by day, in every way, I am getting better and better."

Our teeth are so important in eating that dental problems, badly fitting dentures, and even temporomandibular joint syndrome (TMJ) can adversely affect your whole digestive system because of increased pressure and inflammation in your jaw. If you have trouble chewing because of one of these problems, you may gravitate toward a less healthy soft and sweet diet instead of a healthier one consisting of hard vegetables and tough whole grains.

TMJ occurs when the jawbone, which attaches in front of the ear, goes slightly out of joint. The causes are many, including having a great deal of dental work with your jaw wide open for long periods of time. Stress that leads you to grind your teeth at night can wear down your back teeth and cause a shift in the joint. TMJ is the second most common cause of facial pain (after tooth pain), and it makes chewing a real pain. Proper treatment consists of wearing a bite plate at night that you get from your dentist; it can stop the annoying clicking that is common with TMJ and also stop the pain.

Acupuncture can be a very useful treatment for TMJ. See Chapter 12 for more on the benefits of sticking very tiny pins into your body.

Sidestepping proper chewing

Okay, we agree, almost nobody chews food 50 times per bite — some people don't even chew it 10 times. The downside to not chewing properly is that the stomach has to work overtime to break down food that falls into the stomach in lumps. Each step of the digestive process makes the food ready for the next. If the stomach doesn't do its job properly, valuable nutrients locked inside the food lumps may not be available to be absorbed into the bloodstream.

To make matters worse, food that is not properly digested by the time it hits the large intestine becomes a feast for bacteria, resulting in symptoms of gas and bloating. We talk about the billions of bacteria that live in your gut later in this chapter and in Chapter 4.

Flushing food down with water or any beverage dilutes the enzymes in the mouth and also the digestive juices in the stomach. It can also push food out of the stomach before it has a chance to be fully broken down. Drink water between meals, but only sip it when you eat.

During a meal, if you find that food seems to have a difficult time passing into your esophagus, before trying to flush with a beverage, get up and move around. You can even stand on the balls of your feet and gently bounce a few times, and you should feel the food move along. However, if you repeatedly feel food getting stuck during swallowing, make an appointment to see your doctor.

Poor eating habits and lack of nutrients can cause a deficiency in stomach acid and in the enzymes required for digestion. We are what we eat, and as nutritional educator Dr. Jeffrey Bland says, "If you eat junk, you are going to look and feel like junk."

Peeking inside the stomach

The esophagus is a hollow tube that moves food from the mouth to the stomach (see Figure 3-2). But that statement doesn't capture the whole picture: The esophagus is more than just a hollow tube because people can still swallow food when they are upside down. How? A team of muscles in the esophagus propels the food down the throat, through the chest, and into the stomach for the next part of the digestive journey. Once in the stomach, the food is trapped behind a special valve called the *esophageal sphincter*.

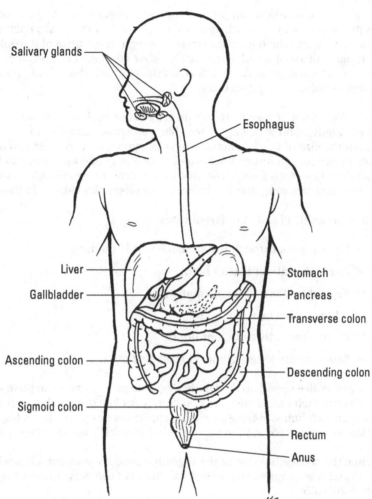

Figure 3-2:
The
digestive
system.

Food in the stomach must be broken down by gastric acid, which is released
by special glands in the stomach when they know there is a job to do. The
same sensors that perceive food and pump acid also close the esophageal
sphincter (the opening between the esophagus and stomach) and open the
ileocecal sphincter (the opening between the small intestine and the large
intestine). It makes a lot of sense to make room for the food coming in by
opening the door to move the waste out. We get to the ileocecal sphincter
shortly.

Gastric juice breaks down protein very effectively because it contains hydrochloric acid. It's as dangerous as it sounds. Certain stomach cells produce this acid, which is concentrated enough that a drop of it would eat through a piece of wood. Fortunately, other stomach cells produce your very own bicarbonate of soda, which coats the stomach lining and protects it from harm — unless you get an ulcer.

How big is your stomach? Here's an easy estimate: Hold out both hands, fingers together and little fingers touching, and make a basket of them — that's about the size of your stomach. This measurement also gives you an idea of the maximum amount of food you can eat at any one time and still feel comfortable. Too much food in the stomach doesn't leave enough room for the mixing and churning that has to occur for stomach acids to do their work.

Different foods digest at different rates:

- ✔ Liquids pass through the stomach within minutes.
- ✔ Fruit takes about half an hour.
- ✔ Vegetables take about 45 minutes.
- ✔ Whole grains take two hours.
- ✔ Protein takes three to four hours.
- ✔ Fats take the longest time, at least six hours.

Tea and coffee speed up the whole digestive process and can push foods out of the stomach before they are completely broken down. They can also irritate the stomach lining. Having a relaxing cup of tea or coffee after a big meal can relax your digestive system so much that you don't actually digest your meal.

When the stomach phase of the digestive process goes amuck, a whole host of symptoms can make life miserable. Many of these symptoms are associated with IBS:

- ✔ If the sphincter between the esophagus and stomach (the esophageal sphincter) doesn't work properly — if it's not tight enough — acid reflux and heartburn are the direct result. Some of the intestinal contents of a big meal can cause food mixed with acid to rise up into your esophagus and cause a burning sensation that we call heartburn. (See the sidebar "Treating heartburn.")
- ✔ If the esophageal sphincter is very loose, food can rise all the way up into the back of your throat. In severe cases of acid reflux, some food can even be inhaled into the lungs as it travels up the esophagus. This problem can result in pneumonia.
- ✔ Overeating can lead to incompletely digested meals, which become food for bacteria and yeast in the large intestine. And, surprisingly, you can be malnourished in spite of the excess foods because you aren't able to absorb what you eat.

TIP

Treating heartburn

To treat heartburn and acid reflux, antacids are used to keep the acid content down, but they have the added negative side effect of letting food go into the intestines undigested. When the stomach acid is neutralized, it may neutralize some of the discomfort of heartburn, but the work of the acid is also neutralized. As a result, your undigested dinner becomes a gourmet meal for bacteria and yeast, which results in gas, bloating, and diarrhea. Plus, the bacteria and yeast get the benefit of food nutrients — not you.

Some antacids, which are made of a type of calcium called *calcium carbonate,* are promoted as calcium supplements as well. (You've probably seen the commercials.) However, stomach acid is required to make calcium available for absorption. These antacids neutralize stomach acid, which means the calcium carbonate is not absorbed and can often cause constipation as calcium is excreted in the stool.

Instead of relying on antacids, we suggest the following:

✔ Try a product called DGL Licorice, which is a dietary supplement that coats the stomach, tightens the esophageal sphincter, and helps prevent heartburn and acid reflux. The chewable, wafer-like tablets taste like licorice.

✔ Eat only the amount of food you can hold in your two hands. (Please don't *actually* measure your food this way — especially in a fancy restaurant!)

✔ Chew your food well.

✔ Don't drink large amounts of liquids with a meal.

✔ As a digestive aid, try putting one teaspoon of organic apple cider vinegar in 4 ounces of water and sip with your meal.

✔ Try not to eat by the clock. Instead, eat according to how you feel. If you still feel like you're digesting your last meal, you just may be doing that. It takes as much as four hours to digest protein and six hours to digest fat. Adding another meal on top of the last one in your stomach and small intestine can make it difficult to digest.

However, if you ignore hunger, the central nervous system signals an emergency "we're starving to death" response. This chemical message stays in the blood even after you've gorged. Thus, you can feel hungry even after you're stuffed, and you keep on eating, further stretching your poor stomach and leading to undigested food reaching the large intestine.

Slipping into the small intestine

When the stomach has finished its work, a mass of acidic sludge (which was your last meal) slips into the small intestine. Immediately, special mucus cells in the lining squirt copious amounts of mucus onto the walls of the small intestine to protect it from the acid.

Another bicarbonate mixture, this time containing digestive enzymes that digest all types of food, is sent in from the pancreas. Bile that is made in the liver and stored in the gall bladder is squeezed out from the gall bladder and enters the mixture to help digest fats.

We haven't yet talked about what happens to sugar. Sugar molecules, such as lactose, sucrose, and maltose, have to be broken down just like any other food. Specific enzymes that come from cells in the intestinal wall break down sugars, which end up as simple sugars: glucose, fructose, and galactose.

Transforming food into you

Next, food is transformed into you. All the mixing and churning in the small intestine finally breaks food down into molecules that are building blocks or energy for tissues throughout the body. They can now be absorbed into the bloodstream or lymphatic circulation and are disseminated throughout the body. Vitamins and minerals are also worked on and absorbed, mostly in the small intestine.

We are all intimately aware of lymphatic tissues but usually know them as swollen glands — those knobs of pain under your chin that swell up when you have a sore throat. They are connected by tiny passages much like blood vessels. But the lymphatic circulation doesn't have a heart to pump it and depends entirely on body movement to do its job right.

According to Deepak Chopra, body tissues and organs are in a constant cycle of growth and repair. For example, the stomach lining is replaced every two to three weeks. Old cells are broken down and replaced by new ones. In the time it takes for you to read this sentence, 50,000 cells will die and be replaced. That means that if you can remove the causes of an intestinal condition and give it the right building blocks, you could have a whole new colon in a matter of a week or two!

Unfortunately, numerous things can go wrong at this stage of digestion in the small intestine:

- ✔ Too little bicarbonate from the pancreas can cause ulcers to form just where the stomach exits into the small intestine.

- ✔ Sugar enzymes can be destroyed by a gastrointestinal infection and create a problem with undigested sugars. When sugar is not absorbed into the bloodstream, it remains in the GIT and becomes food for intestinal bacteria and yeast. Sugar is the preferred food for bacteria and yeast, while protein and fat are ignored. The byproducts of bacteria and yeast digesting sugar create gas, bloating, and even diarrhea — all of which are symptoms of IBS.

- Bile can be overproduced or underproduced. Too little bile results in bowel movements that float with undigested fat. Too much bile has a laxative effect that can result in diarrhea.

  Too much fat in the diet can cause very strong contractions of the gall bladder that can cause pain. Gall stones forming in the gall bladder can trigger abdominal pain when the gall bladder contracts.

- Irritation or inflammation from infection and exposure to acidic digestive contents in the small intestine can make the gut wall raw and allow undigested food molecules, yeast byproducts, and bacterial byproducts to be absorbed into the bloodstream. This is called *leaky gut*.

- Yeast organisms all by themselves can invade the intestinal lining and cause a leaky gut, which allows undigested food molecules, yeast byproducts, and bacterial byproducts to be absorbed into the bloodstream. As we explain in the upcoming section "Leaking in the Gut," a leaky gut can lead to an immune system reaction against these foreign substances not only in the GI tract but also in the bloodstream.

- Various stages of malnutrition can occur when nutrients are not properly broken down from food and absorbed for growth and repair of the body. Malnutrition and poor digestion become a vicious cycle.

Processing waste in your large intestine

The large intestine is mainly a waste recycling depot. If the small intestine has done its job properly, most of the nutrients have been removed from the food you eat, and the remaining fiber and other nondigestible waste passes through the ileocecal valve into the large intestine.

The large intestine has three main functions: reabsorbing digestive fluids, generating stool, and moving stool. We discuss each in the following sections.

Recycling and reabsorbing digestive fluids

The quarts of saliva, gastric juices, and pancreatic liquids that travel to the large intestine would make every bowel movement very loose and also cause dehydration if the large intestine didn't vacuum up those liquids and recycle them.

Generating stool

The large intestine creates stool by pulling out as much water as it can but still leaving it soft and well-formed so it's not too hard to pass. Although juicer manufacturers won't appreciate the comparison, think of the waste that is created when you put fruits and vegetables through a juicer. The food is pulverized, the juice (which contains the nutrients) is used for energy, and the waste is dumped.

Just like the esophageal sphincter, the ileocecal valve is a one-way trip into the large intestine with no way back. And that's a good thing, because we don't want yeasts or sugar-loving bacteria going into the small intestine, feasting on sugar, and causing gas, bloating, and diarrhea.

The cells making up the lining of the large intestine secrete large amounts of mucus to protect the lining from being irritated by fecal waste, which usually contains a large amount of potentially irritating undigested fiber. In healthy people, the bulk of stool is composed of *friendly* bacteria, which has many functions, including the breakdown of hormones.

Transporting stool

After it generates stool, the large intestine gently moves the stool up the right side of the colon, across the top of the abdomen, and down the left side into the rectum. Stool gathers in the rectum until it builds up enough pressure that you feel you want to empty your bowels.

How does this movement happen?

The means of transporting food and waste through both the small and large intestines is automatic waves of movement through the GIT that are caused by muscles not under our conscious control. These muscles are called *involuntary* muscles. They react to fullness in the intestine and begin a rhythmic movement of the waste matter to its final end. The intestinal muscles push a meal through the small intestine and finally empty the leftovers into the large intestine.

When a full load reaches the rectum, a certain amount of voluntary muscle action can help push it out, but that's about the extent of our control. Conversely, if you are trying to hold back a rush of diarrhea when you are in the middle of an airport lineup, the only muscles on your side are the voluntary muscles around your anus.

Voluntary muscles are ones that move at our command, for example leg and arm muscles. Involuntary muscles have their own Energizer Bunny that just keeps working on its own. They consist of heart muscle, intestinal muscle, uterine muscles, and muscles in blood vessels. We talk more about the two different kinds of nervous systems that control voluntary and involuntary functions in the body in Chapter 4.

Malfunctioning

What we have learned about IBS is that IBS intestines do not contract normally, as you can see in Figure 3-3. The involuntary intestinal muscles, instead of contracting smoothly in rhythmic fashion, seem to be disorganized and even violent. Like a muscle spasm, they contract in an exaggerated way and can cramp up for hours at a time. When the bowel is locked into a cramp, the fecal matter does not move along as it should, yet the water in the fecal matter keeps getting absorbed into the intestinal wall causing constipation. Air can become trapped inside a section of cramping, causing swelling, bloating, and abdominal pain.

The area of the large intestine just above the rectum suffers the most cramping. When this area doesn't move and all the water is extracted from the stool, the eventual bowel movements have been squeezed into small hard pellets.

In addition to this involuntary action, certain factors within our control can lead the work of the large intestine astray. For example, constipation can occur because of

- ✔ Lack of fiber in the diet
- ✔ Insufficient water intake
- ✔ Failure to observe the call of nature when it comes

If constipation occurs regularly, it can lead to excessive secretion of mucus in the intestines to help protect the lining of the large intestine from irritation.

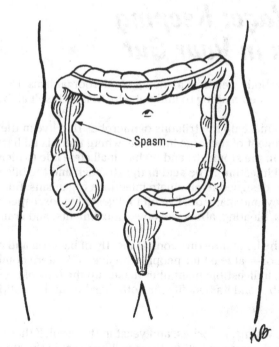

Figure 3-3: An IBS colon.

Spasm

Often adults with constipation link their condition with bathroom habits that they learned as children. Sometimes constipation manifests in a strict classroom environment where the child is permitted bathroom breaks only at scheduled times. Sometimes it manifests when children have to learn to hold it in during long car trips or family vacations. The body learns to conform but leaves behind a disruptive condition like constipation.

Pressure build-up from constipation, as well as straining to have a bowel movement, can cause balloon-like outpouchings of the GIT called *diverticula,* which we talk about in Chapter 7. Also, many people suffering from IBS with constipation have the unpleasant side effect of hemorrhoids caused by the strain. Hemorrhoids are varicose veins that surround the anus and rectum. They are caused by pressure from straining that blocks the surrounding blood flow and causes veins to balloon out.

But constipation isn't the only malfunction that can occur in the large intestine. The first function of the large intestine is to remove excess water from the waste that ends up there. In the case of IBS-diarrhea, often the waste moves through so quickly that there is not enough time to grab up that extra water, and watery diarrhea results.

It Takes a Village: Keeping Good Bacteria in Your Gut

Ten percent of our body weight is made up of microorganisms. Does that make you squirm? Keep reading to find out why that fact isn't all bad.

About 400 species make up the trillions of microbes that live in the warm, protected environment of the large intestine, where there is no harmful acid (such as you find in the stomach) and no harsh alkaline bile (which is found in the upper small intestine). The acid in the stomach and the bile in the small intestine are designed to eliminate infectious organisms. But those that survive the journey, and many do, live off undigested foods, especially sugar, and can cause gas, bloating, abnormal bowel movements, and cramping pain.

The microbes in the large intestine consist mostly of bacteria and make up the bulk of the stool — at least for people who live in Western countries. (In some cultures, indigestible plant fiber makes up the bulk of the stool. We talk more about fiber and its benefits for both diarrhea and constipation in Chapter 10.)

There can also be worms, parasites, and yeast in the stool. If there is an overgrowth of yeast in the large intestine, there will be yeast in the stool as well. Read more in Chapter 4 about yeast growing out of control when we upset the balance by taking drugs and eating too much sugar.

Scientists who devote their lives to studying stool know that a diet low in fiber increases the harmful *putrefactive bacteria* — the ones that produce chemicals called putrescine and cadaverine in the intestines. Many people with IBS talk about a particular odor that accompanies their bowel movements. Perhaps it is the putrescine that contributes to the putrid odor.

In contrast, a diet high in complex carbohydrates (vegetables and whole grains) promotes the growth of beneficial bacteria, which have a much less offensive odor.

What is the purpose of having beneficial bacteria in the GIT?

- **Immune protection:** Just by being there, the microbes in the intestine provide a constant workout for the immune system. Antibodies are continually being made against all bacteria because the immune system is always on guard for a life-threatening invasion.

- **Yeast and parasite control:** The yeast and parasite populations are prevented from overproducing by teams of bacteria who are lords and masters of the GIT.

- **Antibiotic production:** A number of bacteria actually produce their own antibiotics to keep invaders in check.

- **Digestion and elimination:** Most organisms in the gut are *anaerobes,* which means they hate oxygen. Thus, they never grow in stool cultures used in most labs. This makes it especially hard to diagnose an overgrowth of bad bacteria that may be causing symptoms of IBS.

  Lactobacillus acidophilus is a common bacteria in the gut, vagina, and on the skin that protects against dozens of harmful bacteria. It has the special ability to break down sugar into lactic acid. Lactic acid has the special ability to kill yeast.

  Milk sugar, fruit sugar, or plain table sugar that has not been digested in the small intestine (because of intestinal damage, lack of the proper enzymes, or allergy or intolerance to these sugars) usually finds itself in the large intestine. If there is the proper amount of Lactobacilli in the large intestine, they can do their work and snatch the sugar out of the greedy grasp of yeast organisms. In Chapter 9, we talk more about the benefits of Lactobacilli for people with IBS.

- **Production of vitamins:** Tiny amounts of usable vitamin B, vitamin B$_{12}$, pantothenic acid, pyridoxine, biotin, and vitamin K are produced in the large intestine from bacteria, especially the ones that don't like oxygen.

Any time you must take antibiotics for a serious infection, be sure to also take Lactobacillus acidophilus to replace the good bacteria that are indiscriminately killed. Just take Lactobacillus two hours apart from your antibiotics. It comes in capsule, liquid, or powder forms. Plain yogurt or plain kefir may serve the same purpose, except in the susceptible few who are severely allergic to dairy products. Try to eat the kinds that don't have added sugar.

You may also hear about a strange-sounding organism called *Saccharomyces bourlardii.* It's a type of yeast that in numerous experiments has shown the effect of helping to repopulate the GIT with good bacteria while pushing out the bad bacteria. This probiotic, like Lactobacillus acidophilus, is available at health food stores.

Leaking in the Gut

In Chapter 4, we talk about Candida albicans, a yeast organism that is a natural inhabitant of the large intestine, as a trigger of IBS symptoms. Here, we want to talk more generally about what unfriendly yeasts do when they grow out of control. They can grow out of control due to taking one of a number of medications, such as antibiotics, cortisone, and hormones. They also grow out of control if you eat a high sugar diet or have a protein deficiency or immune weakness.

When yeast cells are not kept in check, they change from a round budding stage to a thread-like tissue invasive stage, and they bore into the small intestine. The yeast threads poke holes in the intestinal lining. With this superhighway to the lymphatic system, there is nothing to stop yeast byproducts, undigested food molecules, bacterial toxins, and other chemicals from percolating into the bloodstream.

The irritation due to yeast makes the mucosal surface raw on a microscopic level and damages its ability to block large molecules, allergens, and toxins, which leak into the lymphatic and blood circulations. The holes are not necessarily big enough to allow the yeast itself to get through, so there is no blood infection of yeast — just hundreds of waste products that should be flushed down the toilet, which end up causing symptoms from head to toe.

Triggering a leaky gut

It's not just yeast that creates a leaky gut. Following is a list of other leaky gut triggers that are co-conspirators in damaging the intestinal lining and allowing the absorption of toxins and chemicals from the intestines into the bloodstream:

- ✔ **Antibiotics:** We discuss antibiotics, which allow yeast overgrowth, in detail in Chapter 4.
- ✔ **Bacteria:** Pathogenic or bad bacteria contaminating any food or water source can cause symptoms.
- ✔ **Parasites from any food source:** Parasites favor an environment that also harbors yeast, so cross-contamination with both organisms is quite common in people who have overgrowth of yeast.

- **Viruses:** These are usually acquired from other people's saliva and other secretions; from not washing our hands and then touching the things we eat; and from putting our dirty fingers where they don't belong.

- **Caffeine:** This bitter, toxic substance from the coffee bean stimulates bile production and is used by many people as a laxative. In people with IBS-diarrhea, caffeine may be too much for your sensitive bowel to take.

- **Alcohol:** In Chapter 19, we note that an overdose of alcohol can cause nausea, vomiting, and diarrhea. Severe alcohol poisoning can cause GI bleeding. For someone with a vulnerable gut, alcohol in small doses may cause some of these symptoms to occur.

- **Chemicals in air and water from industry:** Toxicology testing has not been done on even a fraction of the 60,000 chemicals used in industry. Many of them end up in our water supply and are found in air samples and our food — especially in industrial areas. When ingested by susceptible people, these chemicals have the potential to cause clinical symptoms, which include IBS.

- **Chemicals in processed food, such as preservatives, colorings, and trans fats:** Chemicals in our food have even more potential to cause physical symptoms in susceptible people. One of the symptoms of allergic reactions to chemicals is diarrhea.

- **Corticosteroid drugs:** These weaken the gut lining, making it more vulnerable to yeast invasion.

- **Hormone replacement therapy:** Hormones can change the intestinal pH and cause an imbalance of organisms in the intestines — too much yeast and not enough good bacteria.

- **Mercury dental fillings:** Mercury is the second most toxic element on the planet. (The first is plutonium.) When mercury is ingested from fish or from inhaling mercury from dental amalgams, or when it's injected as a preservative in the flu vaccine, it can act as an antibiotic in the intestines, killing off bacteria and leaving yeast to overgrow (see Chapter 4).

- **Mold and fungus in nuts, grains, flour, and fruit:** Mold is a close cousin to yeast and can stimulate yeast growth, as well as cause allergic reactions.

- **Nonsteroidal anti-inflammatory drugs (NSAIDS):** All NSAIDS irritate the gut, and one of their main side effects (even from aspirin) is GI bleeding. If bleeding occurs, it means you also have irritation and leaky gut.

- **Sugar and flour products:** These food products stimulate leaky gut by being food sources for organisms that irritate the gut lining, such as yeast.

It's vitally important to know how to treat leaky gut. We talk about probiotics and herbs that heal the gut in Chapter 9. But most important is to try to avoid the causes of leaky gut whenever possible. Prevention is the best medicine.

Functioning properly

It's important to know the functions of the intestinal lining so we can understand what happens when it malfunctions. When it's healthy, here's what the lining of the small intestine does:

- ✔ It houses enzymes that digest foods.

- ✔ It absorbs food molecules: glucose to be converted into energy; amino acids from protein for growth and repair; and fats for cell membranes, hormones, and energy.

- ✔ It allows nutrients like vitamins and minerals attached to carrier proteins to cross into the bloodstream.

- ✔ It's lined with lymphatic tissue that protects and detoxifies the body.

- ✔ It's surrounded by immune cells that act as the first line of defense against foreign bodies and infection.

- ✔ It's responsible for making 90 percent of the serotonin in the body.

Functioning badly

When the intestinal lining is disrupted from any cause, much more can happen. A leaky gut invisibly but invariably leads to:

- ✔ Incomplete digestion of food, which creates more food for yeast, pathogenic bacteria, and parasites to thrive on. Gas and bloating are a direct result.

- ✔ Faulty absorption of food, which leads to malnutrition and triggers food cravings because even though you may be eating tons of food, your body is not getting the nutrients it needs and craves more. Weight gain is inevitable.

- ✔ The disruption of vitamin and mineral transport into the blood by damaging the carrier proteins. The result is that all the metabolic processes in the body work at a huge disadvantage, because vitamins and minerals are vital for everything that happens in the body. Fatigue is a direct result, and after several months, chronic fatigue syndrome can occur.

Deficiency of one mineral alone — magnesium — leads to heart symptoms, muscle cramps, and low energy. B vitamin deficiency leads to nervous tension, weight gain, skin rashes, diarrhea, and lack of energy. Selenium deficiency lowers the immune response. The list of disruptions in the body is very long and includes about 60 different nutrients. Protein deficiency causes edema, bloating, and water weight gain.

✔ Gut lymphatic tissue being damaged by yeast and then overloaded with the toxins from yeast and abnormal bacteria and partially digested foods. Gut swelling, irritation, and inflammation thought to lead to IBS or inflammatory bowel disease (see Chapter 2) are direct results. The liver is overworked because the gut is not controlling chemicals and waste as it should be, and the body itself becomes toxic, leading to more fatigue, mood swings, anger, and irritability.

✔ Immune weakness resulting from chronic overwork. Chronic immune stimulation causes protein deficiency, leading to further immune weakness independent of IBS. The immune system becomes less responsive, and frequent colds and flus are a direct result.

✔ A ratcheting up of the whole vicious cycle when you succumb to bronchitis or pneumonia and have to take a round of antibiotics. The antibiotics kill off more gut bacteria, allowing more yeast to overgrow. You become more protein deficient, malnourished, and immune-suppressed.

✔ Toxins getting past the gut immune cells into the bloodstream, causing another riot of defense as antibodies are produced against invaders. Antibodies against many yeast and bacterial byproducts are known to cross-react with body organs and can produce multiple symptoms and flare-ups of autoimmune disease, multiple sclerosis, lupus, thyroiditis, and rheumatoid arthritis.

✔ Immunoglobulin A (IgA) molecules, which are normally produced in the lining of the gut, being disrupted by gut inflammation. As a result, they can no longer protect against parasites, bacteria, viruses, and yeast.

✔ A disruption in the balance of serotonin in the body. Damage to the cells that produce serotonin can result in mood swings that no amount of Prozac will treat. (Prozac is a drug that stops the breakdown of serotonin to create a false elevation in this neurotransmitter and hopefully an upswing in mood.)

The solution to all these devastating problems is to heal the gut lining, repair malnutrition, rebuild the immune system, and restore the ecology in the gut.

Solving the yeast situation

Since we have inundated you with information about the horrors of yeast, it's only fair that we give you some solutions. (Note that we touch on what to do about yeast in Chapter 4, and we also address it more fully in Chapter 10 when we talk about improving your diet to fight IBS.) Here are some very important yeast-fighting tips that can be found at www.yeastconnection. com, a Web site where Dr. Dean is medical advisor:

✔ **Boost your immune system:** Yeasts cannot get the upper hand if the immune system is intact. Correcting a protein deficiency is key in people who are malnourished and suffering chronic wasting disease.

✔ **Avoid sugar, wheat, and dairy.** These foods have the greatest effect on yeast. When these foods are broken down into their various sugar molecules, they become easy pickings for the world of yeast living in your intestines. We talk about substitutes for these foods in Chapter 10.

✔ **Take a probiotic dietary supplement or eat organic, sugar-free yogurt or kefir every day.** Stonyfield Farms has the kind of yogurt you should be looking for, and Lifeway brand has the right kind of kefir.

✔ **Take Saccharomyces boulardii:** This is a friendly yeast that can help crowd out Candida albicans.

✔ **If you aren't able to chew your food 30 to 50 times per bite, consider taking a digestive enzyme to help break down your meal.** You don't want undigested food to become food and fodder for yeast and bad bacteria. Digestive enzyme deficiency is the first sign of protein malnutrition; protein is required to produce digestive enzymes.

✔ **Take a natural antifungal formula.** Look for one that contains a combination of yeast killers, such as the following:

- *Caprylic acid* is a fatty acid derived from coconut oil that has natural antifungal properties.

- *Pau D'Arco* is from the bark of a tree that grows in South America. Natives recognized it as an antifungal treatment because, unlike other trees, it won't support the growth of mold.

- *Oregano oil* is a powerful anti-infective herb that has the capacity to treat an overgrowth of yeast, as well as infectious bacteria and viruses.

- *Black walnut* is well known for its effectiveness as a parasite treatment, as well as its antifungal properties.

- *Grapefruit seed extract* in its liquid state can be used to soak vegetables and fruits to kill parasites. In powder form in an antifungal formula, it is effective against yeast and parasites.

- *Garlic* is a true antifungal herb and can be eaten regularly in the diet.

- *Beta carotene,* found in large amounts in carrots, broccoli, sweet potatoes, and spinach, is converted to vitamin A, which boosts the immune system and strengthens the skin and mucus membranes to help protect against yeast infection.

- *Biotin* is a B vitamin that seems to have the effect of preventing yeast from transforming from a budding stage to a tissue invasive state.

✔ **Avoid chemical exposure as much as possible.** This step is important because it takes the pressure off your liver and immune system from having to constantly neutralize excessive chemicals. Following this step could be as simple as changing your perfume, hair products, and cleaning products to ones that are organic, nonpolluting, and nonscented. You help yourself, your family, your neighbors, and the environment at the same time.

✔ **Exercise.** This step in the yeast-fighting plan is important because exercise helps keep your lymphatic circulation moving. The lymphatic system clears waste products from all the tissues in the body.

✔ **Balance your emotions.** Emotions and attitude play as large a role in yeast as they do in IBS. In Chapter 12, we address how to get your moods working for you and not against you to be able to deal with these annoying conditions.

✔ **Work with a knowledgeable and caring health professional.** This is another step in yeast fighting that we wish everyone could follow. We suggest some medical and naturopathic organizations in Chapter 21 that can help you find a great doctor in your area.

How do you diagnose a leaky gut? The cells in the gut have tight junctions between them to let small molecules of food through and keep larger molecules out. *Mannitol* is a small sugar molecule that goes through tight junctions with no problem. But a *disaccharide* (a double sugar molecule) like lactulose is kept out. An Intestinal Permeability test measures how much mannitol and sugar penetrate the cells of the gut. If lactulose is absorbed, this indicates holes in the gut lining and leaky gut. If neither lactulose nor mannitol is absorbed, this indicates a case of malabsorption. To perform the test, you take a heaping teaspoon of lactulose and just under a teaspoon of mannitol in two teaspoons of glycerol. A urine sample is taken and tested for how much lactulose and mannitol are excreted.

Rejecting Foods: Vomiting and Diarrhea

We don't eat foods that smell and look bad, but what happens when we accidentally eat something poisonous? Our gastrointestinal system has a way of sensing problem foods. If we taste something that is bad, we immediately spit it out, but if it gets as far as the stomach, a sensory system in the gut creates a wave of nausea followed by vomiting up the offending food.

Vomiting after drinking too much alcohol is a survival mechanism to get rid of the poison that is building in the body. Similarly, food poisoning can cause such a massive reaction in the GIT that vomiting and diarrhea occur simultaneously.

One of the chemicals that is created when alcohol breaks down in the body is *acetaldehyde.* It is the cause of hangovers. This nasty chemical causes headaches, brain fogginess, muscle cramps, nausea, and vomiting, and it also damages nerve cells.

Protecting the GIT

From the eyes, nose, and mouth to the anus, each of us has many resources that protect the GIT from harm. Our senses — sight, smell, and taste — warn us away from foods that are rancid, moldy, and bitterly poisonous. However parasites, viruses (cold, flu, and hepatitis), and bacteria (salmonella) can be mixed in our foods without our knowing it. These organisms don't wave flags as they stealthily slip into our bodies.

Most of the time, we are not affected by the many microbes swimming in our environment because of all the defense mechanisms built into the body. For example,

- ✔ In the mouth, saliva contains IgA, an immune substance that can bind bacteria and deactivate certain parasites.

- ✔ In the stomach, strong hydrochloric acid kills off foreign microbes and helps break down protein that can produce allergy reactions if it remains undigested.

- ✔ Enzymes from the pancreas that squirt into the small intestine continue working on the protein and can also attack parasites.

- ✔ Any invader that has made it this far is attacked by more IgA made in the gut's lymphatic tissue and lurking in the intestinal mucus.

- ✔ Bile from the gall bladder is also on the offensive. One of its chemicals is strong enough to kill microbes.

Immunoglobulin A (IgA) is a specific class of antibodies that is found mainly in body secretions such as saliva, sweat, or tears (not to be confused with the 1970s rock group of a similar name). It is produced specifically against viruses, bacteria, and parasites that we ingest in our food and drink. It works by preventing the attachment of viruses and bacteria to mucus membrane surfaces from the nose and mouth to the anus.

An *antigen* is any substance that excites your immune system enough to produce antibodies to fight against it. An *antibody* is a protein produced by the immune system in response to the presence of a specific antigen. Antigens may be foreign substances from the environment, such as chemicals, bacteria, viruses, or pollen; or they may be formed within the body, such as bacterial toxins, yeast toxins, or tissue cells.

The immune system fight means antigens and antibodies melt together in a death dance, which usually ends with the antigen being neutralized and eliminated from the body in gobs of mucus from the nose, throat, urine, or stool. Uncontrolled antigen–antibody reactions can trigger many more cycles of immune reactions, escalating inflammation and tissue damage.

Relying on the lymph system

In the 1600s, Dr. Hans Conrad Peyer, while studying the anatomy of the lower part of the small intestine, found an abundance of lymphatic tissue in the lining. This particular area of lymphatic tissue was named *Peyer's Patches* but has since been found throughout the small intestine.

You know about swollen lymph nodes. You get them in your neck when you have a bad cold and occasionally under your armpit or in your groin if you have a cut or infection of your arm or leg. The same type of lymph swelling occurs in the intestines.

Pain also results when the swollen lymphatic tissue presses against a nerve or stretches the wall of the intestines. As we note in Chapter 2, people with IBS can be very sensitive to stretching pressure in the GIT.

We mention lymphatic tissue in the previous section. Now it's time to explain what it is. Lymphatic tissue consists of thin vessels, lymph nodes, and the spleen. It's a complete circulatory system, like the capillaries, veins, and arteries that carry blood, however the lymph system carries white blood cells and picks up waste material throughout the body.

Invading substances or organisms, such as bacteria, viruses, parasites, and developing cancer cells, are picked up by the lymph fluid where the white blood cells attack and neutralize them. These white blood cells also try to prevent incompletely digested food particles from crossing the gut wall and entering the bloodstream. Some cells make antibodies; others try to engulf the antigens.

In the past decade, researchers have renamed the gut's lymphatic tissue and called it MALT, which is not related to a milkshake but stands for *mucosa-associated lymphatic tissue*. When a foreign substance enters the GIT, the MALT sensors are turned on and an attack is mounted against the invasion. The foreign body or antigen is tackled by immune cells or by antibodies in order to neutralize it. But the downside is that MALT reactions, even though they are doing a necessary job, may trigger nausea, vomiting, diarrhea, swelling, or pain.

Loving Your Liver

While not directly inside the GIT, the liver has many necessary functions that impact the workings of the gut. The liver is a miracle organ that, according to Deepak Chopra, performs at least 500 different operations necessary for proper functioning of the body. One digestion function is to produce bile from cholesterol, and bile is necessary for breaking down fatty foods.

The liver is a necessary stop on the journey of food through the body. In the liver, protein, carbohydrates, and fats are processed, and then they are sent to various body tissues to take part in energy production or growth and repair. Some of them may be stored for future use. A large part of the liver's function is to neutralize toxins and dispose of them through the kidneys in the urine; the intestines by way of the stool; or the skin through sweat.

The key to a healthy liver is moderation. The liver can be overworked if it is asked to process too much alcohol, too many drugs or medications, or too much food. Toxic byproducts from yeast, which we talk about in Chapter 4, must also be neutralized in the liver. If all the drugs and toxins in the body are not immediately deactivated by the liver, they can end up circulating in the bloodstream and causing damage to organs before they can be eliminated from the body.

Even when toxins are passing through the intestines, if you have IBS with constipation, these toxins can be reabsorbed repeatedly without being eliminated. Some symptoms of toxic overload are fatigue, rashes, fibromyalgia, nausea, and headaches.

Pleasing Your Pancreas

The pancreas is responsible for two main functions that have to do with digestion:

- Producing bicarbonate to neutralize the partially digested acidic food mixture that is dumped into the small intestine from the stomach
- Producing and releasing enzymes that further break down protein, fats, and carbohydrates

If not enough bicarbonate is produced to neutralize stomach acid, you can develop ulcers where the stomach meets the small intestine. Lack of sufficient pancreatic enzymes results in severe malnutrition even if you eat well.

Beyond digestion, the pancreas has a whole other life. It's not necessarily related to digestion, but it has everything to do with allowing the transformation of sugar into energy. The pancreas produces insulin, which is a hormone that has the unique ability to open up doorways in cell membranes and allow sugar to enter. Sugar then acts as the fuel for metabolic systems that create energy for running all the activities in the whole body. If insulin activity is absent or inefficient (a condition called *insulin resistance*), high blood sugar (diabetes) is a result.

Timing Is Everything

Transit time is the time it takes for food to travel from mouth to anus. The extremes can be several hours to several weeks, but the normal transit time is 24 hours.

A transit time much shorter than 24 hours means the small intestine doesn't have enough time to extract the nutrients from your foods. While the more easily digested carbohydrates may be broken down, protein and fats may not. Your stools may reflect this fact by floating on the surface (because they're filled with fat) or containing undigested strands of meat. Remember, if you are not digesting a food, you are not gaining nutrients from the food — that's what digestion is all about.

Now that we have seen the incredible orchestration necessary to digest a meal, we can recognize the many causes of digestion gone awry:

- Eating too quickly
- Drinking too much fluid with a meal
- Eating large meals
- Not eating enough fiber
- Not getting enough exercise to help stimulate movement in your intestines
- Lacking proper nutrition to make necessary enzymes, bile, and immune factors
- Eating when stressed — stomach tension can shut down blood flow and diminish production of gastric juices, which means that stress ulcers may actually be caused by the back flow of caustic juices from the small intestine

Curious about your own transit time? The *beet test* is the time it takes for the natural red dye in beets to go from one end of your digestive system to the other. If your stool is red within 24 hours, you have a good transit time. If it's much faster, you have fast digestion and may not be getting the best out of your food before it's flushed out the other end. Taking two days or longer to come through is not good either, because you are absorbing toxins from waste that's lying around in your intestines too long. You can do the same test with corn on the cob.

Becoming Stool Savvy

Fecal waste contains undigested food — mostly indigestible plant cell walls from vegetables — as well as bacteria, yeast, intestinal secretions, and debris from dead cells flaking off the GIT lining. Here are some stool facts to keep in mind:

- Stool is normally yellow brown, colored coded in this way by bile salts from the gall bladder.

- Red stool is often due to eating beets.

- Bloody stool is an alarm sign that you can read about in Chapter 7.

- Black tarry stool is caused by bleeding high up in the GIT, which is no longer red by the time it exits.

- Pale colored stool is due to a blockage in the bile duct or hepatitis, both of which keep bile from entering the intestines and lending its normal yellow brown color.

- Stools that are loose and frothy (as opposed to watery) often indicate some form of intestinal malabsorption. Such stools may contain fats, shreds of mucus, and/or bits of recognizable, undigested foods.

- Stools that float are full of fat due to fat malabsorption.

- Watery stools of any type are usually called diarrhea.

- Mucusy stools indicate that excessive mucus is being produced in the intestines and indicate an underling bowel irritation or inflammation.

- Constipation involves stool that is hard and dry and comes out painfully in pebbles. Bowel movements are usually fewer than three per week.

The 1996 National Health Interview Survey found that about 3 million people in the United States have frequent constipation — we would hazard a guess that it's much more than that. Women seem to suffer more than men, as do people over the age of 65. Constipation accounts for 2 million visits to doctors annually, even though the majority of people treat themselves with laxatives. (We talk about the dangers of overuse of laxatives in Chapters 4 and 8.)

Chapter 4

Targeting Triggers

. . . .

In This Chapter

▶ Considering original triggers

▶ Pointing the finger at food and chemicals

▶ Seeing how stress affects the colon

▶ Keeping an eye on other culprits

. . . .

*I*n Chapter 2, we define a *trigger* as a stimulus that sets off an action, process, or series of events. The triggers we talk about in this chapter are all implicated in stimulating symptoms of IBS.

If you read this entire chapter, you'll be introduced to all the possible triggers for IBS that we know about. And if you happen to suspect that your IBS is triggered by something other than what you see here, we want to know about it. You can write to us at ibschristine@shaw.ca.

Identifying Original Triggers

As we explain in Chapter 2, the medical community doesn't yet know what causes IBS in all patients. What we think may happen with IBS is that there is an underlying predisposition to the condition — an original trigger. For example, the original trigger could be

✔ A bowel infection (see Chapter 2)

✔ A family predisposition — bad genes, a bad diet, or both

✔ Antibiotics taken at an early age that irritate the bowels and set up abnormal bacterial and yeast overgrowth

✔ Severe psychological stress, such as that caused by physical and sexual abuse

✔ Inadvertent psychological stress — for example, soiling your pants as a child at school

The previous list is not all-inclusive for circumstances that predispose a person to IBS. A combination of several triggers — a special recipe designed for your own body — may also create IBS.

Here's our theory: Whatever the original trigger may be for you, after it's set in place in your bowel and in your mind, then a food, an environmental trigger, or another stress can create the tipping point that leads to IBS. The process seems simple enough, but on an individual basis there is no way of telling specifically what is causing what.

Getting the Terms Straight

People with IBS think about food all the time. "What can I eat?" and "What can't I eat?" are huge concerns.

Before we discuss specific food triggers that affect many people with IBS, we want to be clear on how we use various terms associated with how people respond to food. In the following sections, we explain the difference between a food allergy, a food intolerance, and a food sensitivity — all of which can be triggers for IBS. These terms are sometimes used interchangeably by people who experience problems with food, but they don't mean the same things.

In short, *food allergy* is defined by the medical community as a reaction to foods involving a specific immune system response. *Food intolerance* is generally used to describe a physical reaction to lactose or to *gluten* (a protein in wheat). *Food sensitivity* is not an allopathic medical term and is difficult to define scientifically, but most doctors agree that it usually involves an inability to break down and digest a food.

Food allergy

Many people use the word *allergy* whenever they notice that their bodies react badly to certain foods. But the medical community is much pickier about how it uses the term. It relies on seeing an immediate reaction, such as hives, asthma, shortness of breath, or swelling, and on finding a certain level of immune cells or antibodies on blood tests.

Medically, the term *allergy* is usually limited to those conditions in which there is an immune reaction on a skin test or blood immunoglobulin E (IgE) antibody test. Your body thinks a particular food is harmful and sets up a massive outpouring of histamines and other chemicals to try to wash it out of your system. IgE food allergy reactions tend to occur within a few hours of ingesting an offending food.

With some food reactions, diarrhea serves to flush out the offending substance. The clue to identifying a food allergy as the culprit for diarrhea is the presence of other histamine hitchhikers like hives, asthma, eczema, and nasal discharge. If you have a double or triple whammy of symptoms after eating certain foods, the simple solution is to give them a pass at the dinner table. (We talk more about how to survive an elimination diet in Chapter 10.)

The most common forms of IgE-mediated food allergens, which doctors believe are true food allergies, are shellfish, nuts, and strawberries. IgE-mediated food allergies, however, are fairly rare. Fewer than 5 percent of all children and 1 percent of adults have these actual food allergies.

Integrative medicine practitioners define food allergies slightly differently from allopathic practitioners. That's because they recognize that it's possible to have a delayed food allergy — one that's mediated by a cousin of IgE, the IgG antibodies. Such a reaction could take up to 48 hours to appear. Because it is next to impossible to remember what you ate two days ago, integrative medicine practitioners routinely order blood allergy tests and have patients remove the foods that have high IgG levels. There is mounting clinical evidence that high levels of IgG antibodies in particular foods are associated with IBS, and removing those offending foods decreases IgG antibodies and IBS symptoms. Common foods with high IgG levels are dairy products, wheat, soy, and corn.

Allopathic medicine is the term given to modern medical practices that focus on finding a diagnosis and offering a drug or surgical therapy that fits the diagnosis. *Integrative medicine* is practiced by allopathic medical doctors who are also trained in nutrition and vitamin therapy and may practice other traditional medicine healing arts, such as acupuncture, herbology, and stress management.

Food intolerance

The medical definition of *food intolerance* is wrapped around lactose and gluten. These two conditions, lactose intolerance and gluten intolerance, are usually inherited but can be acquired, and they involve a deficiency in the enzymes needed to break down these foods. We talk about these two conditions in Chapter 2 and reveal that they are often mistaken for IBS. Although not as well-defined, fructose intolerance also affects some individuals who have symptoms of IBS. (Fructose is the sugar found in fruit.)

So how do you develop a food intolerance? In the case of gluten, the intolerance is genetic and often reveals itself during childhood. But all three types of food intolerance may actually be brought on by a bowel infection.

In Chapter 2, we explain that some people who suffer bowel infections can end up having symptoms of IBS. (We also note that there are steps you can take to try to avoid that fate when you get a bowel infection.) Acute episodes of infectious diarrhea, like dysentery, can scrape off layers of cells from the delicate mucus lining of the gut. That lining contains enzymes that digest wheat, dairy, and fruit. The inability to make these enzymes causes an acquired lactose or gluten intolerance. When wheat, dairy, and fruit aren't properly digested and absorbed, the undigested mush just keeps moving through the small intestine to the large intestine (as we explain in Chapter 3). Fermentation and putrefaction add to the nastiness of the mush and feed bacteria and yeast, which multiply and overpopulate the bowel with millions of gas-forming organisms.

In some people, a bowel infection is severe enough to throw them into genuine food intolerance from protein deficiency, lactose intolerance, and/or fructose intolerance. And, if you have the genetic predisposition for gluten intolerance (celiac disease), a gastrointestinal infection may be enough to bring it out of the closet.

To try to prevent future IBS symptoms or food intolerance when you have a gastrointestinal infection due to bacteria or parasites, stop eating wheat, dairy, and fruit. Usually you can go back to eating these foods after your symptoms subside.

Sometimes when we have flu-like symptoms, we are tempted to turn to our comfort foods. But having a milkshake can keep you sicker, longer when your flu is actually a gastrointestinal infection due to bacteria or parasites.

Food sensitivity

Some people who have neither an IgE food allergy or a diagnosable food intolerance can still find themselves suffering with food reactions. These reactions are usually jumbled up under the heading of *food sensitivity*. (Some people may be diagnosed with a *delayed* food allergy, as we mention in the "Food allergy" section.)

Some foods are just hard to digest and can cause gas and bloating. A plateful of broccoli, Brussels sprouts, cauliflower, onions, and cabbage produces a lot of sulfur in the intestines because this mineral is found in very high amounts in these healthy vegetables. Sulfur foods can produce a very odiferous result, and the gas can trigger an episode of IBS. (Sulfur is essential in the body, especially for liver detoxification maneuvers, so you need to choose the time and place to indulge and only eat small quantities.)

ANECDOTE

Charlene's story

Charlene was at her wit's end with her IBS symptoms. Although she hadn't considered suicide, her days felt like they were not worth living. From her perspective, everything was a trigger for her IBS, from getting out of bed to drinking water. She was unable to work or leave the house, and she arranged her furniture to shorten the distance from her chair to the toilet.

Charlene started keeping a journal of how she was feeling because she seemed to be the only one that believed she was ill. As she was venting in her journal, she talked about the food she ate, the thoughts she was having, and the symptoms she was experiencing. Within a week, she noticed a pattern: Eating certain foods always resulted in a rush to the bathroom, while other foods seemed safe.

Finally, armed with her journal, Charlene went to a doctor who was willing to listen and do some tests. They discovered that Charlene actually had gluten enteropathy or celiac disease. When she was treated for that condition (see Chapter 2), her IBS symptoms subsided. Soon, she was able to resume her life and rearrange her furniture.

Some people react very negatively to pesticides and herbicides found in some foods, or to artificial dyes, colors, sweeteners, and other additives. We talk about some of the worst offenders, such as aspartame and MSG, later in this chapter. Your best defense against food additives is to read labels and not eat anything that you can't pronounce!

As if the above list wasn't long enough, we also have to point the finger at fats. Because fats in the diet trigger a flood of bile from the gall bladder, and bile can have a strong laxative effect on the intestines, for some people with IBS fat is the enemy. The same goes for spicy foods: The heat and irritation they produce can be too much for a sensitive IBS bowel.

Watching What (and How) You Eat

What's food got to do with it? Food has so much to do with IBS that it can make your head — or your bowel — spin. And food is the thing that people with IBS obsess about, because even the act of eating can turn on the valves and gears in your gut and make things move way too fast.

Here are some of the IBS triggers that involve the simple act of eating:

- ✔ **Large meals:** Large meals can overpower your stomach's ability to properly break down foods, creating undigested mush that is fed on by gas-forming bacteria and yeast. (See Chapter 3 for details about how this digestive mishap occurs.)

- ✔ **Eating too late at night:** Eating late can create noises, gurgles, and rumbling in the intestines that in the wee hours of the morning make you worry that something is seriously wrong. (And yes, you're right, worrying just makes things worse!)

- ✔ **Eating foods that cause allergic reactions, intolerances, or sensitivities:** Food allergy, intolerance, or sensitivity can result in alternating constipation and diarrhea; your bowels dance to the tune of your diet.

In Chapter 2, we discuss common food reactions that are often mistaken as IBS: allergies or intolerances to gluten, wheat, lactose, and casein in dairy. In the following sections, we discuss other foods that are triggers for IBS.

The reason we list these food triggers is because eliminating them from your diet may alleviate your IBS symptoms. One study found that a group of IBS sufferers who strictly followed an elimination diet of potentially allergic foods had an 88 percent reduction in painful abdominal cramps, 90 percent elimination of diarrhea, 65 percent less constipation, and 79 percent improvement in miscellaneous allergy symptoms. In various surveys and studies, on average half of IBS patients report having one or more food intolerances.

There are so many different triggers that affect IBS sufferers in different ways and to different degrees. It is important that you know what your triggers are and make every effort to avoid them. Don't let anybody tell you that something should or shouldn't trigger your IBS. You are the expert on what is happening with your body.

Figuring out if fruit is a problem

Lactose is the sugar found in dairy products, and as we explain in Chapter 2 and in the "Food intolerance" section earlier in this chapter, many people have trouble digesting it. But it's not the only sugar that can cause digestive ills. More than a few people have an intolerance to fruit sugars, such as fructose, sorbitol, and mannitol.

We know that fruit packs a great nutritional punch, so most of us assume that eating fruit and using sweeteners made from fruit sugar (fructose) must also be good. Not necessarily. Have you ever overdosed on juicy, mouth-watering peaches or plums only to find yourself running to the bathroom? The same goes for fructose-laced products and especially high fructose corn sweeteners found in many products labeled *sugar-free*. The high density sugar can cause fluid to rush into the bowel, triggering episodes of diarrhea.

The incidence of genetic fructose intolerance is about 1 in 10,000 people. However, a lot more than 1 in 10,000 people with IBS seem to have fructose intolerance. In a study of 80 IBS patients, one-third were not able to digest fructose. When fruit and foods sweetened with fructose corn syrup were eliminated, so were their symptoms.

In a study published by the *American Journal of Gastroenterology,* of 183 patients with IBS symptoms, 101 experienced symptoms of belching, passing gas, bloating, pain, and change in their bowel movements when fed a fructose meal.

Fructose (fruit sugar), sucrose (cane or beet sugar — table sugar), and high fructose corn syrups are all implicated in fructose sensitivity. Avoiding cane and beet sugar may be difficult but will improve your general health; we discuss this topic more in the next section. High fructose corn syrup is now implicated in causing high blood sugar levels leading to diabetes, so you're wise to avoid it as well. Fruit, however, is as an important source of vitamins and minerals. If you must avoid fruit entirely, you want to pay special attention to Chapter 9, where we talk about dietary supplements and IBS.

Staying away from sugar

If you have IBS, refined sugar is not your friend. Refined sugar in your tea or coffee, in baked goods, candy, chocolate, and all manner of pleasurable treats can be the key to triggering your IBS symptoms. As we discuss later in the chapter, *Candida albicans* is a yeast that grows into the vacuum left when antibiotics kill off good bacteria in the gut. Candida albicans can also grow out of control if you eat too much refined sugar or too many refined sugar products.

How much is too much? Considering that we have only about two teaspoons of sugar (glucose) in our blood stream at any one time, and one can of soda has about ten teaspoons of sucrose, even one can of soda is too much!

It costs nothing to give up sugar, but the benefits go beyond the bowel. Increased energy and weight loss can be yours. In Chapter 10 we talk about *stevia,* a natural and extremely safe sweetener that you may want to consider adding to your pantry.

Stopping the sorbitol

Sorbitol is the trade name for a laxative used to treat constipation. Its evil twin, when it comes to IBS, is marketed by the sugar-free sweetener industry as a "safe" sweetener.

Sorbitol is a sugar alcohol that is only partly absorbed in the body. The unabsorbed part pulls water into the large intestine, causing distention that stimulates the muscles of the bowel and translates into the urge to have a bowel movement — sometimes at a moment's notice. (Not what you want when you're in the middle of the Golden Gate Bridge.) Sorbitol also acts as a fuel that bacteria use to create lots of nasty gas.

Some sorbitol products require an FDA laxative warning but, let's face it, the tiny labels on a one-serving dose of sorbitol don't have room to give you details about the gas, painful cramps, bloating, and diarrhea that this two-timing sweetener can cause. The amount you have to consume to achieve the laxative effect of sorbitol is only two teaspoons a day. It's hardly worth it. If you buy a pack of sugar-free candy weighing 40 grams, about 20 grams could be sorbitol. Low-fat cake mixes, maple syrup, toffee, and caramels can all contain enough sorbitol to make your life miserable. Even regularly chewing sugar-free gum laced with sorbitol can be enough to trigger IBS. One doctor found that of seven adults who were given 10 grams of sorbitol, five experienced gastrointestinal symptoms.

The take-home point on sorbitol: Cut it out of your diet before you sign up for the million-dollar workup for your IBS. If you've gone sugar-free in an effort to control IBS or diabetes, this news about sorbitol can be especially important for you.

Reducing fat

Fat can be an IBS trigger because it stimulates the release of bile from the liver (see Chapter 3). Bile can be very irritating to the intestines, especially sensitive IBS intestines. Fatty foods include

- ✔ Cheese
- ✔ Chicken and turkey skin
- ✔ Chocolate
- ✔ Egg yolk
- ✔ Fried foods
- ✔ Full fat dairy
- ✔ Meat
- ✔ Oils and shortening

The phony fat olestra, which is used in low-fat chips and snacks, is well known for causing side effects like diarrhea and cramping. *Sudden leakage from the anus* is a warning that you can find in very small type on some olestra packaging. Even worse, it robs your body of the fat-soluble vitamins A, D, and E by pulling them out of your body along with the fat. Avoid this food.

Battling irritable bean syndrome

Beans just can't help it. High in fiber and loaded with tasty carbs that gas-producing bacteria love, they are excellent gas triggers. And when you have IBS, sometimes any amount of gas can trigger an attack.

All beans, including soy, contain *raffinose,* a natural complex sugar. Some people just don't have enough of the necessary digestive enzymes in the gastrointestinal tract to break down this complex sugar into simple sugars for absorption. With incomplete digestion, raffinose can find itself in the large intestine as food for bacteria and cause an overproduction of carbon dioxide, hydrogen, and methane. The result is — you guessed it — bloating and gas.

If you cook your own beans, be sure to soak them overnight and get rid of that nasty water before you cook them. If you eat beans outside the safe confines of your home, a remedy called Beano contains a special enzyme that breaks down beans and may help you digest them without all the special effects that they usually make!

As with broccoli and other sulfur foods, you don't want to avoid beans in general. They are very healthy foods; just choose the time and place when you pile them on your plate. And when you choose them, chew them well.

And as a last resort, there is always the GasBGon cushion! No kidding. Go ahead and laugh, but there is a special pillow devised for squelching gas. It uses acoustical foam and a charcoal filter to dampen both the sound and the smell of unsociable gas! (Don't let anyone substitute it with a whoopee cushion, which would only add to the sound effects of your already gurgling insides.)

Being cautious about soy

Soy milk is a well-known substitute for dairy products. (Most nondairy baby formulas contain soy.) But for some people with IBS, soy is not a happy choice. Dieticians who promote the benefits of soy (it's a high protein vegetable source, high in fiber, and a good source of B vitamins) think that you can train your raffinose digestive enzymes to do a better job. They say you should start with small amounts of soy and give your enzymes time to develop.

What we're discovering is that soy can block thyroid hormone production, leading to *hypothyroidism* (low thyroid function) or *thyroiditis* (thyroid autoimmune disease). Soy also contains *phytate,* which blocks mineral absorption, unless it undergoes a long fermentation process to neutralize the phytate content. Asian populations thought to derive various health benefits from soy — such as fewer menopause symptoms, low blood pressure, and low cholesterol — use only fermented soy products. They do not indulge in daily soy protein shakes, soy milk, or other soybean products, and they don't take soy supplements.

If you are taking soy as a dairy substitute or as a source of protein, consider eliminating it and then doing a challenge test to see if it suits you. You can learn more about elimination and challenge testing in Chapter 10. If you find that soy is not your friend, you have many other dairy substitutes to choose from. Rice, almond, hazelnut, and oat milk are available in most health food stores and grocery stores.

Feeling the Effects of Blood Sugar

Blood sugar is supposed to stay within a certain normal range, and if it doesn't, lots of bells and whistles go off at central command in your brain.

Balancing insulin and adrenaline

If it goes too high, blood sugar is brought down by insulin. If you eat toast and jam with a coffee saturated with sugar, your blood sugar shoots up like a firecracker, and insulin is rapidly deployed to push all that sugar into the body's cells to be used as fuel for energy production. What can happen is that with too much sugar in the blood, an excessive amount of insulin is released, and your blood sugar suddenly plunges. Without enough blood sugar going to the brain, you begin to feel dizzy and even nauseous, you see little stars, and you may even faint.

If your blood sugar goes too low — such as in the situation we just described — it's hoisted back up by adrenaline. (Your blood sugar may also get too low if you're diabetic and have taken too much insulin, or if you're hypoglycemic.) An adrenaline surge to keep your blood sugar up is a normal response, and so is your body's natural fight-or-flight reaction to excess adrenaline.

Clenching up the bowels

A rush of adrenaline may make you think that you are having an anxiety attack. Your heart pounds, your palms are clammy, you're sweaty and fearful, and your bowels go into a clench as they clamp down in a tight spasm.

Clenching is really a survival mechanism; if you're in a truly scary, life-and-death situation, the last thing you want to do is rush around trying to find a restroom! However, the clenching feeling in the gut may be interpreted by people with IBS as an attack of extreme proportions. For them, instead of shutting down the urge to have a bowel movement, the adrenaline rush can trigger cramps, gas, and diarrhea.

Keeping blood sugar on an even keel

It's very important to keep your blood sugar levels on an even keel. However, people with IBS can get in a vicious cycle with low blood sugar because they tend to avoid eating in order to avoid symptoms. When you don't eat for more than three hours, your blood sugar levels may fall. And if you eat food that is high in sugar, you get a rebound lowering of sugar.

We tell you more in Chapter 10 about the foods to eat and snack on that tend to be soothing for the bowel. Knowing what to eat and what not to eat is the first step in regulating your blood sugar. The second step is to eat frequent small meals to keep your blood sugar in balance.

Running in the Family

In Chapter 2, we explain that genes are not a definitive cause of IBS. However, IBS does seem to run in some families. If not genes, what's to blame?

The bad habits you pick up from your parents may be even more important than what's in their genes. If your mother or father had IBS when you were growing up, you may actually have *learned* how to have the disease by observing it in them. It can be a simple matter of seeing your mother holding her stomach and running to the bathroom following a meal or hearing your father complain of gas and bloating. An unassuming child can learn that this is a natural response to eating. On outings or trips, anxiety in the whole family can be created by a parent frantically searching for a restroom. Such behavior can't help but trigger a sensitivity to bowel issues.

To back up this fact, a number of studies have shown that children of parents with IBS have more doctors' visits and trips to the hospital than other children. These doctor's visits can be for any condition, not just for gut issues. That means environment and social conditioning are part of the development of IBS. We don't know yet whether these children learn to place their stress in their guts or are just more aware of and sensitive to gut symptoms.

In addition, people who use the same family recipes and have the same eating patterns have similar elimination habits. Maybe you're in an eating rut based on your family's habits. Say you eat the same things day after day, such as toast, jam, and coffee for breakfast; sandwiches for lunch; meat, potatoes, and rolls at supper. That's three servings a day of wheat. If you don't chew and digest your meals thoroughly, you could end up with several doses of day of undigested wheat in your intestines. Molecules of undigested wheat can end up in your bloodstream and cause antigen–antibody allergy reactions.

So genetics can't shoulder the blame; IBS is also triggered by our home life and the meals we share — we inherit the bad recipes and bad habits. People share much more than genes; they share the same foods, the same water, and the same indoor and outdoor air, including cigarette smoke, which may also be a trigger for IBS (as we discuss later in the chapter).

Solving the Candida Crime

The yeast called *Candida albicans* naturally makes its home in the gastrointestinal tract; it is kept in tight control by the trillions of bacteria in the intestines. Periodically, under the influence of a variety of factors, such as antibiotics (which we discuss in the next section), the birth control pill, steroids, cortisone, a high sugar diet, and stress, the yeast go wild — literally. We call this type of yeast overgrowth Crook's Candidiasis after Dr. William Crook, who devoted his life to helping people (mostly women) with this condition.

In medical school, doctors are taught that yeast is either a pesky vaginitis or an overwhelming blood infection in cancer or AIDS patients. But Dr. Crook pointed out a condition that dances between those two extremes. This happens because as yeast overgrows, it changes from a cute little bud into a menacing string formation and pokes holes in the mucus lining of the intestines. In Chapter 3, we explain the effects this process can have on your digestive system.

If a trillion bacteria are killed with a week's worth of antibiotics, a trillion yeast can grow into that space. So far, scientists have identified around 180 waste products of Candida albicans. We're not just warning you here about getting a local vaginal infection; this is war!

The waste product that has been studied most is *zymosan.* It's an inflammatory substance found in the capsule of the yeast. Another is *arabinitol,* which has been shown to produce toxic effects on the brain and nervous and immune systems of animals. Alcohol is also a byproduct of yeast overgrowth, so the bad joke here is that your intestines become a brewery. (You can even have measurable blood alcohol levels with a bad case of Candida overgrowth!)

Yeast overgrowth can cause widespread symptoms that range from headaches, head congestion, depression, and anxiety to throat and chronic cold symptoms, swollen glands, coated tongue, gastric upset, gas and bloating, constipation or diarrhea, vaginitis, arthritis, cystitis, muscle and joint aches, and numbness and tingling of the extremities. When you go to your doctor with gas and bloating but describe a whole laundry list of these other symptoms, his eyes may glaze over because he may not think of Candida overgrowth as the common and devastating problem that it really is.

In Chapter 3, we discuss in detail how to prevent or combat an overgrowth of yeast. Here's a hint: First, you starve it by avoiding sugar, bread with yeast, fruit, and fermented foods. Next, you add *probiotics* — good bacteria — to your diet, either by eating yogurt or taking probiotic capsules. Then you move in for the kill, eating lots of garlic, taking antifungal herbs, and occasionally getting an antifungal prescription to finish off the job.

Making the Chemical Connection

You may not realize that every breath you take, every bite you eat, and every drink you swallow is potentially laced with approximately 60,000 chemicals in common use. And it's not just chemicals produced in your own backyard. We now have reports that vicious dust storms that originate in Arab countries and China become mixed with petrochemicals and heavy metals and show up on our doorsteps.

Every body of water ever tested for chemicals turns up positive for medications, pesticides, herbicides, and heavy metals. Although we believe that *any* amount of particularly dangerous chemicals in the environment is unacceptable, scientists have tabulated numbers that represent what they believe to be *acceptable risks* of these chemicals.

Medications are chemicals, as are food additives and even cigarette smoke. Actually, any of the 60,000 chemicals in daily use can have an adverse effect on us, sometimes without us even knowing it. When you are playing the detective game with IBS, anything is a suspect. Even the fluoride in water and the high amounts of fluoride in tea (both green and black) are known to trigger IBS.

In the following sections, we discuss some of the best known chemical triggers of IBS.

Antibiotics

Over the past several decades, the U.S. population has grown dependent on antibiotics to treat even minor infections. Their overuse has resulted in the creation of antibiotic-resistant bacteria that have learned to outfox the most brilliant pharmaceutical scientists.

Antibiotics kill small, one-celled organisms; that's their job. When we take them to stop a bad bacterial infection, however, they aren't smart enough to tell the difference between the good guys and the bad guys. Thus, even the good bacteria get wiped out. The fact that the good bacterial count diminishes with antibiotic treatment isn't the end of the story. In the vacuum left after antibiotics wipe out the bacterial population of the gut, a normal gut fungus or yeast called *Candida albicans* takes up residence. As we explain in the previous section, Candida is another trigger of IBS.

Other medications

Certain antihistamines, antibiotics, antacids containing magnesium, laxatives, diuretics, sedatives, caffeine-containing medications, antidepressants, and mineral supplements containing excessive amounts of magnesium can trigger IBS symptoms.

After it's absorbed into the bloodstream and carried to cells, magnesium is an important mineral for preventing heart disease and muscle spasms and for relaxing the muscles and blood vessels. It also has a relaxing effect on the bowel. However, magnesium inside the gut irritates the gut lining. So if it is not absorbed, it has laxative effects. All magnesium salts can irritate, especially magnesium oxide, and are useful if you are constipated. But people with IBS do better on magnesium glycinate or magnesium taurate, which tend to be absorbed instead of causing diarrhea.

Antidepressants like Prozac and other serotonin reactive uptake inhibitors (SSRIs) can cause nausea, vomiting, dry mouth, constipation, and diarrhea. In fact, any medication that you swallow has the potential to cause GI symptoms. So, if you are on a new medication and you experience increased bowel movements, ask your doctor whether that drug could be to blame.

The irony is that some doctors prescribe antidepressants for people suffering from IBS (see Chapter 8). Make sure that you and your doctors are completely aware of the drug's side effects in case you are prescribed something that actually increases the risk of diarrhea and constipation.

Food additives

Monosodium glutamate (MSG) is an excitotoxin that acts on the brain to make you think something tastes better. *Excitotoxins* are a class of flavor enhancers, such as MSG and aspartame, that can overstimulate the brain, causing neurons to die from exhaustion. (Neurosurgeon Dr. Russell Blaylock has written a book called *Excitotoxins: The Taste that Kills* [Health Press] that implicates these chemicals in many diseases.)

As MSG enhances the flavor of your food, it also can trigger a lot of other undesirable activity. MSG reactions include migraines, headaches, tingly flushing of the face, stomach upset, nausea and vomiting, diarrhea, asthma, panic attacks, heart palpitations, chest pain, confusion, allergic reactions, skin rash, and runny nose. Many of us know about *Chinese restaurant syndrome* and ask our favorite restaurants to hold the MSG.

Read labels to find MSG, but be warned that it is found in products like Accent, bouillon cubes, barley malt, cans of broth, flavorings, seasonings, and hydrolyzed products, and it may not even be listed on the label.

Another food additive to be aware of is *aspartame,* the artificial sweetener whose brand names are NutraSweet and Equal. Included in the dozens of side effects of aspartame are IBS-like symptoms of nausea, diarrhea, abdominal pain, itching, and hives. Here's a substance that's found in up to 5,000 products, including children's medications. Beyond IBS, it's a cause of headaches, mood swings, weight gain, infertility, and about 80 other symptoms.

Mercury

Mercury is the most toxic of the five heavy metals, and when it's in the presence of lead, it becomes more than 100 times more toxic. In the following sections, we explain where you come in contact with mercury and how it can trigger IBS symptoms.

Sources of mercury

Mercury is naturally occurring in the earth and is off-gassed. This is one way it finds its way into the atmosphere. It then comes down with rain and contributes to ground water contamination. It's also found on the ocean floor and is carried along the food chain, accumulating in the fish and sea vegetation.

Also, elemental mercury is used in dental fillings. (Your "silver" fillings aren't silver at all; they are 50 percent mercury mixed with other metals.) Elemental mercury is liquid at room temperature, and you may remember playing with it as a kid when you broke a thermometer or in high school chemistry class. This type of mercury vaporizes at fairly low temperatures. The vapors are toxic and can be deadly to small children. When you have mercury amalgams (fillings), they release vapor every time you chew, every time you brush your teeth, and every time you drink something hot.

Another form of mercury — ethyl mercury — is found in vaccines. This type of mercury, called *thimerosol,* is more neurotoxic than the other forms. After it's injected into you, you may never get it out. This mercury is implicated as the trigger for autism in children.

Many sources of mercury are dumped into the environment. For example, mercury vapor is emitted from crematoriums because mercury fillings are not removed before a person is cremated. Mercury is found in smoke from coal-burning plants, and gold mining produces many pounds of elemental mercury. All this mercury ends up in the food chain, starting with the ocean. Fish, especially the larger ones (tuna, salmon, swordfish, shark) accumulate this mercury in their tissues. The bigger and older the fish, the more mercury contamination it has. There have been documented cases of mercury poisoning in persons who ate even a moderate diet of fish.

The problems it can cause

Scientists have determined a range of mercury levels in the body that are considered acceptable. Here's the problem: The upper limit of this range is where the *majority* of people begin to show obvious symptoms from having too much mercury in their bodies. But many people display mercury symptoms at levels much lower than that.

How is mercury a trigger for IBS? Mercury is a powerful antimicrobial agent. When you ingest mercury, such as from eating contaminated fish, this mercury goes into your intestines. Not all of it comes out with the digested food. Some of it stays in the intestines, and some gets absorbed into your bloodstream, where it filters through the liver and kidneys. The mercury left in your intestines kills off friendly bacteria, which encourages yeast overgrowth.

Also, research shows that mercury in the intestinal tracts of humans and primates causes pathogenic bacteria — those that can cause disease — to become resistant to antibiotic therapy. (Could this be the reason we now have "super bugs," the so-called *stealth* pathogens that no medical antibiotic can eradicate?)

What else can mercury do to your body? According to toxicologists and neurologists we interviewed, mercury — in particular, ethyl mercury — is a neurological toxin that causes brain damage and contributes to symptoms of multiple sclerosis, Parkinson's disease, and Alzheimer's.

Are you a fan of *Alice in Wonderland*? Even wonder why the Mad Hatter was mad? He was mercury poisoned. Yes, it's true. Hat makers used to use mercury to shape felt hats, and they wore no protective gear or masks when doing so. They inhaled the vapors, which eventually caused them to go crazy. Today, we inhale mercury vapors from our dental fillings and have mercury injected every time we get a flu shot or vaccine. We're not much better off than those hat makers. The road toward madness is just a little slower these days.

Ways to reduce exposure

The more people become educated about the problems with mercury, the more they will demand that their governments take action. But limiting mercury in your own environment is something you can begin today. Here are some positive steps you can take now:

✔ Go to www.mercurypolicy.org to read more about mercury and its effects.

✔ Go to www.epa.gov/ost/fish to learn which fish are safe to eat and which aren't. The safest fish tend to be smaller deepwater fish. Larger fish, like tuna, have eaten far too many smaller fish and accumulated all their mercury.

✔ If you must take a vaccine, try to get a single dose vial that is not preserved with the form of mercury called thimerosol.

✔ If you have mercury amalgams in your teeth, go to www.iaomt.org and find a biological dentist in your area who performs a mercury breath test to see if you are releasing mercury vapors when you chew.

✔ Find a doctor who is familiar with the problems mercury can cause. Diagnosing mercury poisoning is difficult and involves more than laboratory tests. The right doctor will consider your history of exposure, your symptoms, and your lab results to come to a working diagnosis.

✔ Never break fluorescent light tubes around your home. They contain toxic levels of mercury that escape in the air, poisoning everyone in the vicinity. Dispose of them properly. Check with your state/local public health or HAZMAT (hazardous materials) organization for instructions on proper disposal.

✔ The same goes for mercury thermometers. Never play with the shiny silver liquid. The amount of mercury in a thermometer, when broken, is enough to require calling a HAZMAT team to your home. If you do break a thermometer, *do not vacuum it up.* Doing so causes vaporization and poisoning of the house and all its occupants — humans and animals. The best thing to do is to not have any mercury thermometers. Replace them with the digital type, and properly dispose of the ones that contain mercury.

✔ In the event that mercury-containing materials are damaged or broken in your home, be prepared. Have the guidelines from your state/local HAZMAT organization on what to do and who to call in the event of breakage.

✔ Replace the thermostat on your heating/air conditioning unit. Most of them — especially in older homes — have a mercury switch. If this breaks, you've got contamination.

Treating mercury poisoning

Even if you don't have dental fillings, chances are that you have had exposure to mercury and other heavy metals and may have some accumulation in your tissues from getting vaccinations, eating fish, and breathing polluted air. If you and your doctor determine that you suffer from some level of mercury poisoning, what can you do to reverse it?

✔ Take safe products that assist in the removal of mercury from the body and support the body's natural biochemical processes. One product that we recommend is called Redoxal NF and consists of an essential sulfur-based amino acid called *methionine,* along with magnesium and other nutrients. Go to www.preventhium.com or call 800-755-1327 to find out more.

✔ Eat plenty of sulfur-containing foods, including garlic and onions, which assist the body in getting rid of heavy metals such as mercury, lead, and arsenic. Foods high in sulfur, such as broccoli, cabbage, Brussels sprouts, cauliflower, and eggs are able to pull small amounts of heavy metals out of the body. Fiber is also important, as it can bind with metals in the GI tract. (However, if you're a woman on oral hormone therapy, do not take fiber at the same time as hormones; the fiber can prevent absorption of the hormones.)

And remember, prevention is always best. Taking adequate minerals, sulfurs, and amino acids can defend against the accumulation of many toxins. Be sure to purchase from a reputable company that knows its products and the origin of its ingredients.

Cigarettes

In the 1800s, tobacco tea was used as a purgative. Yep, it's as bad as it sounds. "Hey honey, let's go down to the new health spa by the creek, drink down some tobacco tea, and spend the rest of the day vomiting and evacuating our bowels!"

We all remember the first time we snuck a cigarette from dad. Most of us got nauseous and sweaty, and if we continued we ended up in the bathroom either vomiting or with diarrhea. That reaction is only natural, because tobacco is a poison, and the body tries to purge it if you keep on taking it. Tobacco is a drug that irritates and stimulates the GI tract causing heartburn, reflux, and IBS. One of the common outcomes of quitting smoking is constipation. (If you are a smoker and have IBS, a little constipation may sound like a great idea right about now.)

If you have IBS, you may not be able to use the nicotine patch when you quit smoking because nicotine is the chemical that causes most of the bowel irritation. Try acupuncture, hypnosis, or the Emotional Freedom Techniques (all of which we discuss in Chapter 12) to help you quit and to help decrease your stress, which is probably why you smoke in the first place.

We have heard of people suffering with IBS with constipation who were using the nicotine patch to get their bowels moving. Do not try this at home!

Facing Up to the Stress of IBS

What if you eliminate all the ongoing triggers we've described so far in this chapter, and you still have symptoms? Does that mean there is an underlying trigger that hasn't been addressed?

Many people argue that stress is the biggest culprit for people with IBS, but does stress itself cause IBS? There is a lot of dancing around this question. Politically correct doctors don't like to say IBS is caused by stress, but on the other hand any excess stress in the life of someone with IBS can cause increased symptoms. (Stress affects many other conditions the same way.)

There are many things at play when we talk about stress. There are our nerves, our adrenal glands, and the games we play in our heads that go by many names: Worry, Fretting, Agonizing, Obsessing. The gut and mind share so many of the same hormones, immune system cells, and neurochemicals that you could say our heads and our bowels share a brain.

Placebo, good; nocebo, bad

We've all heard about placebos — you give someone a dummy pill, and there is more than a 50 percent chance that they'll get better. What do placebos say about us? Are we all just a little bit nutty? We don't think so. Placebos are evidence that if you think something is going to be good for you, chances are it will be.

But what about negative thinking? *Nocebos* can have the opposite effect. If you take something — or do something — that you think will make you sick, it just might.

When you have IBS, you may expect to get sick just because you are going to be out of the house for several hours without a handy bathroom. If you expect it to happen, you may experience more symptoms than if you stayed at home.

The mind is a powerful tool. Learn how to stimulate more placebo responses than nocebo responses in Chapter 12. If it sounds like we are saying that IBS is all in your head, be assured that we aren't. It's just that the mind–body connection is stronger than Western medicine has liked to admit.

Figuring out how your bowels get nervy

Some people wonder if the bowel has a mind of its own; well, it does. We talk about that fact in Chapter 3, but here are the gory details as they relate to stress.

The *autonomic nervous system* (ANS) controls bodily functions like heart rate, digestion, and breathing patterns. We don't have to think about making our heart beat, releasing enzymes for digestion, or remembering to breathe. The ANS does all that for us. The ANS consists of two parts: the sympathetic system and the parasympathetic system:

- The sympathetic system controls the fight-or-flight reactions of the body. In a fight-or-flight situation, the sympathetic nervous system produces a rapid heart rate, increased breathing, and increased blood flow to the muscles that are necessary for you to run away from something attacking you. The sympathetic system gets the body ready for action.

- The parasympathetic system gets the body ready for digestion, rest, and repair.

In a perfect world, the parasympathetic and sympathetic team should be in balance as they react to what's going on. But that balance isn't always possible. If you feel that you are always under attack, you'll be constantly under sympathetic control, meaning that you'll tighten up your muscles and your intestines. The result can be constipation, which periodically releases and causes diarrhea. Too much parasympathetic stimulation can create the production of excessive digestive juices and digestive processes and a tendency toward diarrhea.

Dysautomonia means your body is disrespecting your autonomic nervous system so all the teamwork is lost as the parasympathetic and sympathetic systems vie for control. Symptoms of this imbalance can include frequent, vague but disturbing aches and pains; faintness (or even actual fainting spells); fatigue and inertia; severe anxiety attacks; rapid heart rate; low blood pressure; poor exercise tolerance; gastrointestinal symptoms such as IBS symptoms; sweating; dizziness; blurred vision; numbness and tingling; anxiety; and depression.

So which comes first, the dysautomonia or the symptoms? Some or all of the symptoms of dysautomonia can be triggered by other things. Something as simple as standing up quickly after lying down, exercising, or eating particular foods can trigger symptoms.

Dysautomonia reveals nothing on physical examination. But when the signals to and from the sympathetic system and the parasympathetic system are out of control, the bowel is either too tight, leading to constipation, or too loose, leading to diarrhea. Or you may experience a frustrating combination of both.

Counting on stress

Believe it or not, your mind is directly connected to your gut through the nervous system and the immune system, so that stress and emotional upsets can be reflected almost immediately. The expression "defecating in ones' pants" leaps to mind, but that's a reaction to the extreme stress of a very frightening situation.

Dr. Richard Earle, who co-founded the Canadian Institute of Stress along with world famous stress researcher Dr. Hans Selye, says that being alive means your stress levels go up and down hundreds of times a day. He says that stress is the energy you invest in your life. Sometimes the stress is good and results in satisfaction and a boost of energy, and sometimes stress is bad and results in fatigue, frustration, or frequent illness.

Researchers are pretty clear that stress does not cause IBS all by itself, but it can make IBS symptoms worse. Stress and worry go hand-in-hand and can catapult you into a vicious cycle.

How many times have you worried yourself into running to the bathroom? A phone call from someone special or someone you don't want to talk to can create the same effect. The connection of the mind to the bowel makes it all happen.

Counting the many forms of stress

People with IBS have a unique relationship with stress that can lead to a physical reaction. Therefore, it's important to be aware of the numerous stressors in your environment. In his book *Healing the Planet* (KOS Publishing), Dr. Jozef Krop, board certified in Environmental Medicine, gives one of the most comprehensive lists of stressors that we have seen. They include the following:

- Chemical stressors:

  - Organic substances, such as formaldehyde, phenol, benzene, toluene, and xylene, plus many chemicals derived from gas, oil, and coal

  - Organic chlorinated compounds, including organochlorides, pesticides, chloroform, pentachlorophenols, polychlorinated biphenols (PCB), and various herbicides such as 2,4-D (2,4-dichlorophenoxyacetic)

  - Inorganic substances, such as mercury, lead, cadmium, aluminum, asbestos, chlorine, nitrous oxide, sulfur dioxide, ozone, copper, nickel, illegal drugs, tobacco smoke, medications, and others

- Physical stressors

  - Heat, cold, weather cycles

  - Noise

  - Positive and negative ions

- Electromagnetic radiation (full range of the light spectrum)
- Ionizing radiation (radioactivity from x-rays, atomic explosions, reactor accidents, reactor leaks, food irradiation, radon gas)

✔ Biological stressors

- Bacteria
- Viruses
- Fungi (molds)
- Parasites
- Foods
- Animal dander
- Dust
- Pollens from trees, grasses, and weeds

✔ Psychological stressors

- Prolonged psychological stress in the family (alcoholism, sexual abuse, family disruption, prolonged sickness of a family member, and so on)
- Prolonged psychological stress at work (overwork, poor relationships, job loss, and so on)
- A death in the family
- Loss due to fire, bankruptcy, and so on

Not a pretty sight. If you need some instant relief just from reading this list, turn to Chapter 12 where we talk about stress busters and give you workable tools to deal with any type of stress.

Leaving No Trigger Unturned

As if the rest of the information in this chapter weren't enough, we need to fill you in on a few additional known triggers for IBS symptoms:

✔ **Reaction to gas and bloating:** Someone with a cast iron gut may have no reaction to a bit of gas, whereas the same amount of gas can trigger a bout of pain or diarrhea in a person with IBS.

✔ **Laxative use:** A history of laxative overuse can lead to chronic bowel irritation and the loss of the body's normal reflex to move the bowels.

✔ **Low fiber in the diet:** Low intake of fiber can cause constipation that scrapes and irritates the intestines. A full intestinal load can then trigger an episode of IBS diarrhea.

✔ **Certain drinks:** Alcohol (which we discuss in Chapter 19), coffee, tea, colas, or carbonated drinks can contribute to IBS, mostly because of irritating chemicals in these liquids.

And this chapter wouldn't be complete if we didn't mention the hormonal association with IBS. We go into great detail about this association in Chapter 5, but you should know that women experience more symptoms of IBS than men. Because men do get IBS, female hormones clearly don't shoulder the entire blame for IBS. But there is something at play with female hormones that possibly stirs up the bowel just enough to be a real problem for many women. The cycle that many women are familiar with is slight constipation the week before the period and then slight diarrhea when the period comes. In someone who has IBS, this normal tendency is very much exaggerated.

Chapter 5

Who Gets IBS and Why

*A*t some time or another, everyone suffers from bowel upset, which could be due to overeating, too much alcohol, too much excitement, flu, food poisoning, or even a parasite infection. It's only when the upset becomes a permanent fixture that IBS is diagnosed. (We focus on differential diagnosis in Chapter 7.)

It appears that everybody is susceptible to IBS. For example, a severe bowel infection at any age could be a cause of IBS. (In Chapter 2, we explain how a bowel infection can lead to IBS.)

Fifty percent of people with IBS began having symptoms in childhood, and most people develop IBS before age 35. If someone develops IBS after age 40, chances of the problem actually being inflammatory bowel disease (see Chapter 2) or cancer are greater, and these other conditions must be ruled out. IBS very rarely develops in old age.

Stating the Statistics

The harsh fact is that as many as one in five people may have IBS. IBS is much more common in women; 65 to 70 percent of people diagnosed with IBS are women. But researchers admit that most of the studies and surveys done on IBS focus mostly on women, so current statistics may be biased. (Maybe men just aren't admitting they have a problem. Later in this chapter, we discuss some of the theories that attempt to explain the female predominance of IBS.)

Wishing for a cure

As we discuss throughout this book, IBS has a significant negative impact on school, work, and the social lives of people with the condition. Doctors admit that they don't have enough tools (by which they mean medications) to treat this condition properly. And people with IBS agree. One of the most vocal complaints from people suffering with IBS is that there isn't a drug to make this condition go away.

We talk about pharmaceutical treatments of IBS in Chapter 8, where we tell you the pros and cons of treating a condition that has no definitive cause with medications that are often designed to suppress symptoms. In Chapters 9 through 12, we also give you an array of non-drug tools and remedies to help alleviate your symptoms.

If you saw the movie *Along Came Polly* with Ben Stiller and Jennifer Aniston, you know that men aren't immune. Of the three lead characters, the two male characters had IBS and the woman didn't. (According to the statistics in that movie, more men have IBS than women!)

Up to 50 million North Americans suffer from IBS. Surveys show that 10 to 20 percent of the U.S. and Canadian population admits to the condition, but there could be many more people who keep their symptoms to themselves.

Most people with IBS-like symptoms — about 80 percent — never go to a doctor about their symptoms. Doctors and researchers refer to them as *mild cases,* but that may not be entirely true. While some of these people probably do have only mild symptoms, others suffer in silence, read books to try to get help, haunt Internet chat groups (sometimes getting questionable advice), and end up still suffering.

Only about 20 percent of people with IBS actually pick up the phone, make the appointment, and show up at a doctor's office. Yet, of all the patients who are referred to gastrointestinal (GI) specialists, a very large number (an estimated 20 to 50 percent) suffer from symptoms of IBS. (Just imagine how that percentage would grow if more people with IBS symptoms actually went to the doctor.)

Here's another statistic worth chewing on: In economic terms, diagnosing and treating IBS may cost the U.S. healthcare system in excess of $29 billion per year! The costs due to lost productivity greatly increase that total.

Singling Out Women

A woman's bowel and a man's bowel are essentially identical. Yet, in the Western world, twice as many women admit to having IBS as men, and women go to the doctor four times as much as men for their IBS symptoms.

Men with IBS symptoms often won't even admit to having the condition when presented with a health questionnaire. We know from personal clinical experience that many men underreport their health symptoms. This discrepancy between the occurrence of the condition and reporting makes it difficult to identify the gender basis of IBS.

Analyzing the gender gap

Why do more women get IBS than men? There is an even larger question: Why do more women get diagnosed with diseases that men seem partially immune to, like depression, chronic fatigue syndrome, fibromyalgia, and other autoimmune diseases?

And why do surveys show that women take more medication and get more surgery than men? When you look at the pattern of doctor's visits in general, more women seem to go to the doctor then men. Why is that?

Here is what we think: Many medical services that women require throughout their lives are regulated and controlled by the healthcare industry and available only under a doctor's shingle. From the onset of menstruation, women are encouraged to have an annual pap test. A doctor must provide a prescription for the birth control pill. And, as a woman gets older, she may need a prescription for hormone replacement therapy, a mammogram, or a breast thermogram. Plus, if a woman has children, generally a medical doctor delivers the baby after a series of regularly scheduled checkups.

Bottom line: There are many more opportunities for women to receive services from medical doctors than men. It follows that when you are lying on the examining table with your feet in the stirrups, your doctor is going to ask how you feel. And being an honest person, you will tell him or her what's going on. If you happen to mention that you have gas and bloating and several bowel movements a day, you have a greater likelihood of being diagnosed with IBS and (we hope) of being helped.

Meanwhile, your partner may be sitting out in the waiting room with the very same symptoms, but he's not going to make a special visit to the doctor's office to talk about his toilet habits.

This analysis may be a bit too simplistic, but if men had to go to the doctor every time they wanted to buy condoms, they might talk more about how they are feeling, be more medicated, have more surgery, and be diagnosed with a lot more diseases!

The incidence of IBS in men remains about the same from age 20 to 70 years. In women, IBS peaks at around 20 to 30 years of age and then is as low as men around menopause — providing they don't take hormone replacement therapy (which we discuss in the upcoming section "Cycling symptoms of IBS").

This is an indication that a woman's hormones have an impact on her bowel. At menopause, when the surges of hormones finally stop, so do some of the symptoms of IBS. We discuss the IBS-hormone connection in the upcoming section "Honing in on hormones."

Realizing that the gender gap starts early

Before puberty, girls and boys experience the same incidence of IBS. After puberty, the numbers change, and girls start to visit the doctor more often with complaints of abdominal pain.

Why the change? Girls' abdomens are, for the most part, very closely guarded by their parents. If your little girl has a very painful abdomen, you don't really know if the problem is intestinal or gynecological. If your son has the same complaint, you can rule out the gynecological problem! You may be apt to give him some over-the-counter medication for stomach upset and assume he'll be fine. With a girl, you can't really toss a coin, so you go to the doctor, and her cycle of doctors' visits begins.

Children with IBS may experience weight loss because they tend to avoid eating in an attempt to avoid IBS symptoms. Also, some children may avoid talking about bathroom-related symptoms, especially if they are in a home that frowns upon bathroom talk. IBS can be very frightening for children, as they generally do not have access to the medical information that adults have. We discuss IBS in children in Chapter 15.

Putting up with pain

Margaret Heitkemper is an RN and PhD who specializes in behavioral nursing. Dr. Heitkemper surveyed 700 general practitioners and gastroenterologists, as well as 2,000 women, half of whom had IBS. She found some important information on how big an impact IBS has on women's lives.

As many as 40 percent of women experienced significant abdominal pain that was intolerable and unrelieved by any treatment they tried. Their pain made them miss days from work and meant they had to curb social activities and limit their travel.

Women with IBS take three times as many sick days as their female coworkers who don't have IBS. IBS is also twice as likely to limit the activities of a woman with IBS as one who doesn't. IBS can even make a difference in her choice of career. Having IBS can make it very difficult to hold down a job as a cab driver or a cop, for example.

Honing in on hormones

Doctors and researchers agree that women's IBS symptoms are worse during their menses, which makes some people believe that IBS may be hormonally related. In fact, 40 percent of women with IBS report having painful periods, and 50 percent have PMS. But researchers agree that hormones are not the cause of IBS. After all, men don't have periods, but some certainly do have IBS.

Linking hormones and constipation

The two major female hormones are estrogen and progesterone. Current research shows that estrogen slows down the gastrointestinal tract, which translates into food traveling at a slower rate. A slower transit time means constipation and bloating, especially if you don't take in enough fiber and liquids. With very little estrogen on board, men (who do have *some* estrogen, just like women have *some* testosterone) have a faster gastrointestinal tract and seem to suffer less from constipation in general.

Progesterone, which is more dominant in the second half of the menstrual cycle and produced in massive amounts during pregnancy, also makes the bowel more sluggish. Anyone who has been pregnant can vouch for that. The question is, do estrogen and progesterone make the gut more sensitive? Researchers don't have an answer to that particular question yet. But the speeding up and slowing down of the bowel due to estrogen and progesterone may be enough to make an already sensitive bowel react.

Cycling symptoms of IBS

Holly believed that she had had mild IBS for at least ten years. She was aware of her trigger foods and avoided them. She was also aware that her symptoms worsened around the time of her menstrual cycle. As menopause approached, a routine trip to her gynecologist resulted in a prescription for hormone replacement therapy (HRT), which she took religiously. Within a month, Holly was experiencing more urgent diarrhea and increased cramping. She attributed the change to starting HRT. She switched to taking supplements instead — black cohosh and Vitamin E — which handled her moderate symptoms of menopause. She was greatly relieved that her IBS symptoms also settled down.

Another aspect of IBS and hormones is that to make a woman's period start, estrogen and progesterone drop naturally and dramatically, in unison. This major shift in hormones marks the onset of the worst phase of IBS symptoms in women. Diarrhea, gas, bloating, and pain are much worse during this time of the month.

Postmenopausal women on hormone replacement therapy (HRT) experience twice as much IBS as women not on HRT. Women on HRT experience IBS much like women who are still having their periods.

With or without IBS, most women admit to increased constipation and bloating the week before their periods. Then, with the period comes several days of looser bowel movements. For women who have PMS and severe menstrual cramps, the bowel and hormones seem to create a conspiracy of discomfort and pain. Women with IBS have symptoms all month, but their IBS constipation symptoms are worse the week before the period and jumbled up with their PMS symptoms, while their diarrhea symptoms are worse during their period — mixed in with period pain and cramps.

Fifty percent of women who complain to their doctors about abdominal pain, pain during intercourse, and painful periods also have symptoms of IBS.

Planning for your period

Dr. Margaret Heitkemper's research tells us that women are more likely to have worsening IBS symptoms before and around their periods. But what can be done about an event that is the very essence of being a woman? Some people suggest that women on the birth control pill have fewer symptoms of IBS, but so far no studies have proven this association. And for some women, the birth control pill is a direct route to getting yeast infections. (We talk about yeast and its ability to trigger IBS in Chapter 4.) So you may not want to try to solve one problem by creating another.

The good news is that if you know you are going to be more susceptible to IBS symptoms immediately before and during your period, you can use that information wisely. You can make plans based on knowing your menstrual cycle and knowing that you don't want to be stuck on an airplane in the middle of the worst week in your month. Sometimes you have no choice, but even then you can take advantage of our advice for plane travel that appears in a sidebar in Chapter 2.

Avoiding misdiagnosis

Penny's gynecological exam determined that she had ovarian cysts. The doctors believed that the cysts could be responsible for the pain that accompanied Penny's diarrhea. Penny had experienced IBS symptoms for several years and was hopeful that the removal of the cysts would bring an end to the IBS. The surgery was deemed successful, but to Penny's dismay, her diarrhea symptoms worsened, as did the cramping and bloating. She also found herself with a roaring vaginal yeast infection. Convinced that something had happened during the surgery, she quizzed her doctor about the steps in the procedure. Penny determined that she had been given a strong antibiotic during surgery to prevent infection, and she realized that the antibiotic had wiped out her intestinal flora. Her doctor recommended a course of Lactobacillus — a good intestinal bacteria found in capsule or powdered form, as well as in yogurt and kefir — for three weeks. Penny was amazed that her yeast and IBS symptoms actually improved. (In telling her story, she says that she had to go through ovarian surgery to find the cure for her IBS — Lactobacillus!)

Women's health advocacy groups are concerned that too much surgery is performed on women with IBS, and it's usually gynecological surgery. Hysterectomy and ovarian surgery occur more often in women with IBS than in women without IBS. In order to have gynecological surgery, you must first be referred to a gynecologist. One study found that too many women with symptoms of IBS are being wrongly referred to gynecologists instead of gastroenterologists.

Misdiagnosis can occur because IBS can cause severe abdominal pain that is confused with other conditions, some of them very serious. And since cancer is at the top of the list, doctors want to be especially sure that they rule out that condition. Women are probably subjected to more surgery than men because we have all those extra parts that can get into trouble — ovaries, uterus, fallopian tubes — compared to men who just have bowels in their abdomens. (Even their testicles, the counterpart of our ovaries, lie outside the abdomen.)

One study that looked into women at a gynecology clinic who had pelvic pain found that more than half of them had symptoms of IBS. After all the necessary testing and investigations were done, only 8 percent of the women with IBS also had a true gynecological problem.

Women with IBS can have pain during intercourse, which makes them (and everyone else, including their doctors) think they have gynecological problems. If you have this problem and your gynecologist doesn't remember his or her training in gastroenterology, a diagnosis of IBS may be missed, and off you go to surgery.

People with IBS have higher rates of surgery than the general population. This fact was proven when researchers examined almost 90,000 patient records, which showed that patients with IBS had three times the normal rate of gall bladder surgery and twice the rate of appendectomy and hysterectomy. IBS patients also had a 50 percent higher rate of back surgery.

If you don't want to end up in surgery — and who does? — it's best to get a second and even a third opinion before going under the knife. And just remember how modern medicine works. If you go to a surgeon, you have a greater chance of ending up in surgery than if you go to a nutritionist first. So get a referral to a good nutritionist who knows about IBS before making the appointment with a surgeon.

Associating Other Conditions with IBS

A number of conditions coexist or are often associated with IBS. The coexistence doesn't mean that one condition causes the other or even triggers the other.

First, we want to mention three symptoms (which aren't really conditions) that are very common in IBS and deserve attention:

- ✔ Headaches
- ✔ In women, left-sided abdominal pain during sexual intercourse
- ✔ Fatigue and tiredness

Headaches and fatigue can be caused by the absorption of toxic chemicals from the gut and a corresponding malabsorption of important nutrients. Left-sided pain during intercourse can be caused by direct pressure on trapped gas in the intestine.

The following list of conditions that are associated with IBS may come as a surprise to some of you, but they occur regularly in people with IBS:

- ✔ **Asthma:** Asthma is thought to be caused by inflammation of the lining of the lung that is aggravated by exposure to environmental substances. The incidence of IBS is four times higher in people with asthma, and that incidence is not associated with any side effects from asthma medication. Researchers wonder if the bronchial inflammation experienced in asthma is similar to the bowel irritation in IBS and if some of the same environmental substances may aggravate both conditions.

- ✔ **Poor sleep or insomnia:** Sleep is affected in people with IBS, who have a higher incidence of insomnia than other groups. If you think that a bad day of IBS causes a lot of tossing and turning, you would be wrong. It's actually the other way around. You could have a bad IBS day after a fitful night's sleep.

- ✔ **Premenstrual syndrome:** PMS is the topic of many jokes at the expense of women who suffer hormonal swings that can interrupt their lives on a regular basis. Hormonal shifts and imbalances create disruptive symptoms in an estimated 40 million women. Symptoms of anxiety/depression, food cravings, headaches, and weight gain define the four major types of PMS. Nearly 50 percent of women with IBS experience symptoms of PMS. However, IBS symptoms are sometimes lost in the more than 100 symptoms that have been designated as PMS-related, making an IBS diagnosis very difficult.

- ✔ **Endometriosis:** This painful pelvic condition occurs when tissue from the lining of the uterus is found outside the uterus, usually around the bowel and ovaries. This condition is considered to be the most common cause of pelvic pain in women in their child-bearing years. It may occur in as many as 10 percent of these women, but figures are hard to confirm because in order to diagnose it you have to actually do a *laparoscopy* (a scope through the belly button to look inside) or abdominal surgery to see abnormalities in the pelvis. At the time of menses, pain and cramping in the pelvis can resemble the worsening of symptoms that women with IBS commonly feel during their periods.

✔ **Fibromyalgia:** About 60 percent of people with this condition also have IBS. This is a condition that affects the musculoskeletal system causing muscle aches, stiffness, generalized fatigue, and insomnia. It's a functional disorder and, much like IBS, has no definitive diagnostic tests. A diagnosis is made by excluding other diseases like osteoarthritis and rheumatoid arthritis. Symptoms for more than six months and tender "trigger points" on the body help make the diagnosis. Treatment is often unsuccessful, leaving patients frustrated and in considerable distress — much like patients with IBS.

The term *fibromyalgia* means "fiber and muscle aching." It's becoming a more common condition in our culture. It may be the culmination of stress, toxins, poor diet, lack of vitamins and minerals, yeast, and leaky gut (which we discuss in Chapter 3). The muscles in various parts of the body seem to be permanently in spasm due to a buildup of toxins and tension. We believe that people with fibromyalgia may benefit from the diet and lifestyle changes we suggest in this book, and acupuncture (see Chapter 12) can be extremely helpful.

✔ **Painful periods:** Medically painful periods are called *dysmenorrhoea*. This is a significant problem for many women, but if you have IBS it's even worse because the symptoms of abdominal cramps from IBS and pelvic cramps from your period are all mixed together. Forty percent of women with IBS have painful periods.

✔ **Pain during intercourse:** Painful intercourse *(dyspareunia)* frequently occurs in women with IBS and often sends them to their doctors to find out what's wrong. It most often occurs on the left side. That's the location of the descending colon and rectum, where stool is stored before elimination. During intercourse, poking into this area may cause more pressure and stretching of the hypersensitive intestinal tissues that seem to be a factor in IBS. A slow and gentle approach can relax the area and decrease the pain.

✔ **Urinary frequency and urgency:** Urinary frequency and urgency are more common in women with IBS. In one study, small balloons were used to distend the esophagus and bladder, confirming that a group of women with IBS experienced more pain than other women when this was done. Other studies where balloons were used to distend rectal tissue show that people with IBS need less distention to stimulate the urge to have a bowel movement and experience discomfort at low balloon pressures. The results from such studies make researchers wonder

> if IBS is related to a problem with smooth muscle function, making people more susceptible to irritation where a sense of fullness can be perceived as pain.
>
> ✔ **Acid reflux:** People who suffer from IBS are 2.5 times more likely to also suffer from acid reflux disease. Researchers point to a disorder in smooth muscle function in this association.

Experiencing Psychological Distress

People who have experienced severe psychological distress, including physical and sexual abuse, have a higher rate of anxiety and depression, as well as a higher rate of IBS. Women are more likely than men to have suffered abuse. They also bring complaints of anxiety and depression to a doctor more often than men and, as we note earlier in the chapter, have a higher rate of IBS than men.

Studies have not definitively proven that women with IBS report more anxiety and depression symptoms than women without IBS. When judging stress in people with IBS, we imagine that it is impossible to separate the stress of having IBS — the pain, the frustration, the worry — from stress in general. Therefore, to try to differentiate whether people with IBS are more stressed is a moot point. The answer is *yes,* of course, wouldn't you be stressed by the symptoms we are describing related to IBS?

Abuse and experiencing the stress it creates are associated with IBS. Abuse is not a proven cause of IBS, but it does make the symptoms worse. In other words, someone with IBS who has experienced physical or sexual abuse will have more symptoms than someone who did not experience abuse. We focus on stress in Chapter 12, where we give practical and useful tools to deal with even severe stress such as abuse.

Having Hypersensitivity

Samantha was excited about the birth of her first child. Somehow, Samantha contracted a serious intestinal infection while in the hospital, complete with diarrhea and vomiting. After several days, she was still making frequent and urgent trips to the bathroom to deal with the diarrhea. The severe cramping and abdominal pain were truly debilitating. Samantha told the doctors that the pain was actually worse than the pain that she had just experienced while giving birth. Nobody would believe her, and she was told that she probably was suffering from postpartum depression.

Studies show that women can tolerate more pain than men. For example, women better tolerate thrusting their hands into ice-cold water than men do. But there's no big surprise here: Women, after all, manage to force an 8-pound (or larger) object through an opening that before and after the event is no wider than a few millimeters. When you challenge a man to think about shoving something that size down his urethra through his penis, he almost passes out just at the thought of it. So pain is nothing new to women.

Why, then, do women have more IBS and, apparently, a more sensitive bowel than men? Does a sensitive bowel (called *visceral hypersensitivity*) somehow equal a survival mechanism for women? Or is there something different in a women's bowel that causes the greater sensitivity?

Experiencing ongoing stress

Another aspect of bowel activity is how various individuals handle stress. We talk more about this topic in Chapter 12, but it's important to mention it in the discussion of why women experience more IBS as well. Apparently, some people with IBS, when faced with an acute stress (perhaps even just driving on a freeway), process various stress chemicals differently. The fight-or-flight chemical called *adrenaline* is released along with several others, and they make the heart speed up and drive energy to our legs to allow us to run. These chemicals also have an effect on the gut.

These chemicals cause a short-term lowering of the immune system in the lining of the gut. In Chapter 3, we mention how the gut is lined with lymph tissue that protects it from infection and invasion. During stress, with the surge in stress hormone steroids (like natural cortisone), the lymph tissue shuts down, perhaps to direct the body's energy toward surviving a direct external attack, which is calculated to be more important in the moment than the attack from within. If you think about it, the body is constantly making those decisions and diverting energy and resources to where they are most needed in the moment.

The trouble is that in our society we feel ourselves to be under fairly constant stress. The question must be asked, does the immune system suffer because of chronic stressors lowering its guard and allowing a form of inflammation that may not be detectable even on the most complete medical workup? Such inflammation may be enough to cause symptoms of IBS in susceptible people. Apparently, these susceptible people are women with IBS. Measurements show that they have higher levels of stress hormones and chemicals than women who do not have IBS.

Although there are myriad causes of stress, one your shouldn't have to deal with is the stress of leaving the house when you have IBS. When you are planning an outing, call ahead to find out about the washroom facilities available, or do an Internet search to see if the mall you are going to has a floor plan online. If you can feel assured that your destination has easily accessible facilities, your stress about leaving the house may diminish. We provide lots more tips for getting out of the house in Chapter 13.

Suffering from worry

Worrying is a form of self-induced stress. Worry is not necessarily a diagnosable condition, but it is a symptom of poor coping skills in life in the sense that a worrier always imagines the worst will happen.

A 2000 study of 239 women patients with gastrointestinal problems were asked how they coped with chronic pain and whether they actively worked on solving their problems. It may seem like common sense, but the researchers proved that the better coping skills one has, the better the outcome. Using a series of questionnaires, patients were rated for good or poor coping skills. Those who had good skills had fewer visits to their doctors and had less psychological distress and pain. Women were rated as having poor coping skills if they felt helpless and powerless in the face of their condition. Those women experienced more psychological distress, visited their doctor more frequently, and were bedridden more often.

Coping skills can be learned, and in Chapter 12, we show you some important coping skills to put you on the positive side of this study.

Part II
Getting Medical Help

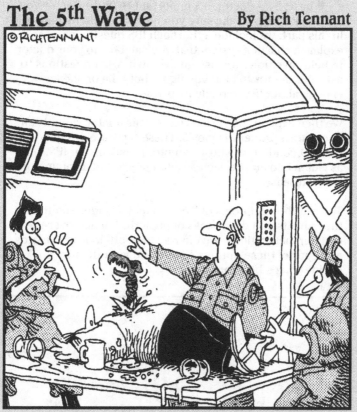

The 5th Wave   By Rich Tennant

"Relax everyone! It's not IBS, not Crohn's disease, just an internal alien implantation."

In this part . . .

Although IBS is not a disease managed on a day-by-day basis by a doctor, it's important to find a doctor you can work with to make sure you have the right diagnosis. In this part, we include a thorough IBS questionnaire and explain a charting system that you can take to your doctor to help save time. We also guide you in what questions to ask your doctor to help you figure out if he or she knows enough about IBS to really help you.

We then explain the various tests your doctor should run to ensure a proper diagnosis. These tests are designed to rule out conditions whose symptoms may mirror IBS, such as gluten intolerance, lactose intolerance, and inflammatory bowel disease.

To treat the symptoms of IBS, you may wonder about the benefits and drawbacks of prescription and over-the-counter medications. We offer an in-depth look at the pros and cons of these options so you and your doctor can decide what's best for you.

Chapter 6

Finding a Doctor

. . . .

In This Chapter

▶ Recognizing alarm symptoms

▶ Asking for what you need

▶ Taking charge of your health

▶ Finding the doctor within

. . . .

Maybe you suspect that you have IBS and want a diagnosis. Maybe you have already talked with your regular doctor and received a referral to see a specialist. Or maybe you've found out that your doctor doesn't know enough about IBS to help you, and you are seeking another health practitioner. We cover all these scenarios in this chapter.

Many of the books and articles on IBS that we've read say that the most important step you can take in managing your condition is to find an IBS-friendly doctor. Such a doctor can help you diagnose your condition and make sure it's not another more serious disease like an inflammatory bowel disease or cancer.

When you find the right doctor, he or she should spend time with you to explain IBS, the treatments available, and the impact of triggers on your symptoms. A good relationship with your doctor doesn't just make you feel warm and fuzzy; it actually translates into needing less office visits. The words you really want to hear from your doctor are, "I know about IBS, and I think I can help you."

With a fluctuating condition like IBS, things often go more smoothly if you know someone is always going to be on the other end of the phone when you need him or her; you breathe a sigh of relief. On the other hand, if you don't have a trusted doctor on your team, the worry and fear factor can tie your intestines into knots.

In Chapter 7, we show you how a good doctor goes about making a diagnosis of IBS. That chapter assumes you have a good doctor to go to who understands IBS. In the event that you don't, in this chapter we help you find one.

But while finding the right doctor is crucial, we actually think the most important step you can take in managing your condition is to take charge of your own body. If you read each chapter of *IBS For Dummies,* you may know more about IBS than most doctors. You will understand how to read your body signs, and you will know what pulls you into IBS symptoms and how to avoid those pitfalls. A knowledgeable and independent patient is actually what most doctors want. So in this chapter, we also encourage you to take charge of your own health.

Knowing When to Get Help

The main reasons people with IBS go to a doctor are much the same as with other conditions:

- ✔ For emergency care
- ✔ For an initial diagnosis
- ✔ For a second opinion
- ✔ For advice on managing their condition
- ✔ To renew prescriptions

In this section, we explain symptoms that often compel someone with IBS to seek medical attention, as well as the importance of being proactive about your health.

Sounding the alarm

Someone with what we may consider mild to moderate IBS may spend months or years dealing with annoying, sometimes painful symptoms without ever mentioning to a doctor what's going on. Diarrhea, constipation, bloating, and other symptoms so common in IBS (see Chapter 2) may make life uncomfortable, but some people choose to live with the discomfort rather than expose themselves to medical experiences they fear may be embarrassing or frustrating.

When someone with this type of history finally seeks help, it's often because of an alarm symptom, and often that person seeks help in an emergency department.

Personal alarms

The following alarm symptoms, many of which actually are *not* symptoms of IBS, signal that you should run, not walk, to your doctor's office. (Better yet, take a cab.)

✔ **Bleeding from the rectum:** Rectal bleeding indicates that something other than IBS is going on. As we note in Chapter 2, rectal bleeding may indicate an inflammatory bowel disease (IBD). Some people experience rectal bleeding if they have eaten lots of roughage, such as nuts, seeds, or popcorn; they scrape open a capillary on the wall of the intestine or at the anus. Hemorrhoids may also cause rectal bleeding. Bright red blood in any amount, or dried blood that turns your bowel movements black, is a special cause for concern; it may indicate a benign polyp that has ruptured, a bleeding diverticuli, or cancer.

The bottom line: If you are bleeding from your rectum, seek immediate medical attention. Don't try to guess the cause for yourself. But before you zoom off to the ER, recall if you ate beets in your most recent meal (which would turn your stool red) or if you have taken Pepto-Bismol (because the metal bismuth in this product can turn stools black).

✔ **Fever:** If you have IBS symptoms and develop a fever, it's not a sign of IBS. Instead, it could indicate inflammatory bowel disease (IBD), diverticulitis, or an intestinal infection (parasites or worms) and should be investigated.

✔ **Nighttime diarrhea:** Diarrhea that wakes you at night is not a symptom of IBS and must be further investigated. It could indicate inflammatory bowel disease or cancer.

✔ **Difficulty swallowing and food sticking in the esophagus:** This symptom is usually related to a growth in the esophagus. (It differs from the emotional symptom where a person feels a sensation of something in the esophagus but can still easily swallow food.)

✔ **Stomach or abdominal pain that wakes you up at night:** IBS does not usually wake you at night. A growth in the abdomen, either benign or malignant, can be painful enough to cause insomnia and wake you at night.

✔ **Abdominal bloating that does not get better overnight:** IBS bloating is usually due to gas, which dissipates overnight. Symptoms that appear like bloating but don't ease at night can be caused by an enlarged liver or spleen.

✔ **Tenesmus:** If you feel that you haven't finished a bowel movement and still feel the urge to go, even though all your stool has emptied out, your rectum and perhaps your large intestine are inflamed. This symptom occurs with any type of colitis, whether infectious or ulcerative colitis.

Alarms for doctors

Some symptoms, which may seem less urgent to you than those on the previous list, serve as red flags to your doctor that something serious may be going on.

✔ **Anemia:** In a patient with symptoms of IBS, anemia may indicate a slow blood loss that may not show up visibly in the toilet. It may point to an ulcer or tumor in the intestines and needs to be investigated.

✔ **Unexplained weight loss:** Suddenly losing more than ten pounds can be an indication of something much more serious than IBS. Cancer is often the cause of such sudden weight loss. However, a serious infection in the gut could cause such a sudden drop in weight as well through loss of fluids.

✔ **Sudden onset in someone over age 40:** Without a history of recent travel or recent use of antibiotics, IBS symptoms in a person over 40 are rare and imply another cause.

Some infectious disease specialists advise all patients with IBD to take a round of therapy for possible parasitic infection even if a thorough gastrointestinal investigation shows nothing. A parasitic infection of the intestines — sometimes called *amebiasis* — can mimic IBS and IBD.

Avoiding the ER

Ideally, you want to seek a diagnosis as soon as you become aware that your IBS symptoms are ongoing, rather than a short-term result of an intestinal bug. Unfortunately, and for a variety of reasons, people often delay seeing a doctor until their symptoms become unbearable or frightening (or both).

Some people with IBS don't seek any help until they end up in the emergency room with excruciating pain. We must stress that this is *not* the way you want to have your symptoms addressed. The more severe your symptoms at the time of your first visit with a doctor, the more likely you are to be treated with drugs to suppress your symptoms. Both you and your doctor may have the impression that you have a more serious condition than you do when your first visit is in the ER.

Identifying the Right Doctor for You

Even doctors who are general practitioners can have areas of specialty, and one specialty can be the manner in which they treat patients. For example, a matter of fact, no nonsense doctor who doesn't have much of a bedside manner may have just the kind of detached attitude that suits a man in a three-piece suit. However, put that doctor in a room with a 16-year-old girl who wants to talk about problems with her period and birth control, and both doctor and patient will probably leave the room trembling.

Let's face it: Not every doctor can deal with every patient or every medical situation. The art of doctoring has a lot to do with people skills, and since these skills are not taught in medical school, you have to hope your doctor was born with them. Otherwise, he or she may not be the person to hear you out about your intestinal problems.

Blinking

In 2005, Malcolm Gladwell introduced the concept of *blinking* in his succinctly named book *Blink* (Little, Brown and Company). Its premise is that people make split-second decisions about others when they first meet.

Doctors are trained — and warned — not to make such snap decisions about patients. They are taught not to ask leading questions such as, "So, Mrs. Smith, you have pain in your lower abdomen, not in your upper abdomen — is that right?" If this type of question is posed, Mrs. Smith, who doesn't want to insult the doctor, will often say, "Yes, that's right." A better way for a doctor to conduct an interview is to first ask, "Do you have pain?" and then continue with, "Where is your pain?"

Our healthcare system has created very busy doctors on tight schedules with only a few minutes for each appointment. They often don't have (or take) the time to find out what's really going on with a patient who has more than one or two symptoms. Because IBS has a number of symptoms, some of them can be left out of the picture when you don't have time to tell your story. It's important, therefore, to bring a list of your symptoms to your doctor so that he or she can get your whole story at a glance. We discuss how to create a useful list of symptoms, and other types of information that may be helpful to your doctor, in Chapter 7.

We must warn you that a few doctors may think that people who bring lists of symptoms to an appointment are obsessed with their health — and not in a good way. Most doctors, however, appreciate the valuable time saved by having the information.

A doctor can only treat your IBS symptoms, not the cause (unless you are still in the infectious stage of your condition, which means an antibiotic or antiparasitic drug can kill the particular organism affecting you). So be specific about the timing and nature of your diarrhea, constipation, or both when you are talking to your doctor. Make sure that your treatment matches your symptoms. (In Chapters 8 and 9, we talk about medications and other treatments available for IBS symptoms.)

Believing in IBS

We talk in Chapter 2 about the credibility gap that plagues IBS. Some doctors just don't believe it's a real condition with serious physical manifestations. And if that describes your doctor's beliefs, no matter how much she may like you as a patient, she just isn't going to put a lot of stock in your symptoms of gas, bloating, pain, and changes in bowel movements.

You want a doctor who is on the same side of the table as you are. You want someone to believe what you say about what you are experiencing. If your doctor discounts the existence of IBS, it's going to be difficult to focus on your concerns.

In cases where a doctor doesn't believe in IBS, you are not just trying to get the doctor to believe that you are suffering and that your suffering is real. You are actually trying to convince the doctor that a well-documented condition, with very real symptoms (and even diagnostic criteria), exists.

And even if you convince your doctor that your symptoms are real, you also need your doctor to make sure that your condition is nothing worse than IBS. As we explain in Chapter 7, he needs to rule out a whole list of other possibilities, either by rational explanations or by rational testing.

A 1999 survey of 1,000 women with IBS and 700 medical practitioners (including doctors and nurses) highlighted some interesting facts. For the most part, doctors did not believe that IBS was a serious medical condition, and though they acknowledged that the condition was distressing, they believed that their patients were exaggerating the pain they felt with IBS.

Women, in turn, felt that their doctors simply didn't understand the extent of their pain or discomfort, which prevented them from discussing their symptoms. Many doctors, including some gastroenterologists, still believe that IBS is primarily a psychological condition.

Working with a primary care physician

Your primary care doctor may be an allopathic doctor in family practice or general practice, or you may have a naturopathic doctor for your primary healthcare needs. Each may have a very different take on IBS.

First, let's define our terms:

- ✓ An *allopathic* doctor treats disease using modern Western medical processes and procedures. Allopathic, drug-based, scientific medicine has been in control of medicine since approximately the 1920s.

- ✓ *Naturopathic* doctors do not specialize in drug therapy; they concentrate on nutrition, lifestyle education, and psychological balancing.

While allopathic doctors are covered by most insurance companies, naturopathic doctors or even doctors practicing *integrative medicine* (combining allopathic and naturopathic approaches) may not be covered. There are a few exceptions; some insurance companies offer allowances for acupuncture treatment, chiropractic care, or nutrition.

While each doctor is an individual, and we encourage you to have an open mind when meeting a doctor for the first time, the following sections offer a broad perspective of the differences between many allopathic doctors and naturopathic doctors.

Educating your allopath

Some doctors have the impression that if they didn't learn it in medical school, it doesn't exist; what they learned in medical school is untouchable and undeniable. Changing such a doctor's mind is a difficult proposition. A patient only has to see the gleam of disbelief in a doctor's eye for a fraction of a second to know that she isn't going to get a fair hearing. (Consider this: An allopathic doctor who has been in practice 25 years was taught in medical school that a patient with *irritable colon* [as it was called then] is a nervous, anxious person with a long history of bowel symptoms but without weight loss.)

The 1999 survey of doctors and women with IBS (which we introduce in the previous section) reported that 87 percent of doctors said they need better education on the topic of IBS. However, 58 percent of doctors surveyed indicated that IBS is easy to diagnose (although most did not follow the Rome II Diagnostic Criteria for diagnosing IBS — see Chapter 2). A majority of women surveyed saw three primary care physicians before getting a valid IBS diagnosis.

If you have any doubts about your doctor's stance on IBS, bring him a copy of the Rome II criteria that we show you in Chapter 2 and a completed symptoms questionnaire from Chapter 7. An article that shows the incidence of IBS, as well as a copy of this book, will let your doctor know that you mean to get to the bottom of your symptoms and you're willing to do a lot of the leg work involved.

Bringing these solid pieces of evidence about IBS will help persuade your doctor that you are a knowledgeable patient with legitimate concerns about your health. The attitude you want to develop is one of teamwork where together you tackle this problem situation.

A growing number of allopathic doctors are very concerned about the epidemic of chronic illness. They are studying traditional medical modalities and bridging the gap for their patients. A name had been adopted for this type of practice — *complementary alternative medicine,* or CAM. (We like to think that traditional medicine has equal footing with modern medicine, so we don't call it alternative.) Some people call it *integrative medicine.*

Involving your naturopath

Naturopathic doctors in many states and provinces are considered primary care doctors. By the very nature of their training, they are aware of the body–mind interplay of illness. They are also trained in nutrition and diet. They know about lactose intolerance, gluten enteropathy, food allergies, and Candida overgrowth, and generally are aware how important it is to distinguish them from IBS.

If you are looking for a naturopath, many of them have Web sites that describe their areas of specialty, their philosophies, and the types of treatments they use. Ask your friends, your massage therapist, or a yoga instructor about naturopaths in your community. Often your local health food store will have information about practitioners in your area. In Chapter 21, we provide some information on locating a naturopath or naturopathic clinics.

Most naturopathic doctors have an association with a specialty lab where they can send tests to determine lactose intolerance, gluten enteropathy, food allergies, and Candida overgrowth. Naturopathic doctors do not specialize in drug therapy; because they specialize in nutrition, lifestyle education, and psychological balancing, they do not reach for the pill bottle to treat your symptoms. In fact, their license does not allow them to prescribe drugs, so they have become experts in prescribing diet, exercise, dietary supplements, and psychological support.

If we're painting a rosy picture of naturopathic medicine, that's because it does shine in the diagnosis and treatment of chronic functional conditions. As you see in Chapter 8, IBS is not a condition that can ever be *cured* by medicines. Because drugs are the main modalities of allopathic medicine, it follows that allopathic medicine actually plays a secondary role in the treatment of IBS.

Asking lots of questions

If you go to the emergency room for your first IBS treatment, the doctor is going to be asking most of the questions. But if you are doctor shopping (a phrase most doctors don't like to hear), you have more of an opportunity to ask some questions yourself.

Before you launch into questions with a doctor, first find out how long your visit is scheduled to be. The office receptionist should be able to tell you. Your appointment time could be 5 minutes or 50 minutes, and you have to adjust your Q & A accordingly. (Frankly, a doctor who can spend only 5 minutes on an initial visit may not be the best one for you.)

Most doctors run behind schedule. If you don't want to spend lots of time in the waiting room, try making an appointment first thing in the morning or in the early afternoon as soon as the doctor returns from lunch.

You may have to ask only one or two questions to get a feel for your doctor and know whether you are going to be able to work with her. So be ready to drop your questions at any time and either move on to the next stage of the appointment (where you may have a physical exam or be given a list of tests) or politely exit the office.

When you ask these questions of your allopathic doctor or naturopathic doctor, your goal is to keep the conversation friendly and not confrontational. The last thing you want is a doctor on the defensive. That being said, some doctors don't like to answer questions — mainly because of the time constraints they work under.

The following questions are geared toward a primary care physician.

- ✔ **Do you have patients with IBS?** This may be the only question you need to ask. If the doctor says that he doesn't have patients with IBS, that answer doesn't make sense when you consider that up to 20 percent of the population suffers from IBS. If your doctor says he sees nobody with IBS, he may have selective vision.

  If the answer to this question is negative, most patients with IBS symptoms won't think twice before they are out the door looking for a doctor they can partner with. If the answer is yes, you can go on to the next question.

- ✔ **What do you think causes IBS?** By reading this book, you are gaining great information about the causes, triggers, and conditions associated with IBS. You will probably know more than your doctor, so go easy here. A simple answer like "We don't know the actual cause, but there are many triggers that involve diet and stress" would let you know that your doctor is on the right track.

  Be very aware and wary of a doctor who insists that there is a specific cause of IBS. If you read Chapter 2, you know that identifying the cause of IBS isn't that simple. Do not be intimidated into believing that *this* doctor is the *only one* that knows the true cause. There are no absolutes when it comes to IBS.

  If a doctor tells you that she knows the specific cause, ask where she got her information or whether that is her personal opinion. For example, a naturopath who has experience with IBS may have noticed that most patients with IBS have certain common triggers. This observation is different from the cause of IBS.

- ✔ **How do you diagnose IBS?** You will have hit the jackpot if your doctor says he goes by the Rome II criteria (see Chapter 2) but investigates alarm symptoms. That statement alone would let you know that your doctor is well informed (and probably has read *IBS For Dummies* cover to cover!). You also want to know if he will help sort out food triggers and food intolerance.

- ✔ **Do you check IBS patients for lactose intolerance?** If your doctor says no, that IBS is not caused by lactose intolerance, you are back to square one. True, IBS is not *caused* by lactose intolerance, but the two conditions can be easily mistaken for each other. The only way to find out if you have lactose intolerance is to do a hydrogen breath test, which we explain in Chapter 7.

✔ **Do you check IBS patients for gluten enteropathy (celiac disease)?** If your doctor gets uncomfortable and says she has to leave the room for a minute, you may have a problem. It may mean she is going out to consult her medical dictionary to remind herself what celiac disease is all about. If she says that celiac occurs only in children and requires a small bowel biopsy to diagnose, you know she is living in the Dark Ages. (We explain the test for this disease in Chapter 7.)

Sometimes, to spare the patient an intrusive test, doctors minimize the importance of celiac disease. And sometimes, to spare themselves the embarrassment of not knowing about a disease, doctors minimize its importance.

✔ **What do you know about fruit intolerance and IBS?** This subject is not taught in medical school. Most doctors learn that allergies to food are mainly IgE-mediated acute allergic reactions to shellfish, peanuts, and strawberries, to name the most common offenders. Many doctors say that fruit is very good for you and does not cause adverse reactions. But as we note in Chapter 4, fruit intolerance can be a very real problem for people with IBS. (A naturopath will likely be aware of fruit intolerance.)

✔ **Does Candida albicans have a role in IBS?** This is an opportunity for your doctor to shine and talk about gastrointestinal infections, antibiotics, and the overgrowth of Candida yeast that can set up an irritation in the gut leading to symptoms of IBS. If he dismisses Candida albicans as a fad disease that has no scientific basis, you may have to move on. A naturopath is likely well aware of this condition and its widespread effects.

✔ **Do food allergies play a role in IBS?** You want to have a discussion about leaky gut (see Chapter 3) and the absorption of undigested food molecules into the bloodstream, which are then treated like allergy-causing substances. This is not mainstream medicine. But a naturopath or a CAM practitioner is going to know about this condition and give you the information you need.

✔ **How do you rule out Crohn's and ulcerative colitis?** Your doctor's answer will usually be that if you have any of the signs or symptoms of these inflammatory bowel diseases, a colonoscopy by a gastroenterologist is in order. She may also say that there are blood tests in specialty labs available to help rule out these conditions based on immune factors. (A naturopath is more likely to know about these immune function tests than an allopathic doctor.)

✔ **How do you treat IBS?** The answer you want to hear is that your doctor is willing to work with you to determine what's best for you. What you don't want to hear is that drugs are the only answer.

Your doctor's answer to these questions should let you know if you can work with him or her to help diagnose and manage your condition.

Deciding on a specialist

In the previous section, we focus on general practitioners, but a GP may not know enough about gastrointestinal disorders to help you. Your GP may not know about celiac disease or all the latest studies on IBS. If she hasn't heard of the Rome II Diagnostic Criteria for diagnosing IBS, chances are she's not up on IBS. That may be your clue to ask for a referral to a gastroenterologist.

If your doctor is an allopath and says your symptoms don't warrant referral to a gastroenterologist, and he doesn't seem to know that IBS is a condition affected by a combination of diet, stress, and bowel infection, you need to find another doctor who will make that referral. Integrative medicine doctors or complementary alternative medicine (CAM) doctors are trained in allopathic medicine, but they bridge the gap between allopathic medicine and naturopathic medicine. This may be the type of doctor you need to see for treatment or to get a referral to a specialist.

Seeing a gastroenterologist

Your general practitioner may refer you to a gastroenterologist who specializes in IBS so that person can help you identify possible food triggers and food intolerance. Or you may be referred because you have an alarm symptom such as fever, bleeding, or severe pain and need to rule out inflammatory bowel disease, cancer, or diverticulitis. We discuss all these diseases and their differentiation from IBS in Chapter 7.

You can be sure that your gastroenterologist knows about the Rome II Diagnostic Criteria, either by hearing about it at a conference or reading GI medical journals. Fifty percent of people visiting a GI specialist have symptoms of IBS, so this condition is actually a gastroenterologist's bread and butter. That doesn't mean this is automatically the perfect doctor for you (especially if he doesn't realize that bread and butter may contribute to IBS), but chances are he does know more about IBS than a general practitioner.

Gastroenterologists see many people with lactose intolerance and celiac disease. They have access to the latest tests — the hydrogen breath tests — to diagnose these diseases and distinguish them from IBS. (We explain hydrogen breath tests in Chapter 7.) But your gastroenterologist may pooh-pooh fruit intolerance, food allergies, and Candida albicans, so you may get only a partial diagnosis. If your lactose test and gluten test are normal but you still have symptoms, we encourage you to look further by visiting either a naturopath or a nutritionist. (You don't need a doctor's referral to see a naturopath.)

Seeing a dietician or nutritionist

You may ask your general practitioner for a referral to a dietician or nutritionist who is knowledgeable in the treatment of IBS to help you sort out your diet and even go on a food elimination diet.

There is no point in seeing a dietician or nutritionist who is not familiar with all the food issues in IBS, as well as the Candida albicans correlation. The main help you want here is support for a food elimination and challenge diet. If you are a junk food eater and your fridge is mainly stocked with beer and condiments, you are going to need a lot of hand-holding.

What's the difference between a dietician and a nutritionist?

- ✔ A *dietician* is usually a hospital-based practitioner who follows the basic food guide produced by the government. Dieticians also usually follow the recommended dietary allowance (RDA) for nutrients. They tend to advocate using dietary supplements just to prevent deficiency — like using the minimum amount of vitamin C to prevent scurvy — rather than for therapeutic purposes. Their training is in sciences, food science, and food preparation.

- ✔ *Certified nutritionist* and *certified clinical nutritionist* are titles given to people who have taken hundreds of hours of courses in nutrition that go beyond the basic food sciences into practical clinical application. (Someone with one of these titles may or may not have an undergraduate degree.) They also learn about the use of dietary supplements in the prevention and treatment of disease.

A dietician who is also a nutritionist is probably the best person to look for when seeking help with your IBS diet. If you have not ruled out lactose intolerance, celiac disease, food allergies, and Candida overgrowth, such a person will be able to help you create an elimination diet. In Chapter 10, we talk more about the elimination and challenge diet, which involves avoiding possible offending foods and then reintroducing them to see if your symptoms return.

A dietician/nutritionist can also talk with you about necessary supplements to help boost your immune system, heal your leaky gut, and help eliminate a possible imbalance of bacteria and yeast in your intestines. Usually a series of three to six visits is enough to get you sorted out and on your way to feeling better.

Seeing a medical acupuncturist

Some medical doctors specialize in acupuncture, but they often just use this modality to treat symptoms. Acupuncture may treat IBS symptoms such as cramping, abdominal pain, tension, and anxiety. But it is also superb for treating the stress that is involved with this condition. And acupuncture can also successfully treat the underlying disruption of the nerves and intestinal muscles that creates disrupted intestinal movement (either too slow, causing constipation, or too fast, causing diarrhea).

However, if your IBS is related to some of the triggers that we talk about in Chapter 4, acupuncture alone can't eliminate the symptoms; you must eliminate the triggers.

Seeing a Chinese medicine doctor

The true experts in acupuncture are the doctors trained in acupuncture, herbs, and pulse diagnosis. They say that using acupuncture without herbs is not true acupuncture. And without pulse diagnosis, they say that it is not possible to really know where to put the needles or what the body really needs.

Chinese medicine doctors can read the pulses of the body and determine such esoteric things as the heat, cold, or dampness in the body. By looking at your tongue, they can determine how you are digesting your food. They know all about IBS, but they also know it can be produced by heat, cold, dampness, kidney deficiency, food stagnation, and a dozen other imbalances in the body.

A symptom of too much heat would be explosive diarrhea that has a strong odor and burns the anus. Dampness would mean sticky bowel movements and a white-coated tongue. Food stagnation has associated symptoms of heartburn and nausea. A Chinese medicine doctor also talks about IBS caused by infection or internal disruptive factors, such as self-blame and guilt, that can lead to internal tension and bowel symptoms.

A Chinese medicine doctor will also prescribe diet therapy, which usually involves avoiding possible food triggers and intolerances.

Chinese medicine is extremely well suited to the treatment of chronic, functional conditions. The focus of treatment is to bring the body back into balance and remove the energy blocks created by a bad lifestyle and stress.

Seeing a hypnotherapist

Some people with IBS just want the pain and bloating to go away and will do anything to make that happen. Seeing a hypnotherapist is sometimes an option, but only after you have ruled out physical causes and triggers of your IBS. Even though hypnosis can help eliminate symptoms, they may just come back if you are gluten intolerant and keep eating wheat, for example.

If you feel that your IBS is psychologically triggered — for example, if you experience IBS symptoms when you have to travel or be in a large crowd without quick access to a restroom — hypnosis may help you break that vicious cycle. (In Chapter 12, we introduce you to some other stress-busting modalities you can safely use that may have the same results as hypnosis but are totally under your control.)

A 2003 paper published in the journal *Gut* found that of 204 patients who used hypnotherapy for their symptoms of IBS, 71 percent responded well initially. Of that number, 81 percent maintained their improvement over a five-year period. Even the 19 percent whose symptoms returned said they relapsed only slightly. To go along with their increased well being, these subjects had fewer doctors' visits, less medication, and much less anxiety and depression.

Relying on the Doctor Within

The most important aspect of managing IBS is taking charge of your condition. IBS has a lot of symptoms, a lot of ups and downs, and you need to be on top of what's going on. You don't have the time, money, or energy to go to your doctor every time you have a symptom. But you do have the time to read this book and get clear about what IBS is and what you can do for yourself.

Assuming power

It's actually much more empowering to be in charge than to think that your doctor knows more about your body than you do. In fact, the attitude of being empowered may help turn off the stress trigger of IBS. You may be tempted to just turn the responsibility for your health over to someone else. Maybe with a different condition or disease (and especially if you have to have surgery), it makes sense to turn over the power. But when it comes to a functional condition like IBS, you need to be in charge.

Before doctors' offices were on every corner, people took care of themselves and each other. In the West, women were the main healers in earlier times — they were the midwives and herbalists, and many of their remedies are experiencing a resurgence as more and more people become disillusioned with the adverse reactions to so many pharmaceutical medications.

Managing your IBS

Managing your IBS *may* be something you can do on your own, as long as you know the rules.

The rule with GI symptoms is to watch for alarm symptoms (which we list earlier in the chapter) and see your doctor if you have them. Otherwise, we believe that people should become more responsible for their own self-care. We should learn more about our bodies, what feeds them, and what messes them up. But this approach comes *after* you find your doctor and get a diagnosis — not before. If you are in denial about severe GI symptoms and keep telling yourself it's just IBS, you could be missing a more severe condition.

Allopathic doctors are very good at emergencies, surgery, and reattaching limbs. They often just don't have the time to deal with chronic conditions that relate to diet, lifestyle, and stress. Therefore, it's wonderful that you are reading *IBS For Dummies* to understand the ins and outs of IBS and how to manage your own condition on a day-to-day basis.

Improving your eating and exercise habits

The first step in managing bowel symptoms is to watch what you eat. In Chapter 7, we talk about making a journal to take to your doctor. But you should also make this journal for yourself. If there is a food or drink that makes your symptoms worse, you can draw the conclusion that it is bad for you. You don't need to pay a doctor to tell you what you already know.

We devote Chapter 10 to information that can help you become smarter about what and how you eat.

Taking steps to improve your eating habits is up to you. Nobody else can make diet changes for you. But change is a hard thing to do. Sometimes we are more comfortable in a bad place that's familiar than a new place that seems scary. If you find yourself feeling overwhelmed by what you think you should be doing, try some of the stress-busting techniques that you find in Chapter 12.

Much the same can be said for exercise: It's up to you to do it, and the benefits are enormous. Don't wait for your doctor to tell you to exercise. Often doctors don't recommend what they don't do themselves! Chapter 11 gives you the whole scoop on exercise and its benefits for IBS.

Dealing with stress

The connection between stress and IBS is fascinating, unless you're the person trying to sort it out. Then it can be downright frustrating, which doesn't help your case one bit. Why do people have such a tough time eliminating stressors that can lead to IBS symptoms? We devote Chapter 12 to the issues of stress, but one challenge is that the relationship between IBS and stress is not always obvious.

If you find that Monday morning is the worst time for your IBS, you may have an easy time figuring out that stress is the culprit. After all, many people find that after a relaxing weekend, they just don't want to go back to the grind of work. But what if your IBS symptoms seem to occur any time (or all the time)?

We often hear people with IBS say something like, "I can't eat a thing without bloating or having excruciating pain and diarrhea." If you have ongoing IBS episodes and can't seem to figure out what triggers them, you may think that *everything* you eat is problematic. When that happens, your physical problems get all mixed up with the psychological aspect of IBS. You may become afraid of eating anything. Plus, you become afraid of leaving the house because you're afraid of having symptoms in public. (We deal with this topic in-depth in Chapter 13.)

Think about the last time someone snuck up behind you and scared the living daylights out of you. What happened? Your heart leapt to your throat, you held your breath, and your intestines tightened in a knot. *Chronic* fear does the same thing; it makes you breathe shallowly and suck in your intestines and tighten them up. After a while, you don't even know you're doing it.

Right this minute, take a deep breath. Fill your lungs deeply, and make your abdomen expand. If you can't do that, or if it feels tight and uncomfortable, you have abdominal tension that translates into intestinal tension. And it only makes sense that if you are trying to hold in gas and diarrhea, you are going to have a tense abdomen as well. In Chapter 11, we show you a host of antistress exercises, including breathing exercises.

Paying attention to your body

To successfully manage your IBS, you have to see your IBS symptoms as signs of things that have to change. You got the IBS symptoms for a reason, whether it be infection, food, or stress. The first step in getting rid of your symptoms is to acknowledge why you got them in the first place. Sticking your head under the sand like the ostrich is not going to help.

It's better to identify what's triggering your symptoms than to just go to a doctor and say, "I have no idea why my bowels are acting up. Can you give me a pill?" (As we explain in Chapter 8, pills are another thing that your bowels may react against.)

It's your body, and you are in charge. You may not know where the owner's manual is, but you are learning, and you can apply what you learn. IBS is very much a condition that people experiment with. After all, you feel awful, nobody seems to have the one answer to how to feel better, and you have to experiment to find out what works for you. Just be sure you experiment with the right information and tools so that you can come out on the other end winning the battle against IBS.

Developing a healthy skepticism

As you make strides toward taking control of your IBS, you're bound to read or hear about miracle "cures" that other people with similar symptoms have found. While we encourage you to read as much as you can about IBS and to talk (whether in person or online) with others who share your situation, we urge you to be cautious about applying all the information you get. Sometimes even people with the best intentions may give you suggestions that don't help.

Consider this situation: You take a new vitamin or mineral supplement, or you try a new diet, and the results are amazing. Your IBS symptoms disappear, and you are just busting to tell everyone about it. A dozen or so people are so inspired by your story that they try your miraculous cure. Maybe one-third of them also get good results, and the other two-thirds experience no change. The people who are cured keep spreading the word. This is how health fads start.

One man's food may be another man's poison. In Chapters 8 and 9, we talk about the medications and dietary supplements that are used to treat IBS. Each one may work well for some people but not for others. And each one may cause side effects in some people that far outweigh any benefits. The same is true for diets; what works wonderfully for one person may cause another person even more problems.

When it comes to IBS, everyone's causes and triggers are very different (see Chapters 2 and 4). Therefore, what can help eliminate IBS symptoms differs from one person to the next.

For example, what if you thought for years that you had IBS but find out it's really celiac disease? You may tell everyone you know that all the symptoms you suffered for years were due to eating gluten foods, and you will warn everyone about the dangers of toast. But someone else's IBS symptoms may be caused by fruit, or the effects of taking an antibiotic, or stress. Eliminating gluten won't do that person any good.

The only way to deal with IBS is to follow a systematic approach, methodically checking through every condition that is mistaken for IBS (with the help of a doctor) and every trigger for IBS (with the help of this book). Only by doing so will you determine the source of your symptoms.

Because many people with IBS symptoms aren't getting the help that they need from allopathic medicine, hundreds of chat groups and online resources are available for this condition. You may find some of them very useful. But *buyer beware:* You could be getting advice from someone who knows less than you do. Reading this book is the first step to getting the full scoop on IBS and sorting out the realities from the myths. And in Chapter 21, we offer suggestions for other reliable sources of information on IBS.

Chapter 7

Making a Diagnosis

*W*ith most conditions or diseases, a doctor starts the diagnostic process by asking about the patient's symptoms and looking for signs. What's the difference between a symptom and a sign? A *symptom* is something that you say is happening to you — it's a subjective experience you have. A *sign* is something objective that a doctor observes or finds on physical examination. With knowledge of the symptoms and signs, the doctor conducts *investigations* — she uses certain processes and procedures to diagnose a disease, syndrome, or condition.

For example, the *symptom* of a heavy cough produces a *sign* of green sputum, as well as other signs of congestion such as lack of air entering part of a lung when a doctor listens with a stethoscope. The doctor wants to rule out pneumonia, so the list of *investigations* includes a sputum sample, a chest x-ray, and blood tests for infection. The doctor just goes down a list of the appropriate investigations for the given signs and symptoms, checking each item off. At the end of that exercise, you can be fairly certain of your diagnosis.

Sounds straightforward, right? So why is it so hard to get an accurate diagnosis for IBS? Because IBS is not a disease; it's a *syndrome* — a collection of symptoms that can be mistaken for diseases or other syndromes. That means all those other diseases, syndromes, and conditions need to be ruled out before IBS can be ruled in.

In Chapter 2, we explain that it took ten multinational groups of doctors more than four years to arrive at the Rome II Diagnostic Criteria, which are used to diagnose IBS based on symptoms. Developing this criteria was a very important step forward in the diagnosis of IBS because it means that you can be diagnosed based on symptoms alone. (The diagnostic criteria are also a validation of the existence of the condition.)

Sometimes, your doctor can make a diagnosis very easily if you are able to provide a complete picture of your symptoms and health history. Your health history and a physical exam may be all that is necessary. But in other cases, you may need blood tests, stool tests, fiber-optic scans, and/or x-rays, all of which we talk about in this chapter.

Preparing for Your First Appointment

In Chapter 6, we describe the situations that would prompt you to see a doctor about your IBS symptoms, whether you need to start with a general practitioner, request a visit to a specialist, or make a trip to the emergency room.

If you suspect you have IBS and have the luxury of not needing to seek emergency care, you will benefit greatly by taking some responsibility for helping your doctor make a diagnosis. We're not suggesting that you waltz into the doctor's office and announce "I have IBS." Your doctor may not take kindly to that approach and may even try to prove you wrong.

What we're saying, instead, is that you should always go to the doctor's office prepared to provide concise and complete information about what you're experiencing. Instead of assuming that your doctor will ask all the right questions to elicit the right information, take time before you arrive at the office to consider what the right information is. In the following sections, we offer our suggestions.

Filling out a questionnaire

It's often very useful to arrive at your doctor's office with a completed IBS questionnaire, such as the one we provide in this section. The questionnaire can be a real time-saver in your appointment because your doctor doesn't have to go fishing for information; instead, she can spend more time telling you what to do for your IBS.

Describe your symptoms. Check all that apply.

❑ Abdominal cramping

❑ Abdominal pain on the left side

❑ Diarrhea

❑ Bloating

❑ Constipation

❑ Straining with a bowel movement

❑ Feeling like your bowel movements aren't complete

❑ Gas

❑ Other _____

How long have you had these symptoms?

❑ A few weeks

❑ About 12 weeks

❑ About 6 months

❑ Less than 1 year

❑ Less than 5 years

❑ 5 to 10 years

How often do you have these symptoms?

❑ Once per month

❑ Once per week

❑ Every day

❑ Several times per day

❑ Constantly

Does your abdominal cramping and pain subside after a bowel movement? Check all that apply.

❑ Yes

❑ Yes, but not completely

❑ Yes, but only after several movements

❑ No

Describe your stools

❑ Mucus in your stools

❑ Blood in your stools

❑ Hard, lumpy stools

❑ Loose, watery stools

❑ Undigested food in your stools

❑ Black color in your stools

Have you missed time from school or work because of your symptoms?

❑ Yes

❑ No

If yes, approximately how much time? _____

How are you managing your IBS symptoms?

❑ Prescription medication

❑ Acupuncture

❑ Hypnotherapy

❑ Over-the-counter laxatives

❑ Over-the-counter muscle relaxants

❑ Herbal remedies

❑ Other _____

Which of the above have helped your symptoms? _____

Charting your symptoms and diet

In addition to filling out the questionnaire, we recommend keeping an IBS journal. Your doctor isn't going to have time to read it, but by keeping a journal, you can learn a tremendous amount about your symptoms and your possible triggers (which we discuss in Chapter 4). In your journal, you can keep a record of your symptoms, your diet, and your sleep habits. You can also create a list of questions to ask your doctor. Then, before your appointment, you can transcribe your notes into a brief summary that will be useful for your doctor.

While the questionnaire is helpful so the doctor can see at a glance the types of symptoms you're experiencing, a journal gives you the opportunity to provide more detail. You can create a daily chart in your journal that lists your major symptoms on the left side and lists the days of the week across the top. For example, you might keep track of

- **Abdominal pain or discomfort:** For each day, note your level of pain on a scale of 0 to 5.
- **Bloating:** You can take waist measurements before and after meals and list those on the chart.
- **Constipation:** Simply note if you have no bowel movements on a given day.
- **Diarrhea:** Record the number of episodes each day and qualify your diarrhea (from completely watery to soft).

Save some space to make notes about the type of stool you're having — loose or hard — as well as any other information you think may be helpful.

In addition to your symptoms, also chart or write down everything you eat and drink. Especially pay attention to alcohol intake, sugar, dairy, wheat, and processed foods. You may discover connections that you would rather deny, but if after every Saturday night pizza party with the neighbors you have an attack of IBS, that should tell you something.

(It may help you to realize that the department of public health works the same way. This agency monitors complaints about food poisoning; if it gets enough reports about the same place, it can be fairly certain that the restaurant is serving contaminated food. A similar thing may be happening to you, but in your case, food that is perfectly safe for someone else may be toxic to your body.)

Bringing previous test results and family history

If you are like many people with IBS, you have seen many doctors in the past about your symptoms. When you meet a new doctor, bring copies of previous lab tests and the results of investigations that have been done. These can help your doctor develop a picture of you and your condition.

You also want to ask your parents and even your grandparents if they have suffered with bowel problems. These problems may be all too evident, but some people hide their symptoms very well and need to be interviewed. As we mention in Chapter 4, IBS is not necessarily passed along in the genes, but it can be triggered by the dietary habits of a family.

Really think about your family gastrointestinal history before going to your doctor. Your parents or family members may have experienced a GI disorder but never had a formal diagnosis. So find out about any signs, symptoms, and suspicions of IBS or an inflammatory bowel disease (see Chapter 2) in your family. Give your relatives a call. And if your father's bathroom visits have assaulted your senses on a regular basis, realize that he may have been experiencing IBS symptoms. Even if he was never diagnosed, let your doctor know about his habits.

Packing for your appointment

Okay, we've given you lots of assignments to complete before you see your doctor. Here's a handy checklist of the things you need to bring to your doctor's office for your appointment:

- ✔ A completed symptom questionnaire
- ✔ A list of questions to ask your doctor
- ✔ A list of medications, supplements, and herbs you are taking. (Bringing the actual bottles is usually the best way for your doctor to see the dosage and ingredients.)
- ✔ Your symptom and food journal
- ✔ A notebook
- ✔ A friend for support and to make sure you don't forget anything

Talking to Your Doctor

Even with a completed questionnaire, a summary of your symptoms, and a food journal in hand, you still have to do some talking when you meet your doctor. In the following sections, we help you prepare for the conversation.

Getting over the embarrassment

Many people who are living with IBS are embarrassed by having to talk about their bowel movements. Maybe you even bought this book because you want the information about IBS but don't want to talk to anyone about it.

When you see a doctor for your IBS, it is very important to be specific, detailed, and yes, even graphic. Simply saying "There's something wrong when I go to the bathroom" won't get you very far. If that's your approach, your doctor has to begin the detective work by first finding out whether your bowel or your bladder is the culprit. When that gets sorted out, a long list of questions begins with "What's wrong with your bowel?" If you answer, "I go to the bathroom a lot," you and your doctor are going to be talking for a long time before you get to the bottom of your problem.

Believe us when we say that your doctor has probably heard it all, so you don't need to tiptoe around this topic. Just spit it out and get it over with. Imagine that you are talking to yourself, and don't give it a second thought.

Stating your symptoms

While your doctor is looking at the written materials you've provided, he'll most likely ask you to tell him about your symptoms as well. Just tell your story, keeping in mind the Rome II Diagnostic Criteria for IBS that we list in Chapter 2.

Here's an example of how your speech might go:

> *On and off, but for about 12 weeks, my bowel movements have changed in frequency and appearance. I get constipated for a few days and have hard, lumpy stools. Then I have diarrhea, which starts out soft then turns watery by the end of the day. I have about six movements a day for a few days. I have bloating and abdominal pain after I eat, and often the abdominal pain goes away when I have a bowel movement. I also pass mucus in my bowel movements, but I haven't seen any blood. The pain and the bowel movements sometimes keep me from going to work or out at night.*

Noting your onset of symptoms

Troy had always been able to eat whatever he wanted, and his diet included a lot of meat. But when Troy met Pam, who was a vegetarian, his meat consumption dwindled, and he found himself eating lots of pasta, breads, and yogurt and fruit smoothies. Troy never felt very satisfied following these meals, but Pam convinced him that his body was adjusting to the new diet and he would feel better soon. When he started having diarrhea, Pam insisted that he was clearing out his system. However, the diarrhea persisted for several months and was accompanied by cramps, bloating, and a lot of urgency. Finally, Troy visited his naturopath, who quizzed him about changes to his diet. They identified the onset of the diarrhea as coinciding with the change in his diet. Troy eliminated wheat, dairy, and fruit smoothies for three weeks. His IBS symptoms disappeared.

As this example shows, *when* your IBS symptoms started is an important piece of your story. It's one thing if you have had these symptoms on and off since you were a child and quite another if you started complaining after a camping trip or a vacation to Mexico. Post-infectious IBS is a category all its own and is a lot easier to nail down than symptoms that just seem to come out of the blue. (See Chapter 2 for a discussion of post-infectious IBS.)

As Troy's case shows, sometimes, just by telling your doctor specifically when your IBS symptoms started, the two of you can identify what may have caused or triggered it. We discuss possible causes of IBS in Chapter 2 and triggers in Chapter 4. Following is a brief overview of the reasons why IBS symptoms may occur:

- ✔ **Bowel infection:** Food poisoning, traveler's diarrhea (bacteria or parasites), and stomach flu with diarrhea can irritate the gut, causing incomplete digestion of food and symptoms of IBS.

- ✔ **Symptoms after taking antibiotics:** Diarrhea and/or constipation are common after taking an antibiotic, which can cause an overgrowth of yeast in the gut.

- ✔ **Radical change in diet:** Eating lots of dairy, wheat, or fruit when you are not used to it can overburden your enzymes and lead to symptoms of IBS.

If you are able to tell your doctor that your symptoms began after any of these situations, it makes diagnosis much easier.

Ruling out red flag symptoms

As we explain in Chapter 6, the following symptoms are not associated with IBS, and if you have any of them, you should tell your doctor immediately. They act like a red flag warning that there is something more than IBS going on:

- ✔ Bleeding from the rectum

- ✔ Chronic, painless diarrhea

- ✔ Difficulty swallowing, and food sticking in the esophagus

- ✔ Stomach or abdominal pain that wakes you up at night

- ✔ Abdominal bloating that does not get better overnight

- ✔ Unexplained weight loss

- ✔ A sudden onset of symptoms over age 40

- ✔ Tenesmus — the sensation of having incomplete bowel movements

- ✔ Fever and chills, especially shivering

Differentiating Your Diagnosis

Your doctor needs to know how long you have had IBS symptoms, how many bowel movements you have a day, what they look like, whether you have blood or mucus in your stools, whether you have pain, and whether you have gas and bloating. With that information in hand, as well as your age, your doctor sifts through what's called the *differential diagnosis* for diseases that are common for your age group and your symptoms.

Differential diagnosis is a medical term that refers to making a comparison between various diseases and conditions to rule them in or out.

With the information you have so nicely laid out, your doctor mentally sifts through your symptoms and cross-indexes them with the symptoms of IBS, as well as the symptoms of the following diseases and conditions:

- **Appendicitis:** A low-grade smoldering infection in the appendix can mimic IBS. In some people, the appendix is in an unusual position and does not involve the classic pain in the lower right abdomen.

- **Bowel infection:** This condition has an obvious onset with an acute episode of severe diarrhea, either while traveling, after eating a questionable meal, or from a stomach flu.

- **Cancer:** A tumor from intestinal cancer or ovarian cancer can cause a blockage in the intestines.

- **Celiac disease:** The distinguishing features of this disease are chronic symptoms of fatigue, weight loss, and anemia, as well as IBS symptoms. Older patients can have osteoporosis because both iron and calcium are not absorbed properly. This condition is often missed because in medical training, doctors have learned that this disease is most common in children. (We hope that the younger crop of doctors is learning more about this common disease.)

- **Crohn's disease:** The main distinguishing features of Crohn's disease are blood in the stool and unrelenting diarrhea. But in some people symptoms can fluctuate between constipation and diarrhea, both with pain. You can also have mouth sores and anal fissures.

- **Diverticulitis:** Chronic constipation can cause pouches to form in the intestines that can become infected and cause abdominal pain.

- **Fibroids:** Women can have benign growths in the muscular layer of the uterus that can cause pain and cramping. The fibroids can push against the intestines and also cause intestinal symptoms. A pelvic examination and an ultrasound can usually differentiate this condition from IBS.

- ✔ **Food allergy:** As we explain in Chapter 4, a food allergy differs from food intolerance. Long-term symptoms include diarrhea and/or constipation, along with acute allergy symptoms of hives or skin rashes. A food diary, food avoidance, and blood testing can help differentiate.

- ✔ **Food intolerance:** Usually someone with food intolerance experiences long-term symptoms of diarrhea and/or constipation. To find out if food intolerance is the culprit, the patient needs to keep a food diary, go on a food avoidance program, or have blood testing. (See Chapter 4 for more information.)

- ✔ **Intestinal polyp:** This benign growth in the form of a mushroom can grow large enough to block the bowel and cause spasms as stool passes by. It can also get torn from intestinal roughage and cause bleeding.

- ✔ **Kidney stones:** The cramping, colicky pain of passing a kidney stone along the ureter from the kidney into the bladder is usually localized and goes into the groin. However, if there is a stone at the juncture of the kidney and the ureter, it can cause abdominal pain that mimics IBS.

- ✔ **Lactose intolerance:** This condition features lifelong symptoms of alternating diarrhea and constipation, gas, and bloating. Some people can acquire lactose intolerance after an infection or protein deficiency; when these conditions improve, so can the lactose intolerance.

- ✔ **Malabsorption:** Undigested food in stools indicates maldigestion and malabsorption that can mimic IBS but is a vicious cycle that deteriorates without proper diagnosis and management.

- ✔ **Ulcerative colitis:** The distinguishing features of ulcerative colitis are blood in the stool and unrelenting diarrhea.

As we explain in Chapter 2, Crohn's disease and ulcerative colitis are not the same disease. However, their primary symptoms are the same, so tests are required to distinguish between them. We discuss these tests later in this chapter.

Having a Physical Examination

A physical exam can actually be a very reassuring experience. Most doctors are comfortable with performing this procedure and strive to make patients feel comfortable as well. What they learn from very simple physical signs may surprise you.

Here are examples of signs that some integrative medical doctors look for and what they indicate. (As we explain in Chapter 6, an integrative medical doctor is one who bridges the gap between allopathic and naturopathic medicine.) Unfortunately, not all general practitioners and family physicians are trained to do the following nutritional evaluation; however, most internists and gastroenterologists are. You can assess your own physical signs and see if they apply to you.

- ✔ Thinning, dry, and brittle hair indicates a deficiency of essential fatty acids and fat-soluble vitamins such as vitamin A and vitamin D. Such a deficiency can occur in celiac disease or due to malabsorption of nutrients in leaky gut syndrome (which we talk about in Chapter 3).

- ✔ Pale complexion can be a sign of anemia common in celiac disease.

- ✔ Lack of small blood vessels in the whites of the eyes is a sign of anemia found in celiac disease.

- ✔ A white coated tongue may be due to yeast overgrowth (Candida albicans).

- ✔ Skin rashes may be caused by fungal infection or food allergies.

- ✔ Dry, rough, and bumpy skin on the backs of the upper arms is associated with vitamin A and essential fatty acid deficiency, which may indicate either celiac disease or a malabsorption of nutrients in leaky gut syndrome (see Chapter 3).

- ✔ White spots on the nails are a sign of mineral (especially zinc) deficiency, which can occur in malabsorption due to leaky gut syndrome (see Chapter 3).

- ✔ Tender areas over the abdomen can indicate trapped gas in the intestines.

The final part of the physical exam (which many patients actually wish doctors would do first, to get it over with) is the rectal examination. The doctor is looking for hemorrhoids that could explain some bright red blood that may appear on the surface of a bowel movement. For men, the rectal exam also gives the doctor the opportunity to examine the prostate for size and tenderness.

You can make the rectal exam much easier on yourself if you can relax. You will be asked to lie on your side facing away from the doctor and to curl your knees up in the fetal position. Then you will take a deep breath as your doctor slips a lubricated, gloved finger into your anus. Tensing up your anal sphincter just makes the whole experience more uncomfortable. Don't forget that you pass stool much wider than the doctor's finger all the time, and you do it by relaxing the anal sphincter.

A routine physical exam may not discover any noticeable signs of IBS. As we explain in Chapter 2, IBS is a syndrome without any specific physical manifestations, except maybe some abdominal tenderness or pain on deep pressure. Even bloating, which most people with IBS complain about, is not really evident to an observer. *You* know that your pants are much tighter since you ate your last meal, but you would have to bring before and after measurements to prove it to your doctor.

All the signs of various types of bowel disease race through your doctor's mind during your physical exam. For example, weight loss and the paleness of anemia are signs of celiac disease. A very tender abdomen around areas of inflammation and scarring is a sign of Crohn's disease or ulcerative colitis.

Responding to Your Situation

After taking a thorough history from you and conducting a physical examination, your doctor may be able to reassure you that your bowel symptoms are not part of a serious disease. Having seen thousands of people with IBS symptoms, many doctors are able to reassure patients even on the first visit, especially if you have done all the homework before your appointment (which we detail earlier in the chapter in the section "Preparing for Your First Appointment").

However, each patient is different, and your doctor will be guided by the severity of your symptoms and the amount of disruption in your life. Especially if your symptoms came on suddenly, your doctor will go to the next level of diagnosis.

You and your doctor want to have an accurate diagnosis for two reasons:

- ✔ To rule out more serious conditions (which doesn't diminish the fact that IBS is very difficult to live with and has very real symptoms)
- ✔ To determine the best way to treat the problem

Often people avoid going to the doctor to get a diagnosis because they are worried it will be something awful. However, the stress of *not* having a diagnosis can actually make IBS symptoms worse.

What may lead you or your doctor to believe you are experiencing something more than IBS or more serious than IBS? The following symptoms indicate the need for appropriate investigations:

- ✔ **Recent bowel infection:** If a bowel infection seems to be the culprit, your doctor will order stool testing to check for yeast overgrowth, bacterial overgrowth, and parasites, as well as blood tests to check for yeast, bacteria, parasites, and HIV.
- ✔ **A food-related problem:** If your diet history indicates an association between eating certain food groups and IBS, your doctor should instruct you to try food elimination and reintroduction, and she may order a lactose tolerance test and celiac blood test.

✔ **Blood in the stool:** This red flag symptom prompts further testing to rule out inflammatory bowel disease (Crohn's and ulcerative colitis), as well as cancer or parasite infection with ameba (called *amebiasis*).

We discuss your doctor's likely response to each of these three situations in the following sections.

Having blood in your stool does not automatically mean there is something seriously wrong with you. An episode of blood in the stool after eating a lot of nuts, popcorn, or other roughage may be ascribed to a small tear in the lining of the rectum. Blood on the outside of a bowel movement is a common sign of hemorrhoids. However, you should always talk to your doctor to let him determine whether the blood is a sign of something serious or not.

Investigating infections

As we note in Chapter 2, we know that the one true cause of IBS in some individuals is a bowel infection that somehow never quite goes away. Bacteria and parasites are the two major infections of the bowel that your doctor will be investigating. However, yeast infection in the gut is also a trigger for IBS symptoms. We talk about the yeast trigger in Chapter 4 and about leaky gut in Chapter 3.

Checking your stool for blood and infection

Your doctor will likely check your stool for blood or infection. A simple test done in the doctor's office can rule out microscopic blood in the stool, which can be a sign of inflammatory bowel disease. All you are asked to do for this test is to bring a stool sample to the doctor's office. The nurse puts a small amount of stool on a special indicator paper, and it changes color if blood is present. The rest of the stool sample is then sent out to test for bacterial, fungal, and parasitic infection.

Proper testing for infection, which should include a stool–white blood cell smear and culture for parasites, is a lot more difficult. We talk about parasites in Chapter 2 as one of the true infectious causes of IBS. Parasites cling to the walls of the intestine and don't usually commit suicide by diving into your stool for a one-way ride into the sewage system. That means that stool samples are notoriously poor for picking up parasites. Stool samples that are sent to an outside lab are usually put into a preservative solution that can actually destroy parasites and make them even more difficult to find.

To ensure you are getting a proper stool sample, you may have to go to a clinic that specializes in tropical diseases and have a rectal swab taken. A rectal swab should not be a painful procedure. It's done in much the same way as a rectal exam, but there is some instrumentation involved. Women are familiar with vaginal speculums, which allow a doctor to take a vaginal swab.

A rectal speculum is much the same, only mercifully smaller. It's well lubricated — and hopefully warmed up! — and inserted with a fair bit of lubrication. Then a cotton swab is rubbed against the upper walls of the anus just past the speculum.

That swab is then rinsed out in water, and drops of the water are viewed immediately under a microscope. The doctor looks for live parasites and eggs. This method is highly accurate, but it does depend on a skilled doctor or technician reading the slide.

Parasite cleaning kits are very popular items sold in health food stores. But be careful about doing a parasite cleanse on your own if you have IBS, because these kits usually contain laxatives.

Checking your blood for infection

Infection in the blood *(systemic blood infection)* is very rare. It usually happens in the hospital when someone is very debilitated from surgery or other infections. A high fever (up to 102°F) usually is the key sign.

More common is a very low grade infection that may be lurking in your bowel. It may be so minor that it doesn't even cause inflammation. Using specialized blood antibody tests, your doctor can diagnose this situation. A lab that specializes in immune system testing can analyze a vial of your blood for antibodies to bacteria, parasites, and yeast.

Bacteria and parasites are recognized causes of post-infectious IBS, which we talk about in Chapter 2. Yeast (Candida albicans) is a lesser known trigger of IBS that can be caused after treatment with antibiotics. Your doctor can check for yeast antibodies in your blood, but this type of testing is most often done in a specialized laboratory; it's not a routine test in most doctors' offices.

We talk about yeast in Chapter 4. If you haven't taken the Crook's Candidiasis Questionnaire yet, do so to find out if yeast could be part of your IBS problem. The questionnaire helps put a solid number on the likelihood that you have yeast. You can find the questionnaire in the latest edition of *The Yeast Connection and Women's Health* (Professional Books) by Dr. William Crook and Dr. Carolyn Dean, as well as at www.yeastconnection.com.

Eliminating food factors

In Chapter 10, we talk about treating your IBS symptoms by eliminating potentially aggravating foods from your diet and reintroducing them consciously. You can do this even before you see your doctor. Eliminating foods from your diet and testing them by reintroducing them is a valid diagnostic procedure.

If you have post-pizza attacks, for example, your doctor may ask you to simply avoid wheat and dairy products for three weeks to see if some of your symptoms settle down. If they do, you may have the answer to your IBS symptoms: the answer being abstinence from wheat and/or dairy! Okay, it's not so simple, but we give you the support you need to accomplish an elimination diet in Chapter 10.

Lifelong avoidance of certain foods is a challenge, so you want to make sure that you have a particular food intolerance or allergy before you commit to that dramatic change. Here, we outline the foods that need specific attention — dairy, fruit, gluten, and wheat — and the testing that helps diagnose a problem with them. If you suspect food is a culprit, you must eliminate each of these foods for at least three weeks to gain an understanding of the role they play in your symptoms.

Detecting a problem with dairy

Dairy can play havoc with your life in several ways. You can have lactose intolerance or lactose allergy, or you can be allergic to *casein* (milk protein). We cover lactose intolerance in Chapter 2 because it is often mistaken for IBS, and we discuss dairy allergy in that chapter as well.

The diagnostic test for lactose intolerance is called the *hydrogen breath test*. If lactase enzymes do not properly break down lactose, an excessive amount of hydrogen is produced. The proper procedure for this test is the following:

- ✔ Fast for eight hours overnight.
- ✔ Breathe into a machine to obtain a baseline level of hydrogen measured in parts per million.
- ✔ Drink a lactose sugar liquid dissolved in water.
- ✔ Breathe into a machine every 30 minutes for up to 3 hours.

A rise of greater than 20 parts of hydrogen per million within the 3 hours is diagnostic of lactose intolerance.

If you have been avoiding dairy for three weeks before the hydrogen breath test because you read *IBS For Dummies* and decided to do an elimination experiment, and you feel much better, you are going to be in for a shock when you eat dairy again and that lactose hits your intestines. That experience, more than anything, will tell you whether your symptoms are related to lactose intolerance rather than IBS. The treatment for lactose intolerance is avoidance. In Chapter 10, we give you lists of foods and medications that lactose hides in to make it easier for you to avoid them.

If your hydrogen breath test comes back negative, which means you don't have lactose intolerance, you could still have a dairy allergy. If you notice that your symptoms improve when you avoid dairy, you may want to pursue further allergy tests. The definition of *allergy* in conventional allergy testing is tied to finding an elevation of IgE antibodies and a positive reaction on a scratch test for a particular substance. The IgE antibody is associated with hives, asthma, and immediate and acute reactions to foods, which can include the sudden onset of diarrhea.

A new breed of allergist, one who looks into the nutritional aspects of health and disease, is finding a correlation between delayed reactions to foods and antibodies IgG and IgM. Blood tests for IgG and IgM food antibodies often come back positive for people who feel they may have food allergy reactions but whose IgE antibodies or scratch tests for foods are negative. The delay in reactions can be as much as 72 hours, which means it may be tough to connect your symptoms to what you've eaten. (Sometimes it's impossible to even remember what you ate for breakfast!) Therefore, you may want to have your IgG and IgM food antibody levels tested to see if your symptoms — which can include fatigue, bloating, gas, diarrhea, constipation, mood swings, hay fever, skin rashes, or many others — are caused by foods.

Feeling out fruit

We all think of fruit as being very healthy for us and providing us with necessary nutrients. That is indeed the case *most of the time*. But if you have fruit intolerance, and if it is causing you to have diarrhea, you are probably losing a lot of nutrients.

Fruit intolerance can be diagnosed in the same way as lactose intolerance, with a hydrogen breath test. The same procedure (outlined in the previous section) is followed except that a fructose drink is ingested.

You may also have blood tests to test for fruit allergies. An IgE test will detect an acute fruit allergy, and an IgG and IgM test will detect a delayed fruit allergy. The three tests will give you a very clear picture of what you can and can't eat. Otherwise, food avoidance and food reintroduction, which we talk about in Chapter 10, are the best way to proceed.

Concentrated fruit juices can be very irritating for an IBS bowel. Check the labels on juices, because some of them contain extra sorbitol, which can be an IBS trigger (see Chapter 4). Remember that prune juice is a laxative all by itself. You may not know that grape juice and apple juice can cause cramping and diarrhea. If you already have a problem with heartburn (see Chapter 3), orange juice, with its high citric acid content, may make it worse.

Also, some people get itchy, scratchy throats when they eat fruits that have been heavily sprayed with pesticides. If you are able to eat fruit, try to make it organic.

Gauging your gluten tolerance

Cynthia had never heard of celiac disease until she was trying to uncover the secret behind her gut-wrenching symptoms. Finally, following an intestinal biopsy, she was diagnosed with celiac disease and learned that it is a genetic disorder. Her mother had always complained of stomach troubles but had never had a diagnosis. Naturally, Cynthia was concerned for the health of her own children but, at the same time, was not eager to put them through a biopsy. The children's pediatrician banished Cynthia's worries when he told her that most testing for celiac is now done by a simple blood test to identify whether antibodies are present.

As we discuss in Chapter 2, gluten intolerance (celiac disease) causes symptoms that are difficult to distinguish from IBS. As we write this book, the more we talk about celiac disease, the more people tell us that they have it and were just diagnosed as adults. Fortunately, there is a simple blood test that can provide a diagnosis. Another test your doctor may run is a simple hemoglobin test to see if you are anemic, which is a sign of celiac disease. Osteoporosis, which shows up on bone density tests, is another clue to the disease in adults.

The celiac blood test actually measures four different aspects of celiac disease. The first measurement is of *gliadin protein,* which is found in gluten. The other three measurements are of body enzymes and tissues that are affected by gluten: transglutaminase enzyme, intrinsic factor, and parietal cells.

If you have a positive celiac test, avoiding gluten is the only way to treat this disease. Fortunately, many companies make gluten-free products and a host of gluten-free grains that you can try (see Chapter 10). Be aware, however, that for some people with gluten intolerance, even a few molecules of gluten could trigger your symptoms.

We met and interviewed the director of a lab that does most of the specialized immune testing for infections and foods in the United States. Located in Los Angeles, the lab is called Immunosciences Lab, Inc. Go to www.immunosciienceslab.com or call 800-950-4686 to find out more. Many of the tests we talk about in this chapter can be ordered by your doctor from this lab.

What about wheat?

Gluten isn't the only protein in wheat that can cause allergies. If your gluten blood test is negative but you still think you are sensitive to wheat, you can get IgE, IgG, and IgM blood tests for wheat allergy. As we mention in the earlier section "Detecting a problem with dairy," many nutritionists and nutritionally-oriented doctors are aware that food allergies are not just acute reactions to IgE antibodies. The IgG and IgM antibodies also attack food protein and can cause symptoms that can be mistaken for IBS.

Considering other food culprits

Any food can cause a reaction in the body. The reaction may not be defined by conventional allergists as a true allergy, but that doesn't make a food reaction any less real. Some people get migraines from eating carrots or rashes from eating sugar.

If you stop eating a food and your symptoms abate, and if you reintroduce the same food and symptoms come back, you have done a controlled experiment and proven scientifically that a particular food is poison for you.

Testing for Crohn's and ulcerative colitis

We know that IBS is not associated with cancer, but the line between IBS, Crohn's, and ulcerative colitis is not as clear. Early stages of Crohn's or ulcerative colitis, which are inflammatory bowel diseases (IBDs), may be mistaken for IBS. In fact, one writer who has Crohn's wonders if there is a continuum of illness from IBS to IBD. We discuss her theory in Chapter 16.

Testing and investigations are important to make sure an IBD is not missed. Just as important is to rule out cancer, and doctors use the tests we discuss in this section to be on the alert for this disease as well.

The most common ways to investigate the intestines, and thus diagnose an IBD, are by using special x-ray procedures and scopes, which we discuss next. However, in the past decade, immunologists have been developing highly specialized blood tests to differentiate between Crohn's disease and ulcerative colitis. This testing is available at Immunosciences Lab, Inc. (www.immunoscienceslab.com).

Taking a picture

A *barium enema* is a type of bowel x-ray where you are given an enema that coats the inside of the large intestine with a chalky barium liquid. Multiple x-rays are then taken with several views of the abdomen. The chalk shows up white on the x-ray, and the surrounding tissue is grey or black. Irregularities in the bowel show up as lumps or craters. A lump could be a tumor (benign or cancerous) or scar tissue; a crater could be an ulcer or a diverticuli.

Diverticulitis is a condition of the large intestine that usually occurs in people who have a history of constipation. Spending too much time straining to go to the bathroom can cause weakness in the wall of the intestine, and tiny pouches *(diverticuli)* are formed. Diverticulitis occurs when the diverticuli become inflamed. This condition can cause severe pain, along with constipation.

An *upper GI x-ray with small bowel follow-through* is a procedure that is used to check the small intestine for Crohn's disease. In this case, you swallow a white chalky substance, and a series of x-rays are taken over a period of several hours as the chalk makes its way through your system.

Getting a scope

Fiber-optic scopes that can look into the bowel have been around only since the 1970s. They were used in industry to snake around obstructions in drains and pipes before someone got the bright idea to use them to get a peek inside the human body. They have mostly taken over the field of bowel diagnosis from x-rays.

If your doctor orders a bowel x-ray instead of a scope, and if the x-ray shows a possible problem, you usually have to follow up with a fiber-optic scope anyway. The scope confirms whether a problem exists.

With scopes, there is the added benefit of no risk of radiation. X-rays are used extensively in medicine for diagnostic purposes, and people assume that they must be safe. But x-rays emit ionizing radiation, which accumulates in the body and at any dose has the potential to cause gene mutations. Any time you get an x-ray, you must weight the benefits against the risks.

A fiber-optic scope called an *endoscope* consists of a tiny camera on the end of a flexible tube, which is inserted through the anus or esophagus. There is also a light source that illuminates the bowel as the scope takes its journey. The doctor looks through the scope or simply watches the picture projected from the camera onto a video monitor. Still pictures can be shot of areas of concern to be studied later.

An endoscope that is inserted through the esophagus looks into the stomach and can help find ulcers. Endoscopes inserted through the anus that get views of the rectum and the final part of the large intestine, where stool collects (the *sigmoid colon*) are called *sigmoidoscopes*. A *colonoscope,* also inserted through the anus, can pass all the way through the large intestine to the small intestine looking for signs of ulceration, polyps, and tumors (see Figure 7-1).

Fiber-optic scopes have really helped in diagnosing gut disorders and are especially useful in ruling out diverticulitis, polyps, ulcerative colitis, and Crohn's disease. They are not pleasant experiences, but they aren't painful either. Usually, you are given sedative medication or drugs that induce amnesia so that you are relaxed for the procedure and don't remember anything afterward.

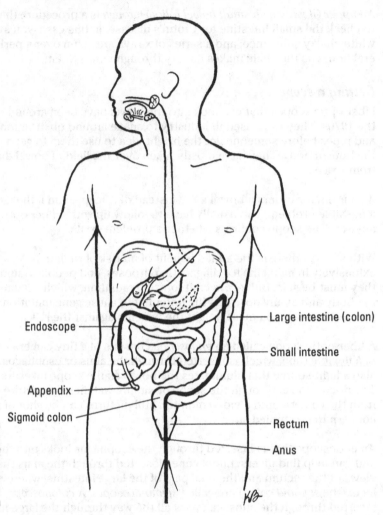

Endoscope —

Appendix —

Sigmoid colon —

— Large intestine (colon)

— Small intestine

— Rectum

— Anus

Figure 7-1:
The route of
a colon-
oscopy.

KB

Prepping the bowel

You definitely have to be prepared for a scope or a barium x-ray. Your colon
has to be completely empty. Otherwise, an area of feces could be wrongly
mistaken for a lump or bump. Usually, you take a laxative drink the night
before the procedure. Be prepared to stay close to the bathroom after you
take the drink. (It's ironic that to get a proper diagnosis of IBS, you are given
the symptoms of the condition.)

Molly was quite certain that she had IBS, but she became concerned when she went from having mostly diarrhea to experiencing constipation that lasted for up to eight days. She consulted her doctor, who agreed that the change in her symptoms might be cause for concern. They scheduled a colonoscopy.

Molly followed a liquid diet for two days and, following her doctor's recommendations, consumed fruit juice and diet soda. Molly's constipation quickly turned to diarrhea after she consumed these beverages, and although she was sure that her bowels were empty, she still had to take a laxative the night before her colonoscopy. She was up all night, and as she was getting ready to go for her procedure, she had leakage from her bowel that caused her to turn back to get cleaned up. Molly had to cancel her colonoscopy because she couldn't be away from the bathroom long enough to get to the hospital.

The same thing happened when Molly rescheduled, so finally she had to be admitted to the hospital the night before the procedure and given the laxative there. Molly was finally diagnosed with IBS with triggers from fruit and aspartame — the very things she took for her bowel prep!

Chapter 8

Medicating IBS Symptoms

● ●

In This Chapter

▶ Focusing on medication for short-term relief

▶ Weighing benefits against side effects

▶ Treating symptoms of diarrhea and constipation

▶ Controlling the pain of IBS

● ●

*1*n Chapter 6, we explain some differences between *allopathic* medicine (which uses modern Western processes and procedures, including prescribing drugs) and *naturopathic* medicine (which focuses on nutrition, dietary supplements, lifestyle education, and psychological balancing).

Allopathic practitioners are tops in emergency care, surgery, and drug therapy — that's what they study and focus on. One weakness of allopathic medicine, however, is in the treatment of chronic functional conditions like IBS. Diet, lifestyle, and stress are key factors in chronic conditions, which also include chronic fatigue syndrome, fibromyalgia, acid reflux, and even obesity and diabetes. Medical experts don't yet know the causes of all these conditions, so they can only treat the symptoms. Because their focus is not on lifestyle, they often overlook it as a possible contributing factor.

The allopathic approach to treating symptoms of IBS generally involves prescribing drugs. Drug therapies have a high *placebo response;* about 47 percent of patients feel better for a while because they think they are taking something that will help them, even if it is a placebo (a pill that doesn't contain active medication).

But drug therapy isn't the only way to treat IBS, and research indicates it's probably not the best. Treatment approaches such as diet, supplements, exercise, behavior modification, stress intervention, and psychotherapy appear to have better long-term results. However, you and your doctor may determine that medication can play a role in your overall treatment program.

In this chapter, we explain the benefits and potential side effects of the medications most commonly prescribed to treat IBS symptoms. In the next chapter, we turn our attention to the naturopathic approach. One of your authors,

Carolyn Dean, is a naturopathic doctor as well as a medical doctor, so we can provide an overview of both types of treatments.

While we strongly encourage you to consider the types of therapies we explain in Chapter 9, you may find that a drug therapy, either alone or in combination with other therapies, makes sense for you. Our goal is to offer a comprehensive overview of what's available to you, so you can make an educated decision about what's best for your symptoms and situation.

Considering the Effectiveness of Drug Therapies

No single drug is effective in relieving IBS over the long-term. That's not great news, we admit, but you can learn how to use medications to your advantage in short-term situations and look at diet, dietary supplements, and lifestyle changes for the long-term.

Before we discuss specific drug therapies that are available for IBS symptoms, we offer some food for thought. As we explain in this section, many people with IBS have had limited or no success with medications. But if you go to an allopathic doctor and ask for help with your symptoms, you'll likely walk away with a prescription in hand. Before you do, you may want to mull over the information in this section.

Documenting limited success

At the 2003 annual meeting of the American College of Gastroenterology, new drug treatments for IBS were of such interest that a special symposium was held to capacity crowds. Clearly, doctors want to help their patients with IBS symptoms. The question is: Are drug treatments the best answer?

Drugs therapies for IBS consist of

- Laxatives for constipation
- Bulking agents for constipation and diarrhea
- Antispasmodics for pain
- Antidepressants for stress

Unfortunately, for the majority of people with IBS, most of these treatments don't work. Some people with IBS don't respond at all to these medications. Others respond initially, but their symptoms recur. Doctors and researchers admit that there is no cure.

A survey conducted by the International Foundation for Functional Gastrointestinal Disorders asked 350 patients with IBS about their experiences with drug therapy. Fewer than one-third of people surveyed who were using medications reported that they were satisfied with the results. Most people surveyed were dissatisfied with the medications' lack of effectiveness.

A common complaint in the IBS community is that not enough research has been done on IBS to find a cure. Prescribing for IBS is distressing for both patients and doctors because finding the right combination of medications to help someone is a hit-and-miss proposition.

When someone with IBS musters the courage to see a doctor, she expects to see some beneficial results from treatment. Patients are often surprised to find that allopathic medicine has few options for treating IBS. Even though up to 20 percent of the North American population suffers IBS symptoms, no definitive treatment protocol has been established, taught in medical schools, and passed on to the public. (A recent survey reported that people with IBS are using a total of 281 different treatments to control IBS symptoms.)

With so much frustration surrounding drug therapies, why don't more doctors recommend lifestyle changes, such as improving diet? The problem is that most people with IBS symptoms tell their doctors that they have already tried dietary changes and that they didn't work. Therefore, they and their doctors assume that medication is necessary. As we point out in several chapters of this book, diet is a rich field to explore. We encourage you to read Chapter 10 about diet before looking for medication.

Assuming it's all in your head

When laxatives, bulking agents, and antispasmodics don't fully work, many doctors seem to assume that the cause of IBS symptoms is psychological. That's where antidepressants come in.

Anxiety and depression in a person with IBS is a chicken and egg situation. Does the anxiety come first, and then the IBS? Or does the stress of having IBS cause the anxiety and depression? Research indicates that anxiety and depression do not *cause* IBS. But that doesn't prevent some doctors from treating the condition as if it were psychological, especially when other medications don't work.

We should note that antidepressants can, for some people, be a useful treatment for pain. (We discuss antidepressants later in the chapter.) But before you fill a prescription for an antidepressant, we encourage you to try to identify what's triggering your IBS symptoms (see Chapter 4).

Reviewing clinical trials

In 2002, under a grant from Novartis Pharmaceuticals, a group of ten eminent U.S. gastroenterologists hand-picked from the American College of Gastroenterology (ACG) were given the formidable task of reviewing and reporting on the current status of effective treatments for IBS. (The group's name was the ACG Functional Gastrointestinal Disorders Task Force. We'll just call it the ACG Task Force, to save you some eye strain!) Their work entailed reading all the published clinical trials on IBS treatments. Among the treatments they reviewed as significant for IBS were

- ✔ Antidepressants
- ✔ Antidiarrheal drugs (Lomotil and Imodium)
- ✔ Antispasmodic drugs
- ✔ Behavioral therapy
- ✔ Bulking agents (like fiber)

We offer some of their findings throughout this chapter. Notice that the experts did *not* review diet modifications.

The ACG Task Force strictly adhered to its mandate to study current scientific, clinical trials on the treatments for IBS. The fact that there have not been many, or any, scientific clinical trials on the relationship of lactose intolerance, gluten intolerance (celiac disease), and fructose intolerance to IBS means that these conditions (which can be mistaken for IBS) did not get attention from this group.

The lack of research on these dietary factors in no ways means they aren't important. It indicates, instead, that no one has come up with the funding to do such studies. (In addition, such studies would be very hard to do. A placebo control study for lactose intolerance, for example, would involve giving one group a meal of cheese and another group a meal of fake cheese.) In Chapter 10, we talk about a food elimination diet to test your own tolerance of different IBS trigger foods and be your own experiment!

Medicating IBS-Diarrhea

A survey by the International Foundation for Functional Gastrointestinal Disorders found that 90 percent of people with IBS use prescription drugs. About 65 percent use over-the-counter antidiarrheal medications. Antidiarrheal medications take several forms:

✔ Drugs that slow down the intestine (such as Lomotil and Imodium)

✔ Bile salt inhibitors (such as Questran)

✔ Bulking agents (such as psyllium and polycarbophil)

✔ Serotonin blockers (such as Lotronex)

Here, we offer details about the use and effectiveness of each one.

Lomotil

Lomotil (diphenoxylate hydrochloride) has been around for decades. It slows down intestinal movements, which means it stops the rush of intestinal contents that are still in their liquid state. This minor traffic jam allows more water to be absorbed from the intestines, as it should be, and makes the stool more solid.

Lomotil should be used only in the short-term and not at all if you suspect you have a bowel infection. It is classed as an opiate drug with addictive properties. At high doses, this type of drug can cause physical and psychological dependence. In other words, if you use it daily for preventing episodes of diarrhea, you may think you need it all the time. To lessen the possibility of addiction, drug companies add atropine to Lomotil as a deterrent. (Atropine causes symptoms of dry mouth and dizziness if you take too much.)

You don't want to use Lomotil all the time. It's far better to find out what triggers your IBS symptoms and just use Lomotil to get you through a plane ride or an evening out. The more you use it, the more susceptible you will be to the following side effects: dizziness, drowsiness, dry skin, itching, nausea, and vomiting.

Imodium

Like Lomotil, Imodium (loperamide hydrochloride) is designed to slow down intestinal movements, allowing the reabsorption of water. However, that's not really what transpires. Researchers have found that Imodium appears to enhance the resting internal anal sphincter tone. What does that mean? Imodium keeps the anus tight when you are at rest. For that reason, it helps to improve stool leakage at night, which is helpful for some people with IBS who have that problem. (For some people, leakage is such a problem that they must use adult diapers.) It would be even more helpful if it worked during the day for other symptoms. Unfortunately, Imodium does not have any effect on abdominal pain or distention. Fortunately, it is less addictive than Lomotil because it doesn't cross from the bloodstream into the brain.

Imodium can cause worsening of constipation. In fact, this medication can throw you from diarrhea into constipation and could possibly cause the type of IBS that involves alternating diarrhea and constipation. You should not use Imodium if you suspect you have a bowel infection. Other side effects include abdominal pain, dizziness, dry mouth, nausea, and vomiting.

The ACG Task Force found three adequate studies that examined the use of Imodium in IBS patients with diarrhea. It found that in general, stool frequency and stool consistency are improved, but bloating and abdominal pain are unaffected. It concluded that Imodium is not recommended for use in IBS.

Questran

Questran (cholestyramine) is a bile acid binding agent. It prevents bile acids from stimulating the colon. In this roundabout way, it slows down the movement of intestinal contents, allows the reabsorption of water from the intestines, and relieves diarrhea. It is not the first line of treatment for IBS-diarrhea but can be called upon if other treatments don't seem to be helping.

Questran is mixed with water and may be taken several times a day. This drug is more commonly used in the treatment of high cholesterol. It must be taken three hours before or after other medications so it does not interfere with the absorption of other medications.

Side effects of Questran are related to the interference with bile. One side effect is a degree of malabsorption that occurs when bile is bound up and removed from the body. Other side effects, unfortunately, may be similar to the symptoms that the medication is intended to treat: abdominal pain, bloating, constipation, gas, a feeling of fullness, and nausea.

Bulking agents

The usual bulking agents include fiber, bran, and psyllium laxatives. They work by helping to move waste through the intestines. They do tend to cause gas and bloating, so for a colon that is hypersensitive to gas and bloating they may not be the ideal treatment. However, judicial use of fiber can help absorb excess fluid that is the main component of diarrhea. The main bulk-forming laxatives for diarrhea include psyllium and two synthetic substances, methylcellulose (Citrucel) and polycarbophil (Fibercon).

The ACG Task Force reviewed the following bulking agents: wheat bran, corn fiber, polycarbophil, and psyllium. It considered none of the 13 trials it analyzed to be adequate and determined that there are only slight indications for the benefits of fiber on IBS symptoms. The ACG Task Force concluded that fiber is appropriate for treatment of constipation but may not be recommended for treatment of IBS-diarrhea.

Lotronex

Lotronex (alosetron) is used to treat diarrhea and abdominal discomfort that occurs in some women with IBS. Lotronex blocks particular serotonin receptors in the gut. Serotonin is a neurotransmitter that affects the brain and the bowel. A vast amount of serotonin is produced in the gut — about 95 percent of the body's total. Some researchers have shown that high amounts of serotonin in IBS patients may be a factor in abnormal activity of the muscles and nerves of the GI tract (see Chapter 16).

Researchers believe that serotonin and its receptors control sensations of pain, contractions of muscle, and the build-up of fluid in the intestines. When these problems intensify, the result can be diarrhea.

Although researchers admit that the exact cause of IBS is unknown, they know that stress, food, medications, and hormonal changes can trigger an excessive release of serotonin. Patients with IBS seem to experience an exaggerated response to serotonin, resulting in pain and diarrhea.

Within ten months of its approval by the U.S. Food and Drug Administration (FDA), Lotronex was withdrawn from the market because of a life-threatening gastrointestinal side effect called *ischemic colitis.* Ischemia is a lack of blood and nutrients to part of the body. It appears that in some individuals, Lotronex shuts down blood flow to a section of the bowel and causes it to die.

But that wasn't the end of Lotronex. In June 2002, it again passed the FDA approval process. However, its use is restricted to women with severe IBS-diarrhea who have failed to respond to conventional treatment for IBS. It should be used only with great caution and under the direct supervision of a gastroenterologist. (As you surely realize by now, there is no agreement in the medical community regarding what "conventional treatment for IBS" is.)

What you don't know may hurt you when it comes to the so-called inactive ingredients in medications. For example, Lotronex has the following inactive ingredients: lactose, magnesium stearate, microcrystalline cellulose, and pregelatinized starch. (The coating that covers each tablet contains several other unpronounceable ingredients as well.) We've heard complaints from people with IBS who are also lactose intolerant that this medication made them much worse.

Constipation is the most common side effect with Lotronex. Patients are advised to stop taking the drug if the constipation is severe but are told they may resume after the constipation has cleared.

Medicating IBS-Constipation

IBS-constipation is defined by infrequent bowel movements, episodes of straining, and hard or lumpy stools. Constipation in general may be the result of not enough fiber or fluids in the diet and a lack of regular exercise. It can also occur in people who are in poor health, who use certain medications with the side effect of constipation, or who abuse laxatives, which over time can stretch and damage the delicate intestinal muscles, preventing them from doing their job.

Focusing on triggers first

A survey by the International Foundation for Functional Gastrointestinal Disorders found that 79 percent of people with IBS take over-the-counter laxatives. Most people with constipation just want to have a bowel movement, and they use laxatives to achieve that end. However, if the trigger for constipation is one or more of the things we talk about in Chapter 4, treating the symptom of constipation instead of the trigger can be a losing proposition.

Increasing your intake of dietary fiber is the first approach that doctors recommend for IBS-constipation, and we show you how to do so in Chapter 10. (You want to be sure that you're mostly increasing your soluble fiber intake; insoluble fiber is much tougher on your digestive system. We explain the two types in Chapter 10 and give you a list of soluble fiber foods in Appendix A.) We would add that you should also try diet changes and avoidance of food triggers, which we talk about in Chapter 4, before taking over-the-counter or prescription laxatives.

Knowing your options

If you're going to take a laxative, we recommend trying bulk laxatives before osmotic or stimulant laxatives because the latter two have more potential for abuse and dependence and actually hurt the gut over time. (We explain each kind in this section.) Keep in mind that most advice about laxatives is based on doctors' clinical experience because there have been no controlled trials with laxatives in patients with IBS.

The list of drug treatments for IBS-constipation is not long. They are mostly laxatives that can be taken by mouth in various forms — tablet, liquid, granules, gum, and powder. Some of them depend on chemically irritating the intestines to get things moving — *not* what someone with IBS wants to have happen. In fact, dependency on laxatives to get things moving means you need greater and greater dosages of the laxative to create a bowel movement, and over time your intestinal muscles stop working on their own.

Heeding the call

A simple, often overlooked step in overcoming constipation is obeying nature's call. By that, we don't mean that you have to hightail it to the nearest outhouse. But when you get the urge to defecate, you must obey. Suppressing bowel movements leads to mixed signals in your body.

Some people can associate their IBS-constipation to suppressing nature's call when they were kids too engrossed in play to waste time eliminating waste or too afraid to ask a teacher to leave the room.

Read the label on the laxative that you are taking. The label often says "for occasional constipation," which means the medication is not meant to treat a chronic condition. Some doctors, researchers, and people with IBS believe that the use of chemical laxatives for IBS-constipation can actually throw people into IBS-diarrhea and contribute to the incidence of the alternating diarrhea and constipation form of IBS.

There are five different types of laxatives and more than 100 products on the market. Here are the five types and some examples of brand names:

✔ **Bulk-forming laxatives:** Fiber is a laxative in this category; we talk about dietary fiber in Chapter 10. Bulk-forming laxatives work by absorbing liquid in the intestines to help form a bulky stool that is soft enough to pass without effort. These laxatives are generally considered the safest but can interfere with absorption of some medicines. They can also stimulate gas and bloating in the intestines. If you don't have excess liquid in your intestines, you must take these laxatives with sufficient water to do the job. Otherwise, they can cause serious gut blockage.

Some common brand names of bulk-forming laxatives include

- Citrucel

- Konsyl

- Metamucil: Made from psyllium seed, this laxative requires large amounts of water to do its work properly.

- Serutan

Sometimes drinking water can relieve mild constipation. Many people experience chronic mild dehydration without realizing it. Be sure you're taking in at least 64 ounces of water every day. That means two glasses of water when you wake up, another during the morning, one at lunch, one in the afternoon, one at dinner, and one at bedtime. See, it's not that hard at all! You need more water if you drink dehydrating beverages like coffee or alcohol, or if you sweat a lot with athletic activity.

✔ **Osmotic laxatives (saline, lactulose, sorbitol, and polymers):**

- *Saline* laxatives use a sponge-like action to draw water into the colon to loosen up fecal matter and help flush it out. They are called saline laxatives because the fluid they attract is salty water. The label on these laxatives usually carries a warning that says "for occasional constipation." If you have IBS-constipation, it's not an occasional happening.

  Keep in mind that saline laxatives work by increasing fecal bulk in the intestines and taking over the work of the intestinal muscles. You can become dependent on them to the extent that your own muscles get weak and ineffective. In the worst case scenario, a bowel that no longer moves needs to be surgically removed.

  Some common brand names of saline laxatives include Citrate of Magnesia, ExLax, Haley's M-O, and Milk of Magnesia.

- *Lactulose* (a synthetic sugar) and *sorbitol* (a sugar alcohol made from glucose) are sugars that feed bacteria and yeast. In fact, that's how they work. The byproducts of yeast and bacteria draw water into the intestines, which moves the stool. This activity causes gas and bloating — symptoms you really don't want to add to your repertoire.

- The *polymers* (polycarbophil) soften the stool and increase the number of bowel movements. But they are recommended only for short-term use.

✔ **Lubricant laxatives:** These products grease or oil the stool, enabling it to move through the intestine more easily. Mineral oil is the most common lubricant, but it's not a safe choice because it's too heavy for the delicate bowel mucosa and becomes sludge in your intestines.

The side effects of mineral oil include malabsorption of vitamins A, D, E, and K. If used in the long-term, mineral oil can create severe vitamin deficiency symptoms. In Chapter 9, we discuss vitamins and how important they are to good health and the treatment of IBS.

✔ **Stimulant laxatives:** These chemical laxatives irritate the bowel lining, which stimulates muscle movement along the length of the intestine, hurrying stool along to its end. Most drugs in this class of laxatives are recommended only for short-term use because using them can lead to dependency. Therefore, they are not a great deal of benefit to people who have life-long symptoms of IBS.

Recent studies indicate that *phenolphthalein,* an ingredient in some stimulant laxatives, is associated with cancer. The FDA has proposed a ban on all over-the-counter products containing phenolphthalein. Most laxative makers are in the process of replacing phenolphthalein with a safer ingredient.

Common stimulant laxatives include

- Correctol
- Dulcolax
- Feen-A-Mint
- Purge
- Senokot

✔ **Emollients (stool softeners and lubricants):** First, a clarification: Emollients are not actually laxatives. We include them here because they are often used by people who mistakenly believe they treat constipation.

Stool softeners provide moisture to the stool and prevent dehydration. The emollients are mostly forms of *docusate,* which is basically a detergent that is not absorbed by the body. As you know from washing dishes, a detergent dissolves grease in water. In the body, a stool softener traps dietary fat and then mixes it with the stool, making hard stool much softer. It does not attract water like some bulking agents, and it does not stimulate the bowel like some laxatives.

Docusate is not very helpful for constipation but can be useful during pregnancy and after surgery. It also takes time to work: The effect is usually seen one to three days after the initial dose.

The side effects of docusate include nausea, mild abdominal cramps, bloating, diarrhea, rumbling sounds, severe abdominal pain, and vomiting.

Some brand names of docusate include

- Colace
- Dialose
- Surfak

Never take a laxative or emollient if you are experiencing symptoms of appendicitis or bowel inflammation — in other words, if you have severe abdominal pains, fever, diarrhea, nausea, vomiting, or bloody stools. Instead, see your doctor immediately.

Zelnorm

One treatment for IBS-constipation beyond laxatives is a group of drugs that manipulate serotonin in the gastrointestinal tract (which accounts for 95 percent of the body's total serotonin). Zelnorm is a *5-HT4-receptor agonist,* which means it blocks the action of serotonin in the GI tract. As a result, intestinal contractions increase and help relieve constipation.

Zelnorm is limited in its application: It is approved only for short-term use for the treatment of chronic constipation, which seems to be a contradiction! So even though your constipation may be life-long, this drug should be prescribed for only four to six weeks. Zelnorm received FDA approval based on the results of clinical studies that lasted only 12 weeks, so researchers don't yet know if there are long-term side effects.

Some doctors will prescribe an additional four- to six-week course of treatment if you do well on the first course. When Zelnorm works, it can decrease constipation, abdominal pain, and bloating. However, after you stop taking it, your IBS-constipation and other symptoms tend to return.

Here's another limitation of Zelnorm: It does not work for men and works for only some women. Plus, only 25 percent of people with IBS have IBS-constipation; most people with IBS experience diarrhea. Studies show that Zelnorm is effective in 11 percent of patients with IBS, whereas a placebo (a dummy pill) is effective in 5 percent of those patients.

Zelnorm also has side effects, some serious. For some people, such severe diarrhea can occur that they experience dehydration, low blood pressure, and fainting. In 2005, the FDA and Novartis (the maker of Zelnorm) issued a revision to the warnings and precautions on the drug's label. Doctors and patients are warned of serious diarrhea that occurred during the investigation period of the drug and has continued after its release into the general population. The most extreme cases are diagnosed as *ischemic colitis,* where blood circulation to the bowel is lost and bowel tissue dies.

Zelnorm should be immediately stopped in people who develop low blood pressure or fainting. And it should be avoided in patients who have diarrhea or a history of diarrhea. The FDA advises that the drug be discontinued in patients who develop symptoms of ischemic colitis, such as rectal bleeding, bloody diarrhea, or new/worsening abdominal pain. Another troubling side effect is a slight increase in gallbladder surgery.

In clinical trials, the following were the most common side effects of Zelnorm: abdominal pain, back pain, diarrhea, flu-like symptoms, gas, headache, indigestion, nausea, sinusitis, upper respiratory tract infection, and urinary tract infection.

Dealing with IBS Pain

Pain is an important defining feature of IBS. If there was no pain associated with IBS, it would be a completely different condition. Most people can put up with diarrhea and constipation alone. But when they have to also deal with gripping, spasming pain, they can't cope so easily.

Pain from spasms can promote diarrhea, or ineffectual spasming can result in constipation. A build-up of gas and bloating can also cause pain as sensitive areas are stretched and twisted. In the following sections, we discuss common medications prescribed to help patients with IBS deal with pain.

Treating spasms

Even though the cause of intestinal twisting and contorting is unknown, doctors offer patients antispasmodics to try to suppress the symptoms. These drugs inhibit smooth muscle contraction in the GI tract. There are two main types of antispasmodics: anticholinergics and smooth muscle relaxants. Their action is focused on the lungs and the gut.

Smooth muscle relaxants have not yet been approved by the FDA and undergone sufficient clinical trials, so they are not currently available for use in the United States. However, we talk about the safe and natural smooth muscle relaxant magnesium in Chapter 16.

Anticholinergics work by diminishing the effects of *acetylcholine,* a neurotransmitter. A neurotransmitter is a chemical that transmits messages throughout the nervous system. In Chapters 2 and 12, we talk about the brain–bowel connection and how the various neurotransmitters help and hinder our guts. Acetylcholine is released by nerves and acts to stimulate muscle tissue. If too much acetylcholine is released, muscles can go into spasm. What makes a nerve cell give up its acetylcholine is an electrical signal from another part of the body. That signal could be produced by a reaction in the gut to a particular offending food or a reaction in the brain to stress and emotion.

The following anticholinergic medications can be used to help prevent or relieve painful cramps and intestinal spasms. They're especially useful when taken 30 minutes before a meal to help prevent cramps that occur with eating:

- Hyoscyamine sulfate: Brand names Anaspaz, Levsin, Cystopaz-M, NuLev, and Levbid
- Dicyclomine hydrochloride: Brand name Bentyl
- Clidinium, which is often used along with Librium or Librax
- Donnatal, which combines anticholinergics and phenobarbital. Its benefits are outweighed by its tendency to cause heavy sedation.

These drugs inhibit smooth muscle contraction, but they also seem to dry up secretions in the intestines. In the process, they can cause side effects of dry mouth, blurred vision, drowsiness, nasal stuffiness, rash, itching, decreased sweating, and inability to urinate. This type of medication may make constipation worse.

The ACG Task Force reported that only three studies on the use of anticholinergic agents met the required standards for its report, and only one study showed a significant improvement in IBS symptoms. The other two studies showed no benefit at all compared to a placebo. The Task Force concluded that it does not recommend these drugs for the treatment of IBS based on available data.

Using antidepressants

Antidepressants can block the way the brain perceives pain, so they are sometimes prescribed in the treatment of IBS. Antidepressants have an effect on neurotransmitters, which play a role in modulating pain. Fortunately, lower doses of these drugs are required to relieve pain than to relieve depression, and lower dosages mean fewer side effects.

Neurotransmitters are chemicals that occur throughout the nervous system that help transmit messages by stimulating cells. Each cell has a receptor, usually on the outside membrane, which selectively receives and binds to specific chemicals like neurotransmitters. After transmitting its message, a neurotransmitter goes back into the cell to be recycled and used again and again.

Some people with IBS may also suffer from depression, but IBS does not cause depression. If you are offered antidepressants for your IBS symptoms, that does not necessarily mean that you are depressed.

Blocking the perception of pain

There are a variety of antidepressants, and doctors may use one of several types of antidepressants depending on your symptoms. Researchers know that from 40 to 60 percent of people with IBS who seek out medical intervention also have symptoms of anxiety, panic attacks, and depression. (Among people who don't have IBS, 25 percent have these symptoms.)

Researchers have taken interesting pictures of the brain when the intestines are irritated with a toxic stimulus. The pictures show a particular brain response. Part of the brain that perceives this stimulation is activated, and the perception of pain is amplified. Antidepressants can act to decrease pain perception. The antidepressant is not curing the pain, just depressing your perception of the pain.

Antidepressants alter intestinal transit time whether or not they alter mood. Some drugs, like Tofranil, can slow down the bowel, which can lead to constipation. Tofranil is a member of a group called *tricyclic antidepressants,* which, in general, are known to cause symptoms of constipation. (Dry mouth and impotence are also common side effects of these drugs.) Other antidepressants called *serotonin reactive uptake inhibitors (SSRIs),* such as Prozac, appear to cause more diarrhea. (The most common side effects associated with SSRIs are nausea, headaches, insomnia, and sexual dysfunction.)

Reviewing research on antidepressants

The ACG Task Force analyzed six studies on the use of the older tricyclic anti-depressants, like amitriptyline and desipramine. It found these drugs to be no more effective than a placebo for relieving all IBS symptoms. However, the drugs did relieve IBS abdominal pain. At the time the ACG Task Force was working (in 2002), SSRIs such as Prozac or Zoloft had not yet been studied adequately in IBS patients, so the Task Force could not form an opinion about them.

A 2004 review of clinical trials of therapies used in the treatment of IBS found that low doses of tricyclic antidepressants are effective in alleviating chronic — even severe — abdominal pain in IBS patients. But because some of the studies were poorly designed, the authors gave a guarded recommendation for the use of antidepressants. They stressed that the serious side effects of antidepressants mean they should be given only to patients with severe IBS symptoms, such as patients who have daily or persistent pain.

Part III
Healing and Dealing with IBS

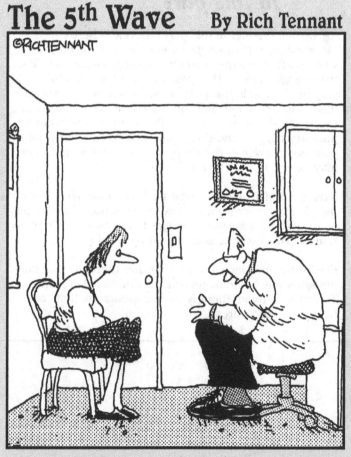

The 5th Wave   By Rich Tennant

"A change in diet can also help your IBS. The next time you're at a restaurant, go ahead and order those probiotics, and treat yourself to some digestive enzymes."

In this part . . .

The first chapter in this part introduces herbs and homeopathic medicines you may want to consider when putting together a treatment program for your IBS. We also recommend that you place a lot of attention on your diet, so in this part, we show you how to eat an IBS-friendly diet and give you a few simple meal plans to follow. We also walk you through the process of avoiding potential triggers and then reintroducing them to see how your body reacts — the simplest way to determine what may be causing you pain.

Exercise is also key to alleviating IBS pain, especially for people who suffer from gas and constipation. We offer lots of suggestions for great exercises to try, as well as motivation to make exercise part of your daily routine.

Finally, we introduce a wealth of other therapies you may not know much about, such as the Emotional Freedom Techniques, hypnotherapy, and acupuncture, that can help you reduce stress.

Chapter 9

Considering Dietary Supplements and Homeopathy

*T*he naturopathic approach to treating IBS symptoms involves making positive lifestyle changes rather than using medications to mask the problem. These lifestyle changes include eating healthy foods, exercising, stopping smoking, and reducing alcohol consumption. (We devote the next two chapters to diet and exercise.)

Two additional tools that naturopaths rely on are dietary supplements and homeopathic treatments, which are the subject of this chapter. As with the medications we discuss in Chapter 8, not everyone with IBS symptoms benefits equally from these treatments. You may find that a certain supplement makes a world of difference for you, but that doesn't mean it'll have the same profound effect on a friend of yours who also has IBS. That's because, as we say many times in this book, the causes and triggers of IBS vary from person to person. The most effective treatments will therefore vary as well.

However, unlike the medications we discuss in Chapter 8, the herbs and other supplements we discuss in this chapter tend to have few side effects. We feel comfortable saying that you can safely try these supplements (in the dosages recommended on the packaging or by a naturopathic doctor) without having to fear serious repercussions. (You may find that you already have some of them in your kitchen cupboard!) And while you can do your own research and buy these products in just about any health food store, working with a naturopath or an *herbalist* (someone who specializes in prescribing herbs and herbal formulations) may add an extra layer of comfort when you first consider which supplements to try.

Perhaps the safety factor is the reason more and more people with IBS symptoms are turning their attention to these types of therapies. Recent surveys indicate that more than half of people with IBS use supplements and other traditional (nonpharmaceutical) therapies to seek relief.

Treating Symptoms with Supplements

The mission statement of the Office of Dietary Supplements at the National Institutes of Health (NIH) in the United States is to study the science of using supplements to prevent deficiency diseases. We know that bureaucracy is often decades behind the times, and this mission statement is a prime example.

The science behind dietary supplements is light-years beyond using vitamin C to prevent scurvy. While the NIH expresses concern about the safety of dietary supplements, research shows that supplements are safer than food: About 100 people die annually due to peanut allergy. In contrast, only the rare person has an adverse reaction to dietary supplements and only if she massively overconsumes them.

The study of dietary supplements as treatments for disease is mainly hampered by the lack of funding for nonpatented medicine. But there is a centuries-long history of using herbal medicine and food-based nutrients for anything that ails you.

Healing with herbs

Herbs have been used for centuries for the treatment of digestive complaints. Historically, they have been used in combination with other herbs — in formulas that enhance the properties of all the ingredients. In modern times, we have fallen in line with the scientific method: We study one herb at a time, and most people take only one herb at a time.

We can't guarantee that each of the herbs we discuss here will affect your intestines in a positive way — some may help you greatly, and some may not. However, there are wonderful herbal combinations for the intestines and some specifically for IBS. One herbal formulator we interviewed, Heather Von Vorous, has had IBS since she was 9 years old. This inspiring young woman created her own kit that includes organic herbal formulas for IBS; visit www. helpforibs.com to learn more.

If you decide to try an herbal formula for IBS, here are some things you should consider:

 ✔ **Study the ingredients.** Make sure that you are not taking a laxative herb for IBS-diarrhea, for example.

 ✔ **Choose organic herbs if at all possible.** Avoid herbs grown using pesticides and herbicides because those chemicals can have a negative effect on the body.

> ✔ **Choose liquid herbs or capsules.** Liquids and capsules are more easily digested and assimilated than tablets. Liquid tinctures are usually preserved in alcohol. The usual dosage is about 15 to 30 drops in a few ounces of water.

If you don't experience relief of your IBS symptoms after trying a prepackaged herbal formula, don't give up on herbs yet. Consider making an appointment with a master herbalist who practices Western herbalism or Traditional Chinese Medicine (TCM). After a detailed discussion, a master herbalist will customize a one-of-a-kind herbal remedy for you. Throughout this book, we stress the importance of recognizing that your IBS symptoms and triggers are unique to you, and a unique herbal formula may just be what the TCM doctor ordered.

You can often find a good herbalist, TCM doctor, or homeopath by inquiring at your local health food store or asking your friends. We've also included a list of professional associations in Chapter 21.

One important note for women: The smooth muscle relaxation that most of the following herbs are capable of makes them very beneficial for preventing and treating PMS and painful periods.

Peppermint oil

The action of peppermint oil relies on its ability to relax the intestine and therefore relieves bloating. Three out of five studies confirm the effectiveness of peppermint oil treatment. It is so safe that it can even be given to children with IBS. Enteric coated pills are the ones most recommended because they dissolve in the intestines, where they relax intestinal smooth muscle and also act as a painkiller.

Fennel

Fennel may not be a household word, unless you are Asian or Indian. It is used to flavor some natural toothpastes and has been around for centuries. You may have tasted it in Indian cuisine and been offered fennel as an after-dinner condiment. It has a mild licorice taste, and people who like licorice find fennel quite pleasant. It soothes the bowel by eliminating gas and bloating. It is an antispasmodic herb that increases the production of gastric juices, which aids digestion.

In Germany, Commission E (which we explain in the sidebar of the same name) investigated hundreds of herbs to define their use in the treatment of disease. Researchers found that fennel was safe for daily use and effective for use in gas, bloating, and abdominal pain. Studies on fennel show that it normalizes the contractions in the intestines and relieves colic, heartburn, abdominal pain, and indigestion.

Commission E

Germany's Commission E is an official government agency that performs a job similar to that of the U.S. Food and Drug Administration, only it's specifically focused on herbs. In 1978, the *Bundesgesundheitsamt* (Federal Health Agency) organized a special commission to evaluate the safety and efficacy of medicinal herbs. The Commission E monographs, the outcome of this effort, consist of more than 300 brief articles on the most medically important herbal preparations. These monographs serve as the basis for the medical usage of herbs within the German healthcare system and outline acceptable manufacturing processes on the basis of available scientific and clinical evidence.

One of fennel's primary oil constituents is similar in structure to dopamine, which is a natural bowel relaxant in the body. Fennel also has antibacterial properties, which may make it useful in post-infectious IBS.

Ginger

Many studies have proven the usefulness of ginger for preventing pregnancy-related nausea and vomiting, as well as seasickness. If you take a tour boat into choppy water, the staff is likely to line up all the passengers and give them ginger capsules because it works better than drugs.

Ginger does much more than treat nausea; it is also useful for indigestion, acting as a strong digestive enzyme, and it's also used for the treatment and prevention of gastrointestinal cramps. It's an antispasmodic that normalizes the tone of the gastrointestinal muscles.

Chamomile

Chamomile is one of the most common herbs in use today, and it's been around for thousands of years. It's one of the herbs you are likely to find on most restaurant menus and possibly even in your own kitchen cabinet. But most people don't realize that it's a safe and effective treatment for IBS.

The German Commission E on herbs officially recognized chamomile, citing many studies that describe its action and its effectiveness. It is approved in Germany for gastrointestinal spasms and as an antiinflammatory. We also know from many other studies that chamomile is a very relaxing herb that can be used for anxiety and nervousness. It relieves gastrointestinal tension by calming smooth muscle tissue, therefore relieving indigestion, gas, and bloating.

The only possible side effect of chamomile is an allergy to it. It is a member of the daisy family, which also houses ragweed, a well-known allergen.

Caraway

This is another ancient herb safe enough for squirmy children and colicky infants. Used both as a spice and a medicinal herb, caraway seeds are an aid to digestion, and they treat indigestion, colic, and nervous tension. Chefs add this spice to heavy foods to prevent indigestion.

Like several other herbs in the IBS lineup, caraway increases production of gastric juices, prevents intestinal spasm, and is a natural antibiotic. Researchers have found several chemicals in caraway that relax smooth muscle tissue in the intestines and either prevent or help eliminate gas.

Anise

Anise (pronounced *a niece*) is an herb used as a spice. It has a sweet licorice taste that is much stronger than fennel. An oil in anise seeds helps aid gastric juice production. It relieves gas and bloating, prevents vomiting, and settles colic. It's also an antispasmodic used to prevent and treat gastrointestinal cramping. Anise is appropriate for use in both constipation and diarrhea because it normalizes bowel activity, making it very useful in IBS. It is also a mild sedative and calms irritability and nervousness.

This herb also acts as an antifungal and prevents the overgrowth of Candida albicans in the gut and the gas and toxins that this yeast produces. (We discuss Candida albicans in Chapter 4.)

Oregano

Oregano is a strong-smelling herb used both as a spice and as a medicine. The only drawback is that if you start using it, you may begin to crave pizza because oregano is a common herb in Italian cooking.

Oregano relieves nausea, vomiting, diarrhea, and muscle spasms. The oils in oregano act as antispasmodics and antiinflammatory analgesics. They increase gastric juice production and eliminate gas and bloating. The calming effect of oregano works on the whole body.

Dr. Cass Ingram (also known as *Dr. Oregano* because of his strong support of this important herb) told us that the best form of oregano to use is oregano spice. Dr. Ingram said that oregano boosts the immune system and kills off yeast and other abnormal microorganisms.

Angelica root

Angelica root is also known as *dong quai*. It's cooked and eaten as a vegetable in many countries, including China. But it is also a very effective herbal medicine. Angelica has been called a female herb because it has such a beneficial antispasmodic effect on menstrual cramps. The same can be said for intestinal cramps, gas, and bloating. In Chapter 5, where we talk about the high incidence of women with IBS, we also mention that symptoms of PMS plague women with IBS. By working in both areas, angelica may be very beneficial.

Medical marijuana

If you live in Canada and suffer from IBS, you may be eligible to receive a prescription for medical marijuana. According to www.Diagnose-me.com, "There are quite a few people who use marijuana to control the symptoms of abdominal pain and nausea associated with irritable bowel syndrome. Some make the claim that this helps more than any other thing they have tried." In the United States, the possession of medical marijuana is legal in 11 states, but the U.S. Supreme Court ruled in 2005 that people participating in medical marijuana programs are not exempt from federal drug laws and can be prosecuted. Also, to our knowledge, IBS is not a qualifying condition to warrant application for medical marijuana privileges in any of those 11 states.

Obviously, if you're caught with marijuana in the United States, you risk jail time — not something we recommend! In addition, marijuana has been proven to negatively affect memory and attention. Heavy users of marijuana can suffer a significant decrease in IQ, may experience a decrease of blood flow to the frontal areas of the brain, and may be at higher risk for any diseases normally associated with cigarette smoking. Marijuana users may also tend to have a poor diet, consisting of snacks that are considered to be unhealthy for people who are suffering from IBS.

We recommend sticking to the other herbs we discuss in this chapter, which are better for your health and — thankfully — legal!

The bitter herbs

Bitter orange peel, gentian root, artichoke leaf, areca seed, and dandelion root all have a role in intestinal health. They are bitter, which stimulates gastric juices, and they also increase bile production, which helps digest fats.

Areca seed is contained in the dried ripe fruit of the *areca catechu,* a tree that belongs to the palm family found in the tropics. It is used for the treatment of parasites, abdominal distention, and constipation.

Boosting your body's minerals and vitamins

If you have IBS, especially IBS-diarrhea, you may be concerned that you have a degree of malnourishment. Daily diarrhea can deplete your body of necessary nutrition, nutrients, and liquids. Knowing what to replace is a difficult task that we make much easier for you in this section.

Some folks with IBS, especially those with diarrhea, have told us that synthetic multiple vitamins (also know as *horse pills*) move through their systems intact. Obviously, a supplement that doesn't get broken down in the digestive system doesn't do any good.

Vitamins and minerals come in many forms other than pills; there are green drinks, vitamin and mineral liquids, vitamin and mineral powders, and even sprays. These non-pill forms avoid the problems created by indigestible and even irritating binders, fillers, dyes, coatings, and colors. We recommend that you look for organic sources of vitamins and minerals, because synthetic sources are not well absorbed and may not give your body what it wants.

There are at least 44 vitamins, minerals, and nutrients that the medical community has identified as important for you to consume, whether in your diet or in supplements. In this section, we highlight the most important ones. You can find a complete table of these nutrients at www.supplementwatch.com/supatoz.

A *nutrient* is any substance that can be used by an organism to build tissue, provide nutrition, and give energy.

Minding your minerals

Minerals and trace minerals are drained out of the body by chronic diarrhea. Even if you eat a healthy diet, if you have diarrhea your meal may not stay in the small intestine long enough to release its nutrients. Calcium tends to be the mineral most recommended by doctors who treat IBS, but we think magnesium, zinc, and a multiple trace mineral are also important additions to an IBS supplement program.

Calcium

The minerals that are most important to body structure and function are calcium and magnesium. Calcium is the most abundant mineral in the body. We think of it mainly as the most important component of our bones and teeth, but its activities go way beyond the skeleton.

Calcium is crucial for heart health, normal nerve function, and muscle activity. It also neutralizes acidity in the body, activates enzymes, promotes cell division, and allows the transport of nutrients through cell membranes. Calcium also helps control blood acid–alkaline balance and plays a role in muscle growth and iron utilization.

Yogurt and kefir are good sources of calcium and may also slow down diarrhea.

Magnesium

Chronic magnesium deficiency presently affects about 80 percent of the North American population for several reasons:

- There is very little magnesium in the soil.
- What little magnesium is found in food is often lost during cooking and processing. Magnesium dissolves in water and is lost if you boil your food.
- Few people eating a diet rich in magnesium, which would include whole grains, dark green vegetables, nuts, and seeds.

Magnesium deficiency is even more common in people with constipation. Magnesium deficiency results in constipation because it causes intestinal spasms. And you can also lose magnesium through frequent diarrhea.

While calcium is crucial, magnesium may be even more important. Why? Without magnesium, calcium cannot function. Magnesium is responsible for the proper function of more than 325 different enzymes. It is especially important in enzymes related to carbohydrate metabolism, which creates the energy that drives our cells and our whole bodies. Fatigue is one of the first symptoms of magnesium deficiency. It's not properly tested in the blood because only 1 percent of the magnesium in the body is located in the blood. But if you have been told that you have a potassium deficiency, you likely have a magnesium deficiency as well.

Magnesium is essential for proper heartbeat, nerve transmission, and muscle function. It works in synergy with calcium. But if there is too much calcium and not enough magnesium, you can get muscle spasms or cramps, tics, nerve tingling, nerve pain, premature labor, or preeclampsia of pregnancy, and even angina or a heart attack! The pain and spasm of IBS can be helped with magnesium.

Magnesium comes in many supplement forms. Magnesium oxide has laxative effects; it can be useful for IBS-constipation, but only about 4 percent of it is absorbed. Therefore, we recommend magnesium citrate. Powdered forms such as Mag Max-O and Natural Calm are a great place to start because you can use a very small amount and work up to the amount that is right for you, whereas a capsule is hard to cut in two! If you are troubled by IBS-diarrhea and magnesium citrate seems to aggravate the condition, you can use magnesium glycinate or magnesium taurate, which are a bit more expensive but do not seem to have the same laxative effect.

Zinc

Almost 100 enzymes depend on zinc for their proper function. Zinc, in close conjunction with vitamin A, supports the immune system and is involved with tissue repair and healing.

Vying for vitamins

Vitamins come in two forms: fat soluble (vitamins A, D, E, and K) and water soluble (all the rest). The main vitamins that are recommended for people with IBS are vitamins A, D, E, and K. This is because they are not absorbed as quickly as the water-soluble vitamins and tend to get pulled out more readily in people with IBS-diarrhea.

Vitamin A

The food sources of Vitamin A are yellow and dark green vegetables, fruits, dairy foods, and eggs. The main supplement source is cod liver oil.

Vitamin D

This is the sunshine vitamin. People who live in northern climates need extra vitamin D from cod liver oil during the winter. And now that so many people are slathering on the sunscreen, we may all be getting deficient if we don't have at least 20 minutes of direct sunlight on some exposed parts of our skin every day! Perhaps we all need to take cod liver oil on a regular basis.

Vitamin E

Unless you eat wheat germ or take wheat germ oil, you aren't going to get much vitamin E in your diet. Vitamin E is a powerful antioxidant that protects the body from damage by free radicals. If you take vitamin E, make sure you check the label for mixed tocopherols with both alpha and gamma fractions.

A *free radical* is an unstable molecule that is the product of normal body metabolism formed when molecules within our own body's cells react with oxygen. It has an unpaired electron that tries to steal a stabilizing electron from another molecule, rendering that molecule unstable, which can produce a chain reaction of harmful effects. External sources of free radicals include chemicals (pesticides, industrial pollution, auto exhaust, cigarette smoke), heavy metals (dental amalgam [mercury], lead, cadmium, cosmetics, vaccines), most infections (viruses, bacteria, parasites), x-rays, alcohol, allergens, stress, and even excessive exercise. (See *The Miracle of Magnesium* by Dr. Carolyn Dean [Ballentine] for more information.)

If we consider the potential free radical damage caused by pesticide-contaminated foods, chlorinated public water, incompletely digested food, and yeast toxins in IBS, vitamin E may be a very good supplement to take.

Vitamin K

Vitamin K is responsible for blood clotting. Without enough vitamin K, the blood is too thin; your first clue may be nosebleeds. This vitamin also helps convert glucose to glycogen, which is stored in the intestines. (If it doesn't do its job, there may be a possibility that the extra glucose is devoured by yeast.) Vitamin K is found in leafy green vegetables and is also synthesized in a normal (meaning not IBS) intestinal environment. If you are not eating raw vegetables, you are lacking vitamin K.

Using digestive aids

You may want to consider supplementing your diet with digestive enzymes and hydrochloric acid. You can do a lot of digesting by chewing properly (at least 40 times per bite of food), but taking enzymes makes sure that no incompletely digested food reaches your large intestine, creating fodder for yeast and bacteria that results in irritating toxic molecules that can get absorbed through the large intestine (see Chapter 3).

Using digestive aids can greatly reduce belching and flatulence. Some nutritionists even say that poor digestion causes these symptoms in the first place. Digestive enzymes and digestive supplements may contain various combinations of the following ingredients:

- **Amylase:** For digesting carbohydrates found in the mouth and in the small intestine

- **Betaine hydrochloride:** Hydrochloric acid that enhances digestion in the stomach

- **Bromelaine:** From pineapple

- **Lipase:** For fat digestion

- **Papaya:** A fruit source of protein-digesting enzymes

- **Pepsin:** For protein digestion in the stomach

- **Peptidase:** For protein digestion in the small intestine

Digestive enzymes are best taken in the middle or toward the end of a meal. With these supplements, the proof is in the pudding. You should notice a difference in bloating, belching, and flatulence when you use these supplements.

Probing probiotics

Probiotics are good bacteria that drive yeast and abnormal bacteria back into hiding. You find probiotics in yogurt or kefir, or in capsule and powder form. They have a very beneficial effect on your intestines and your whole body.

Researchers say there are up to 400 different kinds of good bacteria in the gut, and (not surprisingly) many different types of probiotic supplements are available. In supplement form, you are looking for doses in the *billions* of cells. The optimum range for the most common probiotic, Lactobacillus acidophilus, is from 1 to 10 billion active cells daily.

Lactobacillus also comes in many other varieties: casei, rhamnosus, plantarum, and bulgaricus. And nondairy sources of Lactobacillus include Bifidobacteria breve, Bifidobacterium bifidum, and a friendly yeast called Saccharomyces bourlardii. They usually come in a sealed container that requires refrigeration to keep the live cells from being destroyed by heat.

Getting Help from Homeopathy

As we discuss in Chapter 2 and elsewhere in the book, IBS is a *functional* condition (meaning it doesn't cause structural damage in the body) without a single known cause or a single effective treatment. Homeopathic medicine is safe and effective and has a very good track record in the treatment of functional complaints.

In Chapter 15, we have a special section on using homeopathy for children's emotions. The following homeopathic medicine is safe and effective for use with children as well. However, it is very important to understand that children who suffer frequent diarrhea are at risk of dehydration and can become very ill very quickly. Dehydration in a child constitutes a medical emergency requiring hospitalization.

Developing a medicine

Homeopathy was developed by Samuel Hahnemann in the early 19th century. It is a natural medical science that uses mostly plants and mineral extracts, which are diluted in alcohol or water to infinitesimal amounts, to stimulate someone's natural healing response. Research has shown that these medicines, if given in a toxic amount (before dilution), can cause symptoms similar to the problems that the patient is experiencing. But the infinitesimal dose can cure those same symptoms.

After 200 years of practice, homeopathy is extremely successful. When used correctly, it has no side effects, can be used even if you're also taking medications, and can be used safely by pregnant women and infants. Although skeptics may attribute its success to the *placebo effect* (in which a patient's belief in an outcome produces that outcome), among the millions who have benefited from homeopathy are infants and animals — groups that are clearly not susceptible to the placebo effect.

Unlike allopathic medicine, which prescribes different drugs for physical and emotional problems, homeopathic remedies are geared toward treating body, mind, and spirit. Moods and emotions, and even the preference for a certain season, color, or climate, all go into the selection of the right remedy for you.

Knowing the basics

Homeopathic remedies typically come in dosages of 6, 12, or 30 X or 6, 12, or 30 C potency. (The X stands for 10, and the C stands for 100, so the C potencies are much higher.) The higher the number, the greater the dilution, and the more potent the remedy. Usually, you take three pellets or four drops of a remedy several times a day. (We recommend the liquid medications instead of the pellets because the pellets are made of lactose, which can cause problems if you suffer from lactose intolerance.)

While homeopathic medicine is extremely safe, you still have to become educated about this modality before using it. You can find an introduction to homeopathy and a list of about 30 of the most used remedies for general health in Dr. Carolyn Dean's book *Natural Prescriptions for Common Ailments* (an e-book available at www.carolyndean.com). Homeopaths and naturopaths who specialize in homeopathy are also invaluable resources because they are trained to take a homeopathic history and prescribe the remedy suited to you and your body–mind picture. You can find out how to access these professionals in Chapter 21.

For a very acute, painful symptom, a remedy can be taken every 15 minutes. However, if after taking five or six doses of a remedy you experience no change in symptoms, the remedy is probably ineffective, and you should seek a new remedy.

Be assured that treating with the wrong remedy a half dozen times does not cause any negative side effects. Also be assured that homeopathic medicines are recognized by the U.S. Food and Drug Administration. They are inexpensive and available in health stores and many pharmacies.

Listing medicines for IBS

The following homeopathic medicines may help with mild to moderate IBS symptoms as a first-aid approach. However, unlike drugs that just treat the symptoms, the right homeopathic remedy may also be the cure — especially if it's prescribed by a homeopath after taking your case history. Remember, these medicines can be safely taken by anyone, and there are no contraindications with pharmaceuticals.

You can simply try the medicine that seems best suited to your symptoms, but we recommend having your homeopathic case history taken by a trained homeopath. What does such a case history entail? The homeopath will want to know all your quirks and habits to find the remedy that suits your personality and your IBS condition. The homeopath can then prescribe a specific constitutional medicine for you. A *constitutional homeopathic remedy* matches your personality and character traits and is best suited for chronic health problems.

Argentum nitricum

This medicine has the best results for people who are anxious and nervous and have the following gastrointestinal symptoms: bloating, rumbling flatulence, nausea, and greenish diarrhea. It also seems to help people who have diarrhea immediately after drinking water or from eating too much sweet or salty food. These people may crave sugar and tend to have blood sugar problems. Besides being anxious and nervous, a person who improves from this remedy tends to be claustrophobic, overly expressive, and impulsive.

Colocynthis

Taking Colocynthis is useful when you experience cutting pains and cramping that are relieved somewhat by pressure on the abdomen. Cramps are worse just before an episode of diarrhea. They are triggered by eating fruit or drinking water. The emotional component of this medicine is anger and indignation. Additional symptoms such as back pain, leg pain, and gallbladder problems are also treated with this medicine.

Lilium tigrinum

This medicine is useful if you have IBS symptoms of alternating constipation and diarrhea. You may be constipated one day and then the next day be greeted by diarrhea in the morning. You may also sense a lump in the rectum that can make you feel the unsuccessful urge to go. The emotions that are associated with this medicine are irritability and rage.

Lycopodium

This medicine is commonly used for people with chronic bowel problems who have a ravenous appetite and may get up at night to eat. It can treat all the symptoms of IBS, including bloating, gas, stomach pain, and even heartburn. The people who benefit most from this medicine have symptoms that are partially relieved by rubbing the abdomen and are worse in the late afternoon and early evening. The emotional predisposition with Lycopodium is lack of confidence and worry.

Mag Phos

Mag Phos (which stands for *Magnesium Phosphate*) is the greatest antispasmodic medicine and the most commonly used magnesium homeopathic remedy. It is effective to treat cramping of all muscle groups, including those that produce hiccups, leg cramps, writer's cramp, abdominal colic, heart pain, lung pain, and menstrual pain. The cramping may include radiating pains, nerve pains, and all sorts of tics and tremors (even twitching of the eyelids). It works especially well in debilitated subjects who are both mentally and physically exhausted.

Natrum carbonicum

This medicine is often indicated for shy and withdrawn people who don't digest and assimilate food and find themselves on restricted diets. They experience indigestion and heartburn when they eat an offending food. Dairy products seem to give them the most trouble, causing gas, explosive diarrhea, and an empty, gnawing feeling in the stomach. Emotionally, the person who benefits from this remedy is actually cheerful and considerate, but her symptoms can make her feel weak and sensitive with a desire to be left alone.

Nux vomica

This medicine is often used to treat hangovers or overindulgence. It treats abdominal pains and bowel symptoms accompanied by abdominal tension, chilliness, and irritability. The gripping tension in the abdomen may lead to soreness in the muscles of the abdominal wall and pain from trapped gas. This type of pain is somewhat relieved by pressure on the abdominal wall.

This remedy is appropriate for both IBS-constipation and IBS-diarrhea. With constipation, there is an urge and a feeling of irritation in the rectum, but only small amounts come out. With IBS-diarrhea, after a bowel movement the pain is relieved for a short time. The emotions expressed with this medicine include irritability and aggressiveness. The person who benefits most is often a hard-driving, Type A personality who craves spicy foods, alcohol, tobacco, and coffee but usually feels worse from having indulged in them.

Podophyllum

This medicine is indicated when a person experiences abdominal pain and cramping accompanied by a gurgling, sinking, empty feeling that is followed by watery, noxious smelling diarrhea. There may also be alternating diarrhea and constipation, or pasty yellow bowel movements containing mucus. The early morning is the worst time for this person, who experiences weakness, faintness, and headaches following episodes of diarrhea and has accompanying stiffness of joints and muscles. Some relief can be found from rubbing the right side of the abdomen.

Sulphur

This medicine is for people who are woken up early in the morning with a sudden urge to evacuate the bowels. More episodes of diarrhea can occur throughout the day, but this symptom alternates with constipation with accompanying offensive and odorous gas. A characteristic oozing around the rectum with itching, burning, and red irritation is a classic sign indicating the need for this medicine. Other features of a person who needs this medicine are poor posture, back pain, and worsening of symptoms with standing for long periods of time. Sulphur people also experience hot, burning feet that kick off the bedcovers.

Chapter 10

Eating an IBS-Friendly Diet

. . . .

In This Chapter

▶ Removing possible offenders

▶ Letting your body go through detox

▶ Adding foods back one at a time

▶ Taking additional steps to combat IBS symptoms

. . . .

*W*e know you've heard the saying "You are what you eat." For IBS sufferers, another truism is "You suffer from what you eat."

It's no secret that many foods — and even the act of eating itself — can trigger an IBS attack (see Chapter 4). Through a combination of diet, which we address in this chapter, and stress reduction, which we tackle in Chapter 12, we hope to help you put an end to the food–IBS connection.

The goal is to identify the food factors that may be triggering your symptoms, eliminate them, and reduce your symptoms. When your symptoms are under control, you will be in charge — not your food! That's the key to success in the diet we recommend here.

Most diets start out by eliminating foods, and our diet for IBS is no different. In fact, most practitioners or doctors who successfully treat IBS start their patients with an elimination and challenge program. But here's the good news: Great-tasting substitutes for some of the foods that trigger IBS can make the food elimination process much easier to handle.

You'll also note that we don't tout an IBS-diet. Because everyone with IBS has different food triggers and preferences, we make sure we don't cross that boundary and tell you what to eat. Instead, we give you options and help you determine what's best for you.

So stick with us: We know that changing the way you eat isn't easy. But we also know it's possible, and the result may be freedom from your IBS symptoms.

Making Smart Food Choices

Before we explain how to eliminate foods in order to test for IBS triggers, we want to offer some general advice on how to be a smarter eater. You may be surprised at how making small changes to the way you eat can improve the way you feel.

Combining food wisely

Food combining was all the rage a few years ago, and for good reason. There are three types of foods:

- ✔ Proteins
- ✔ Fats
- ✔ Carbohydrates

Carbs fall into two categories: simple sugar carbs (think white bread, cookies, and crackers) and complex carbs (such as vegetables, grains, and beans). All carbohydrates get broken down into sugars in your body, which provide the energy you need to operate. One "liquid sugar" product that many people consume is soda. There are about 10 teaspoons of sugar in a can of soda. This type of sugar is called *refined* sugar.

You digest each type of food at very different rates. Proteins stay in your stomach for about three hours, and fats can hang out in the stomach for about six hours. But the simple sugars in carbohydrates are supposed to float right through your stomach; they actually should get broken down by enzymes in the small intestine.

If you eat simple carbs (especially refined sugar) with protein or fat, the sugar from the carbs gets trapped in your stomach. When sugars hang around in your stomach, they can begin to ferment and create gas. Younger people usually have enough stomach acid to digest the fermentation, but as you get older, the burps and belches begin to develop into a chorus of indigestion. So what do you do? If you're like many people, you take antacids. But in Chapter 3, we explain that antacids aren't the answer because they further deplete your stomach acid and lead to incompletely digested food.

If you have IBS, we recommend a moratorium on sugars, period. (In Chapter 4, we explain why refined sugar and even the sugars in fruit may trigger IBS symptoms.) But if you can't completely eliminate sugar from your diet, we urge you to eat it separately from protein and fat. In other words, don't eat meat, fish, poultry, eggs, cheese, milk, or butter at the same time you eat concentrated sugars like fruit, fruit juice, or refined sugars in pastries, cakes, soda, or candy. As long as fruit isn't a trigger for your IBS symptoms, try to eat fruit about 30 minutes before a meal.

A sugar primer

Sugar comes in many forms. Naturally occurring sugars add sweetness to whole fruits, vegetables, and milk products. Added sugars include sucrose and other refined sugars that appear in processed foods, soft drinks, fruit drinks, and other beverages.

You encounter all sorts of words that refer to various kinds of sugars. Here are a few you may be wondering about:

✔ The term *simple carbohydrate* refers to monosaccharides and disaccharides.

✔ *Complex carbohydrate* refers to polysaccharides.

✔ The most common naturally-occurring monosaccharide is fructose, which is found in fruits and vegetables.

✔ Common disaccharides are sucrose (glucose + fructose), found in sugar cane, sugar beets, honey, and corn syrup; lactose (glucose + galactose), found in milk products; and maltose (glucose + glucose), from malt.

✔ Polysaccharides include starches, such as root vegetables.

Simple carbohydrates take minutes to break down in the body, whereas complex carbohydrates take up to an hour. Therefore, the sugar molecules from complex carbs hit the blood stream with much less velocity and less shock to the body than simple carbs. That's where the glycemic index comes in.

The *glycemic index* is the rate at which foods are changed into sugars and cause a rise in the body's blood glucose. It's a complex system, and some of the results may surprise you. If you are interested in learning more about the glycemic index, go to www.glycemicindex.com. You can even type in one of your favorite foods and find out its glycemic index.

Because it takes three or four hours to move a protein meal out of the stomach, eating dessert right after a heavy meal can also lead to fermentation and indigestion. If you have tummy troubles, it's best to skip dessert with a meal and occasionally indulge your sweet tooth three hours before or after a meal.

Reducing fats

A universal piece of advice we can offer for anyone with IBS symptoms is to reduce the amount of fat you consume. Fat in the diet causes lots of bells and whistles to go off in your body. Enzymes from the pancreas and bile from the liver are both required to digest fat. Large amounts of bile in the intestine can be irritating and cause cramping pain. Fatty foods include full fat dairy, cheese, meat, fried foods, and chocolate.

Not all oils are created equal. Avoiding essential fats is unhealthy. Coconut oil may be the best oil for a person with IBS. Medium chain fatty acids are found in abundance in coconut oil, and they are absorbed more efficiently in the digestive tract than longer chain fatty acids found in some vegetable oils. Also, recent research shows that the longer chain fatty acids found in polyunsaturated oils (soy, corn, and other vegetable oils) are the most harmful oils for people with intestinal problems, leading to inflammation and irritation. Flax, olive, coconut, and sunflower are essential fats that are not long chain but help build and rebuild all body tissue. Coconut oil can be used for cooking, and some people even mix it into their morning protein drinks.

Knowing what's healthy for you

As Jim was recovering from a bout of traveler's diarrhea, he thought that it would be a good time to make some changes in his diet. He replaced some of his staples with healthier alternatives. For example, Jim ate white bread with every meal and decided that he would switch to whole wheat. He also figured that because whole wheat is so healthy, he could eat as much as he wanted. Within a couple days, Jim was making several trips to the bathroom and fearing that he was reliving his vacation diarrhea, with excessive gas and bloating to boot. What he didn't realize was that the travelers' diarrhea had made him susceptible to overreacting to the extra roughage in the excessive amounts of whole wheat bread that he started to consume.

More than a few people have told us that after they began eating "health food," they developed symptoms of IBS. They thought they were doing something good for their health but got blindsided by their digestive tracts! The health foods that most people move to when they make a bid to change their lifestyles include whole wheat bread, soy products, and fruit. (If you've already read Chapters 2 and 4, you probably know where this little vignette is going.)

Here are some ways that healthy foods can cause problems in certain people:

- ✔ Gas and bloating are common symptoms when people start eating more roughage.

- ✔ The extra roughage from whole wheat could start the diarrhea ball rolling in a susceptible individual.

- ✔ Eating more wheat could uncover an underlying case of gluten intolerance (celiac disease, which we explain in Chapter 2), causing either constipation or diarrhea.

- ✔ Soy protein powders, soy cheese, and soy meat products can cause susceptible people to develop gas and bloating. (As we note in Chapter 4, soy is very difficult to digest, especially if it is not fermented.)

- ✔ As we explain in Chapter 4, if you don't have the enzymes to digest fruit, you are going to suffer the intestinal consequences.

What you need to remember as you read this chapter, or any other resource that recommends dietary changes to address IBS, is that your body is different from any other body. A health food for one person may be an IBS trigger for another. Pay attention to your body's signals as you eat different foods, even healthy ones, and at the first sign that a particular food offends your system, cut it out of your diet.

Eliminating Possible Food Triggers

Even if you have only been skimming the chapters in this book so far, you may have noticed that we place a *lot* of emphasis on food triggers for IBS and food allergy or intolerance that is mistaken for IBS. We want to be very clear that unless you do the right tests to determine food allergy or intolerance, or unless you go on an elimination diet to do your own experiment with food triggers, you have not plumbed the depths of IBS.

Most tests require a doctor's prescription, but not so with an elimination and challenge diet. You can take this step on your own, but you have to use your common sense and intuition and look upon it as a clinical trial of one person.

People with IBS use the process of elimination and challenge constantly, although they may not know the name for it. You eat something that you realize (too late) may have triggered a reaction, so you eliminate that food for a while — mostly out of fear! The next time you are faced with that food, you may try it just to see what happens.

The memory of pain is often short-lived, and it is easy to forget that after eating a certain food two months ago, you spent three hours keeping family and friends away from the toilet. That's why we recommend using a structured elimination and challenge experiment, so you can prove to yourself which foods bother you. Plus, people with IBS rarely have just one trigger food, so eliminating just one food at a time may not help much at all. You need a plan that helps you eliminate as many triggers as possible.

If even the thought of eliminating food stirs up stress for you, turn to Chapter 12, where we talk about a unique form of emotional acupuncture called Emotional Freedom Techniques (EFT). You can use EFT to get you through the food cravings.

We have no doubt that you will go off the elimination diet at least once during this process. A birthday party, a holiday, a friend who is jealous of your willpower and waves a cake under your nose — any number of temptations will cause you to stray. It happens all the time, but you learn from the experience and get stronger with the next effort.

If you are conducting an elimination diet and you choose to sample a forbidden food in the midst of it, please do so close to home — and close to the toilet. When you have taken trigger foods out of your diet, even for a few days, sometimes a mere taste can send your bowels into spasms.

Two weeks toward better health

Before you even start eliminating foods, make notes about how you feel. How many bowel movements are you having a day (or a week if you suffer from constipation)? When do you have most of your pain, gas, and bloating? What foods do you think are not your friends? Write it all down, and then make daily entries during your elimination adventure. Journaling your journey is very useful because often you don't remember how bad you felt before you made a big lifestyle change.

If you haven't already done so, you may want to read Chapters 2 and 4 to get a more detailed account of the following triggers, which we think should be avoided completely during an elimination diet. (We include here the food intolerances that are sometimes mistaken for IBS.)

- ✔ Alcohol
- ✔ Coffee
- ✔ Dairy
- ✔ Food additives and all diet products with aspartame
- ✔ Fried foods
- ✔ Fruit
- ✔ High fructose corn syrup
- ✔ Processed foods
- ✔ Spicy foods
- ✔ Sugar
- ✔ Wheat

Eliminate these foods for at least two weeks to get them totally out of your system. By that time, your immune system (which may have been attacking these foods) will have settled down, and all the inflammation and irritation from them should be gone.

Yes, we can hear the storm of protest. Life as you know it is now over! There is nothing left to eat! How can you possibly survive! You are shouting at the top of your lungs, "You have ruined my life!"

Okay, now that that's out of your system, let's deconstruct what just happened. If you say there is nothing left to eat, that means you have been surviving on bread, donuts, and coffee (with cream and two sugars) for far too long! It's time for a change, and that change will all be for the good.

We're tempted to go into a tirade here about the deterioration of our food supply, but we won't. Suffice to say that we need to expand our horizons beyond wheat and add more grains. Dairy is hard to digest for a good segment of the population, and sugar is a non-food that feeds yeast in the intestines. Additives, fried food, alcohol, and coffee can all trigger symptoms of IBS, so you are better off without them.

In the process of eliminating these foods, you also reduce the amount of sugar in your digestive system that feeds yeast. You may or may not have yeast overgrowth (Candida albicans), which we discuss in Chapters 3 and 4, but the elimination diet has the added bonus of being an anti-yeast diet.

What's left to eat?

The idea of giving up wheat and dairy may make you wonder what you *can* eat. And taking away sugar only adds insult to injury!

The foods that you can eat include

- Fresh meats, poultry, and fish
- Vegetables
- Nuts and seeds
- Unprocessed oils — flax, olive, sunflower, and coconut
- Whole grains, such as rice, millet, quinoa, amaranth, and kasha
- Water, lemonade, and herbal teas

You can also check with your naturopath, integrative medicine practitioner, or health food store owner for a meal replacement powder that can be made from eggs, rice, pea powder, or whey. This meal can help take the pressure off digestion, help eliminate toxins, heal the gut, and save time when you are stressed out about what to eat.

A natural sweetener that doesn't cause the problems created by sugar or artificial sweeteners is stevia. It is available in powder or liquid form in health food stores. Stevia is made from the bark of a tree that grows in South America and is 200 times sweeter than sugar.

Later in the chapter, in the section "Translating Your Results into Better Habits," we provide a shopping list and recipes you can use while you're on the elimination diet, as well as afterward (when you realize how beneficial healthy eating can be).

The morning elixir

If you have been a poster child for a junk food diet, you may want to ease into an elimination diet. To do this, keep eating your regular diet for the moment, and start drinking what we call the *morning elixir.* This drink begins a gentle cleansing process in your body, tunes up your liver and digestion, and helps eliminate toxins. (This drink is called the *master cleanser* when it's used during a fast.)

The ginger component subdues any possible nausea that you may feel from changing your diet, and the cayenne gets your circulation going and keeps your hands and feet warm. (Cayenne is red pepper, but it has the ability to heal the intestines as well as stimulate blood flow.) Some recipes for this drink use about 1/8 teaspoon of cayenne, but to start with we ask you to use just a pinch of this powerful healer.

To make the morning elixir, combine these ingredients:

> A quart of water
>
> The juice of one lemon
>
> A pinch of cayenne
>
> The contents of one capsule of ginger

If you find this drink too sour, add 1/8 teaspoon of stevia. (When this drink is used during a fast, the recipe calls for 1 teaspoon of maple syrup to provide some calories and minerals.)

You don't have to just drink this tonic in the morning; most people love it and drink it all day. You can mix it and pack it to go to work, substituting it for water, tea, and coffee.

Detox and die off

There is an aspect to the elimination diet called *detoxing and die off.* The name alone should serve as a caution to people who are eating a very bad diet to go slowly — different things can happen when you stop eating foods you are addicted to. For example, you may know that if you are a regular coffee drinker and decide to eliminate coffee, you can get headaches from the caffeine withdrawal. The headache is a result of detoxing. In this section, we give you some tips on how to make the detoxing process (whether from caffeine, sugar, or other addictive foodstuffs) not so painful.

If your diet consists mostly of bread, dairy, sugar, and coffee with some protein and a vegetable or two thrown in as an afterthought, your body may react when you eliminate the bread, dairy, sugar, and coffee. Part of the reaction is the dying-off process that yeast and certain bacteria go through when you quit feeding them simple sugars. But if you understand what's really happening, you can do something about the detoxing and die off symptoms that you experience.

Here's what happens in your body when you eliminate simple sugars and other addictive foods:

- As yeast are starved and die off in the millions and billions, their 180 chemical byproducts (which we mention in Chapter 4) may be absorbed into your bloodstream. These chemicals may make you feel tired, foggy, headachy, stiff, and sore.

- As you break down fatty tissue in your body, stored *pseudoestrogens* (chemicals from the environment that are similar to estrogen), other environmental chemicals, and other toxins stored in the fat cells are released into your bloodstream. Pseudoestrogens block hormone receptors and can play a role in thyroid problems, PMS, and early menopause.

- Food addictions, with a power similar to tobacco, coffee, and alcohol addiction, are screaming out to be fed.

Not knowing about detox and die off can be the downfall of many diets. You feel so yucky that you just don't want to continue. Feeding the cookie monster seems your only way out, because doing so momentarily stops the headaches, woozy feeling, aches, and pains.

Here are resources you can use to deal with detox and die off, which usually occurs within the first two weeks of changing your diet:

- **Good food:** Later in the chapter, in the section "Translating Your Results into Better Habits," we offer a grocery list and recipes to help you improve what you eat both during and after your elimination diet. Use them. (Specialists tell us that strict vegans can develop IBS that does not reverse until they correct their protein deficiency.)

There are patented, hypoallergenic, meal replacement formulas that can provide you with healing, nutritious meals while you are on an elimination and challenge diet. One such meal replacement formula in a rice base, called UltraInflammX, is designed to restore GI function. It's made by a company called Metagenics and available from a naturopath or integrative medicine doctor.

✔ **Water:** Drink eight glasses of filtered or bottled water every day to flush toxins out through your kidneys. Using the morning elixir is even better.

✔ **Psyllium:** Take psyllium husk capsules or powder to maintain two bowel movements a day and sweep out the dying yeast debris. This advice is mainly for people with IBS-constipation.

✔ **Magnesium:** Use magnesium citrate powder or magnesium citrate capsules (see Chapter 9). Magnesium is necessary for energy, detoxing, muscle relaxation, and sound sleep. It also protects the heart and helps prevent diabetes.

✔ **Probiotics:** Take probiotics (see Chapter 9), which are the good gut bacteria, from the first day of your elimination diet.

✔ **A journal:** Write down what you are feeling when you reach for something that you know you want to eliminate.

Probiotics can be used by people who have either IBS-diarrhea or IBS-constipation. We offer more detailed instructions for when and how to use psyllium and magnesium in Chapters 8 and 9.

Challenging Each Food

Miranda had gone through an elimination diet for two weeks, and her IBS symptoms had subsided. She decided that it was time to reintroduce plain milk into her diet to see what would happen. She enjoyed milk by itself, on her cereal, and with tea. She was hoping that after two weeks, milk would pass the test and prove to pose no problem. She started with a little milk in her tea in the morning and didn't notice anything. At lunch, she drank a glass of milk, and within the hour she felt the familiar rumbling in her intestines. Soon she was in the bathroom, glad that she had tested milk at home and not at work.

After you've successfully followed the elimination diet for at least two weeks and your IBS symptoms seem under some control, it's time to move to the next part of the experiment — figuring out what you can add back. Here are the basic steps you take:

✔ Continue following the elimination diet.

✔ Add back one portion of one new food each day.

✔ Keep a journal of your reactions to the food.

Gas and bloating are big clues that a food is not your friend, and these symptoms usually come quite quickly after eating an offending food. If your symptom is predominantly diarrhea, you may have that reaction within just a few hours. But constipation-predominant IBS takes a lot longer to appear, so the gas and bloating are your first clues. If you actually have an allergy to a food that you've added back, you'll probably experience a rash, stuffy sinuses, and/or headaches.

It's important to follow the recommendation to add only one portion of a new food per day. If that food gives you a reaction, you may have to wait for another day or two to go back to your baseline level of symptoms before testing another food. If you don't have a reaction, the next day you can add another new food. But if a food doesn't give you a reaction, you still don't want to overdo it; eat a non-offending food only every third day.

Rotating your foods every three days is actually the best possible diet. It's a common sense way to keep variety in your diet and to keep away from food allergies and food reactions.

Pay careful attention to your reactions to foods that you are reintroducing. If you try some wheat and just feel a little gassy afterwards, heed this warning sign. A bit of gas following a bit of wheat today can turn into an hour on the toilet tomorrow. Any reaction in your digestive tract is reason enough to stay away from a particular food.

You obviously want to test wheat, dairy, and sugar to see if you can sneak them back into your diet (unless you're committed to just avoiding them altogether). But if you test wheat, dairy, and sugar, be sure to experiment with foods containing only one ingredient. For example, bread contains wheat, yeast, and other ingredients. So if you want to test wheat, don't eat bread; instead, eat plain shredded wheat. Just pour a bit of boiling water on it and enjoy!

What, plain shredded wheat doesn't tempt you? Actually, it's not that bad. Shredded wheat was our dad's favorite food, even though he was allergic to it! When he developed diabetes, we tried to convince him that his lifelong gas, bloating, IBS, sugar cravings, and weight gain were due to wheat allergy. He gave up wheat, and for three months, dad's blood sugars were back to normal. Then, he had an appointment with a dietician. She told him it was perfectly permissible to have six servings of bread a day. Shortly after reintroducing bread, his IBS symptoms came back and his blood sugar went up. He chose to take diabetic medication rather than giving up bread.

If you have a negative reaction to wheat, you have a choice to make as well. It's actually much easier to live without wheat today than it was 15 or 20 years ago. Plenty of other grains are now made into breads or eaten as cereals or side dishes — millet, quinoa, buckwheat, and amaranth are the ones with the least gluten.

Do not challenge wheat, dairy, or any other food if you already know or suspect that you are allergic to it. Even after just two weeks off allergic foods, you may become more sensitive to them.

Translating Your Results into Better Habits

Whether the elimination and challenge process indicates that one food offends you or a dozen are to blame for your IBS symptoms, we hope you use the opportunity (and your heightened willpower after two weeks of sacrifice) to make some lasting changes to your diet. The information in the following sections can help.

Although the current rage is a high protein diet, it tends to be low on roughage and low on liquids. Dairy, meat, and fish are great sources of protein, but they are also very dense foods that don't hold much liquid compared to vegetables, and they don't have as much roughage as whole grains.

Here's another drawback of a high protein diet: You miss out on beneficial bacteria. A diet high in complex carbohydrates promotes beneficial bacteria in the intestines and helps promote *probiotics* — the good bacteria in your gut. A low fiber diet does the opposite.

Substituting good foods

In our experience, it takes about six weeks to switch from an unhealthy diet to one that is healing for IBS. It's not something that you do overnight. In fact, you can upset your stomach and intestines even more if you make an abrupt change in your diet. There are twelve food groups with replacements in the Table 10-1; each week take two of these groups and implement your changes for a slow and gradual transition. Under the "Present Diet" column, we assume that you are probably eating the Standard American Diet (whose initials are, appropriately, SAD). Foods in the "Present Diet" are loaded with chemicals and additives, which are irritating to the bowel. In the "IBS Diet" column, we list the foods that are preferable for you to eat. Note that the "IBS Diet" foods are all allowed during the two-week elimination diet we explain earlier in the chapter.

Table 10-1	Preferred Diet for Someone with IBS
Present Diet	*IBS Diet*
Processed cold cuts, hot dogs	Antibiotic-free meat
Fried fish, farm-raised fish	Wild salmon, shellfish
Pork	Free-range chicken

Present Diet	IBS Diet
Beans, tofu, tempeh, veggie burger	
Sugar, molasses, candy, chocolate, maple syrup, honey	Stevia
Milk, cheese, cream, yogurt, coffee creamer	Rice milk, almond milk
Butter	Nut butters
Fruit, fruit juices	Vegetables
Coffee, black tea, soda	Grain coffee, organic herbal teas, green tea
Diet drinks, alcohol	Mineral, spring, or filtered water
Hydrogenated oils	Organic butter, coconut oil
Light olive oil, lard	Extra virgin olive oil
GMO corn oil, canola oil, vegetable oil	Sesame oil, flax oil
Refined white flour bread, crackers, bagels, tortillas, pizza, cookies, cakes, muffins, pasta, pretzels, Danish	100 percent sprouted-grain breads (made from sprouted grains); Essene, Ezekiel, and Manna breads are examples

By viewing this list, you get a good idea of how much processed food we eat. IBS is a condition created by our present civilization, and people with IBS are a bit like canaries in a coal mine. What do we mean by that? Canaries are carried into mine shafts in their cages. If the canary keels over, the miners know that the air is bad, and they high-tail it to the surface. With conditions like IBS and chronic fatigue syndrome, certain people seem to be more susceptible to medications, environmental stressors, and poor lifestyle than others, and they succumb to these pressures earlier than the rest of us.

For example, at a recent conference, we met a naturopathic student who said she was diagnosed with IBS, but it seemed to flare up only when she went off her organic vegetarian diet. She realized that her bowel sensitivity was due to herbicides and pesticides on non-organic vegetables and fruits.

Planning a menu

Your daily menu should include the main food groups to ensure complete nutrition:

- A whole grain dish (made of a grain you can tolerate after the elimination diet)
- A source of protein, such as fish, chicken, or eggs
- Three or more green vegetables
- Three or more red or orange vegetables
- A source of high-quality fats, such as flax oil, coconut oil, organic avocado, nuts, and seeds

Shopping for health

Following is your IBS shopping list that can help you find foods that will become your new best friends.

Grains

Rice (Lundberg organic), basmati rice, barley, quinoa, millet, kamut, spelt, buckwheat, amaranth, oatmeal, cream of buckwheat (Pocono)

Nondairy milks

Rice Dream rice milk, Pacific Almond milk, oat milk, hazelnut milk

Organic butter/ghee

Kate's, Alta Dena, Horizon, Purity Farms Ghee (clarified butter)

Wheat-free bread

Health Seed Spelt, millet, rice, sprouted grain, Essene, Manna

Soy protein

Tempeh, soy yogurt

Remember: Use only fermented soy products, which are easier to digest.

Sweeteners

Stevia (KAL brand), occasional organic maple syrup, and raw unrefined honey (local)

Salt

Lima Atlantic Sea Salt, Si Salt, Muramoto, De Sousa Rock Salt

Be aware that sea salt does not contain iodine, so you may need to take iodine pills or kelp daily.

Seasonings

Herbamare, Sea Seasonings (Dulse, Dulse w/ Garlic, Nori w/ Ginger, Kelp w/ Cayenne), Braggs Aminos

Canned bean brands

Eden, Pacific, Westbrae, Shari Ann's

Nuts and seeds

Almonds, walnuts, sesame seeds, pumpkin seeds, sunflower seeds, cashews, pecans

Organic oils

Extra virgin olive oil, flax seed oil, sesame oil, coconut oil, sunflower oil

Organic snacks

Guiltless Baked Blue Corn Chips, Bearitos Blue Corn Chips, Kettle Corn Chips, Arrowhead Mills Popcorn

Condiments

Braggs Vinegar, organic soy sauce, Tree of Life Mustard, raw sauerkraut, organic balsamic vinegar, Eden Tamari (soy sauce)

Making good meals

Lots of great resources for healthy menu ideas are available. The following sample meals and suggestions are edited and excerpted from Dr. Carolyn Dean's book *Hormone Balance* (Adams Media). Note that you can use each of these meal ideas during your two-week elimination diet. Another resource for tasty wheat- and dairy-free recipes is *The Yeast Connection Cookbook* by Dr. William Crook and Marjorie Hurt Jones, RN (Professional Books); and www.yeastconnection.com, where Dr. Carolyn Dean is medical advisor.

Breakfast: Homemade whole grain cereal

While you can purchase whole grain cereals at any grocery store, you may find that you can eat only certain types of grains, which reduces your grocery options. An easy solution is to make your own whole grain cereal in a slow cooker.

Have on hand some or all of the following grains and seeds: organic rice, kamut, quinoa, millet, barley, rye, oats, amaranth, sunflower seeds, and pumpkin seeds. If you are avoiding gluten foods, eliminate rye and oats.

Use a quart-size slow cooker. Just before bed, measure out 2 ounces per person of three grains and seeds. (You can rotate your choices throughout the week.) Cover the grains and seeds with 5 ounces of water, and let your slow cooker cook on low overnight. In the morning, you have a delicious cooked cereal. If it's too dry, add hot water and stir.

If you don't have a slow cooker, just soak 2 ounces of grains in 5 ounces of water overnight. In the morning, bring it to a boil, and simmer on low for about 15 minutes. Add more water if it's too dry.

Add 2 tablespoons of flaxseed oil for a good source of healthy omega-3 fatty acids. In the first two to four weeks of the elimination diet, eat your cereal without fruit. Then, if you are not troubled by fruit intolerance or yeast over-growth, add some pieces of pear or apple, or some blueberries.

Lunch: Tempting salads

Purchase a pound of organic mesculin salad mix. (Costco, Trader Joe's, Whole Foods supermarkets, and health food stores carry this salad-in-a-box.) Cut in an avocado and tomatoes. Sprinkle in sunflower seeds, and add a healthy dressing such as this one:

> 1/2 cup of cold pressed olive oil or coconut oil
>
> 1/4 cup lemon juice or apple cider vinegar
>
> 2 cloves of garlic (run through a garlic press)
>
> 1/2 teaspoon dry or dijon mustard

Shake the ingredients in a covered jar. You can use this dressing on salads, cooked vegetables, or fish. Some people with IBS find that coconut oil is easier to digest than olive oil. Try both and see which one suits you best.

Dinner: Soup, fish, or chicken

You have several great options for dinners during your elimination diet. Following are our suggestions for making satisfying soups, fish, and chicken dishes.

Super soup

Trader Joe's, Whole Foods, and health food stores carry boxes of organic vegetable soup, precooked wild rice, 1-pound bags of frozen organic vegetables,
coconut milk, and curry powder. You can make a superb meal in five minutes
with these foods.

Pour a box of vegetable soup into a medium saucepan. Add a 10-ounce pack-
age of precooked wild rice, and heat. Add a 12-ounce can of coconut milk.
When everything is simmering nicely, stir in a bag of organic frozen vegetables and a teaspoon or more of curry powder to taste. (The turmeric in most
curries is a powerful anti-inflammatory.)

Fabulous fish

A frozen filet of wild salmon can be thawed out in a few minutes in its pack-
age in a pan of hot water in the sink. (You can use the time to steam slices of
sweet potato for a side dish.) Cook the fish for a few minutes in a toaster
oven, and pour the healthy salad dressing we suggest in the "Lunch:
Tempting salads" section over everything.

Chicken delight

Use your largest stockpot and put a vegetable steamer tray in the bottom to
elevate the chicken above the steaming water. Place one fresh or frozen
(free-range) chicken on top of the tray (between 3 and 4 pounds). Add 2
tablespoons of curry to the water. Keep about 1 quart of water on a slow to
medium boil, and steam the chicken. If the water boils low, add more.

When your frozen chicken has been steaming for just over an hour (or your
unfrozen chicken has been cooking for about a half hour), add one or two
whole organic yams, two beets, and two onions to the pot. (You don't even
have to cut them up; you only have to peel the onions.) A half hour later, add
two whole potatoes. Fifteen minutes later, add two whole carrots and one cut-
up squash and cook for another ten minutes. In the final five minutes, add
two cups of greens (kale, collards, or spinach).

This dish may take two hours to cook, but it requires only a few minutes of
prep time.

Your first meal is a fabulous chicken dinner with all the trimmings. The rest
you can freeze, including the quart of curried chicken stock, or you can
immediately make a soup with the rest of the leftovers.

To make soup, cook rice in the chicken stock. (Use basmati rice for an interesting taste.) Then add some of the cooked chicken and all the vegetables.
You can add coconut milk, more curry to taste, and any frozen vegetables
you have on hand. We usually make six quarts at a time, freezing some and
eating the rest over the next two days.

If you don't like curry, you can substitute 2 teaspoons of sage in the stock water or other cooking spices that you love.

Taking Additional Steps for Diarrhea and Constipation

Certain foods are beneficial both for people with diarrhea and those with constipation, and some are not. In the sections that follow, we offer information to consider for your specific symptoms.

Weighing soluble and insoluble fibers

Foods that are high in *soluble fiber,* the type of fiber that traps water, can help sop up the excess fluid like a sponge in a GI tract that's moving too fast. Soluble fiber taken with enough liquids can also help soften hardening stool. For that reason, soluble fiber seems to be helpful for people with IBS-diarrhea as well as those with IBS-constipation. Insoluble fiber, on the other hand, may not be good for people with IBS because the rough edges of fibers may irritate sensitive intestines. There are diets based on eating soluble fiber and avoiding insoluble fiber. These diets can be very helpful, but you always have to remember that everyone is different.

High levels of soluble fiber that are beneficial for IBS are found in dried beans, oats, barley, and some fruits (like apples and citrus) and vegetables (such as potatoes). That's great to know, but many people with IBS have trouble digesting beans, which have the reputation of being gassy in even the strongest stomachs. And citrus fruits tend to be too acidic for some people with IBS.

Foods high in insoluble fiber are wheat bran, whole grains, cereals, seeds, and the skins of many fruits and vegetables. That's why you often see people peeling tomatoes and apples because they realize they just can't digest that much insoluble fiber.

In Appendix A, we provide an extensive list of foods and their levels of soluble and insoluble fiber. This chart was created by the U.S. Department of Agriculture (USDA). Studying the soluble/insoluble fiber chart may help you understand why certain foods bug you and certain foods are okay.

One IBS diet lists rice as the food with the most soluble fiber, but the type of rice is important. The chart in Appendix A shows that refined white rice has no soluble fiber, but brown rice does. Probably white rice works in some IBS diets because very few people react to it. It's a staple food in hypoallergenic diets. The same reasoning may be used for white bread — especially if it is sourdough bread, another hypoallergenic food. Our USDA charts say it still contains a high amount of insoluble fiber, yet some people feel it soothes their bowels.

White rice and white flour are not very nutritious, and you don't want to eat them at every meal.

The trick to using soluble and insoluble fiber foods in your diet is to choose the foods that are high in soluble fiber and low in insoluble fiber. Doing that calculation makes oatmeal rise to the top of the list. That's an easy food to make for breakfast or to order when you travel.

Remember, through an elimination diet you may find that certain soluble fiber foods are not your friends and certain insoluble fiber foods are. It's all individual. And a person with IBS-diarrhea may determine that his symptoms are triggered by the same type of food that causes constipation in his friend who has IBS-constipation.

But there are ways in which the two conditions don't overlap when it comes to eating. In the following sections, we offer some additional pieces of advice you can use depending on your specific symptom. And if you have the type of IBS that alternates between diarrhea and constipation, you should play ping pong with these suggestions, using them according to your symptoms on a given day.

Combating diarrhea

People with diarrhea don't do so well with hot and spicy foods, which just seem to add to the gas and burning symptoms. (We've heard people say that chili peppers burn when they come out as much as they do when they go in.) Avoid those foods whenever possible, and consider the following tidbits as well.

Chew, chew, chew

Eating small, frequent meals and chewing slowly and completely are great IBS-prevention habits to adopt. A big meal stretches the stomach and intestines and can set the cramping and diarrhea wheels in motion.

In Chapter 3, we note that the size of your stomach is about equal to your two cupped hands held side-by-side. In any 15-minute period, don't eat more than one handful of food. (*Your* handful, not Michael Jordan's handful!) Just measure out that amount and put it on your plate. Chew slowly, or take a bite and chew about 40 times while you are reading or working on your computer. That way, you won't feel that you have to rush through a meal.

Avoid obvious triggers

If you follow the elimination diet we suggest in this chapter, you can pinpoint what your specific food triggers are. But if you haven't yet undertaken the elimination and challenge process, you can help yourself by avoiding foods that often trigger IBS-diarrhea. Alcohol, coffee and all caffeine products, soda and other carbonated drinks, fried foods, sorbitol (the artificial sweetener), fructose (found in fruits and honey), and high fructose corn syrup are on the list of foods that may make you miserable. See Chapter 4 for details.

Increase food-based soluble fiber

Increasing dietary fiber is the most common recommendation for both forms of IBS. But hiking up the amount of roughage you consume can cause gas and bloating, so you have to start slowly and get your body used to this new experience. It can take a few weeks for those symptoms to lessen.

We know fiber is good for us; we need the roughage and bulk in the intestines. However, for people who have IBS-diarrhea, there is such a thing as having too much fiber. For them, too much fiber may stretch the stomach and intestines, setting off symptoms.

The best forms of fiber for IBS-diarrhea are food-based soluble fibers that can dissolve in water, instead of insoluble fibers that can't. Soluble fibers are partially digested so the intestines hold onto them longer than the insoluble kinds that go in one end and out the other. Foods high in soluble fiber include beans, bran, and barley.

Improving constipation

If you suffer from constipation, you need bulk and liquids to keep things moving. (You also need exercise, which we discuss in Chapter 11.) You must drink eight glasses of water each day, but to make sure fluids don't interfere with your digestive juices (see Chapter 3), save your water drinking for between meals — one hour before or one hour after.

Water without minerals is one thing we all have to be aware of in these days of filtered and distilled water. Minerals are crucial for all body processes, so if you drink distilled water (which contains no minerals), make sure you take a good multiple mineral and trace mineral supplement.

Fiber is an even more appropriate treatment for constipation than for diarrhea. To bulk up your stool, experts recommend consuming between 12 grams and 35 grams of fiber a day. A teaspoon holds 4 grams of fiber, so we are talking about needing 3 to 9 teaspoons a day of fiber. That may not sound like a lot, but 9 teaspoons of dry bran sitting on a plate can seem like a mountain.

Specific carbohydrate diet

A diet that you may come across in your reading about IBS is a diet that has a long history of helping the inflammatory aspects of inflammatory bowel disease (IBD) but can also be used for IBS. We have met Elaine Gottschall, who used her diet to cure her son of IBD and continues to research and write about this condition some 30 years later. She calls it the *specific carbohydrate diet,* and you can read more in her book *Breaking the Vicious Cycle: Intestinal Health Through Diet* (Kirkton Press) or on the Web site www.scdiet.com.

Keep in mind that this is an extremely strict diet and should not be undertaken lightly.

In a nutshell, here are do's and don'ts of the specific carbohydrate diet.

Do's:

- Fresh or frozen beef, lamb, poultry, pork, fish, eggs*

- Vegetables: fresh or frozen, raw*, or cooked (with no added sugar or starch)

- Homemade yogurt fermented at least 24 hours

- Natural cheeses with little or no lactose, such as cheddar, Colby, havarti, Swiss, and uncreamed cottage cheese (dry curd)

- Fruits: fresh or frozen, raw*, or cooked (with no added sugar)

- Salad and cooking oils (including those made from grains)

- Honey, nuts* and nut flours*, spices of all kinds

- Very dry wine, occasional gin, rye, Scotch, bourbon, vodka

Don'ts:

- Grains, including bread, rice, pasta, cereal, and products with corn

- Processed meats: hot dogs, cold cuts, fast food

- Potatoes (or starchy roots)

- Milk, margarine, soy products

- Chocolate, starches, added sugar (including corn syrup, cane sugar, molasses)

- Beer, sherry, cordials, liqueurs, brandy

The asterisk (*) indicates foods that are generally added a few weeks or months after starting the diet. They should not be eaten if diarrhea is active.

Because high fiber foods help move constipation, it follows that foods that have little fiber and little water make it worse. Cheese, meat, processed foods, candy, and ice cream are the worst offenders. All these foods except meat are eliminated in the diet we recommend in this chapter.

Doctors and researchers agree that dietary fiber should be the first line of treatment for IBS-constipation. According to medical research, fiber makes the bowels move but may not have any effect on pain. Researchers also agree that the gas and bloating in the first few weeks of adding fiber can be a real turnoff. That's why we recommend adding fiber and fiber foods very slowly to your diet.

If you know you don't consume enough fiber in your food, you may be tempted to take a laxative to get your system moving. In Chapter 8, we warn about the problems laxatives can cause (especially because they aren't intended for use with a chronic condition like IBS). Instead, try taking bulk fiber pills or powders, such as psyllium, or using a new natural roughage product called areca seed, which we mention in Chapter 9. You can also safely use magnesium citrate powder or capsules to loosen, soften, and move the stool.

Chapter 11

Alleviating IBS with Exercise

*I*f all the benefits of exercise could be put in a pill, it would be a billion-dollar seller. Study after study shows that exercise affects every part of the body. Trouble is, exercise will always be something that you and you alone have to take the time to do.

Even just the regular movement on a boat or ship can be enough "exercise" to create a positive change in IBS-constipation. But buying a yacht is probably the most expensive remedy for constipation that you will ever find. It's much simpler to walk, swim, bike, jog or do yoga, tai chi, or Pilates.

It's a sad fact that more than 60 percent of adults do not move as much as they should. About 25 percent of adults are not active at all. Women are even less active than men. An alarming 50 percent of young people (ages 12 to 21) are not vigorously active on a regular basis. IBS is a younger person's condition, and inactivity could be a contributing factor.

In this chapter, our aim is to motivate you to start — and stick to — an exercise routine that can improve every part of your body, including those parts most affected by IBS.

Defining Exercise

We mostly hear about two types of exercise. The first is *aerobic*, which causes a lot of air to move through your lungs because you are huffing and puffing while running or playing racquetball. The second is *strength training*, which may conjure up images of big, sweaty men lifting weights heavier than you are.

Obviously, aerobic exercise and strength training are great for your health. But people often overlook another type of exercise: stretching, or flexibility exercise. Many people think of stretching as a warm-up for aerobics or weight training, but it's a form of exercise all by itself. In the following sections, we address the benefits of all three types of exercise.

Allowing air in

When they think of exercise, most people think of aerobic exercises like running, swimming, and biking. Perhaps that's why it's so hard to get started on an exercise program; maybe you just can't imagine yourself in a pair of tight shorts with a number on your back doing a 10K run.

Aerobic exercise is focused on your heart, lungs, and muscles. Speeding up your heart and increasing your breathing rate makes your body demand more oxygen. Your circulation increases, and oxygen is driven to every part of your body. You sweat and glow with the effort. This type of exercise gives you an endorphin high and increases your stamina.

But don't think that you have to do a 10K run to receive the benefits of aerobic exercise. A brisk 20-minute walk is all you need to get your endorphins primed and pumped. Add to that a smile on your face, an appreciation of the wonders of nature, and a love of life, and you're on your way toward a positive healing cycle.

Building strength

Muscle burns calories. The more muscle mass you have, the more calories you burn and the more weight you lose. Therefore, strength training has become very popular. Having stronger muscles is not just about losing weight; it also reduces fatigue from daily activities and chores.

You don't even have to lift weights to do strengthening exercises. One exercise program that we talk about later in the chapter, called *T-Tapp*, includes exercises that are designed to hold your muscles in such a way that you are able to build muscle and burn calories without needing weights. (Special T-Tapp exercises also pump the lymphatic system and are extremely beneficial in IBS.)

Finding flexibility

Stretching exercises put special emphasis on your joints. One reason so many people are plagued by back and hip arthritis is they don't give their joints a workout (other than getting in and out of chairs). Stretching exercises can take every joint in the body through a range of motion, and in the process they stretch all the muscles and keep them toned.

Yoga is the main stretching and flexibility exercise that we talk about in this book. That's because yoga is one of the most beneficial exercises for IBS.

Benefiting from Exercise

We've compiled one of the most comprehensive lists you'll find of the benefits of exercise. Regular exercise can

- Improve digestion
- Improve lymphatic flow
- Reduce stress, both mental and physical
- Increase immune system resistance
- Improve posture
- Increase the production of estrogen, progesterone, and testosterone
- Increase sexuality due to the extra energy and increased hormone output
- Increase endorphins — the feel-good neurotransmitters in the brain
- Balance serotonin in the gut — the natural Prozac hormone
- Reduce anxiety, depression, irritability, and mood swings (as a result of endorphins, serotonin, deeper breathing, and improved posture)
- Improve self-confidence and self-esteem
- Increase mental acuity and the ability to concentrate
- Increase metabolism, burn calories more efficiently, and improve the appetite
- Increase core body temperature, which improves enzyme function for digestion and metabolism
- Increase circulation, which increases blood flow and oxygenation, giving your face and skin a healthy glow
- Stabilize the heart rate and strengthen the heart
- Lower cholesterol and triglyceride levels
- Stimulate the nervous system
- Stimulate and condition the muscles
- Improve mineral uptake in the skeleton

As if that weren't enough, a 2004 study at the Harvard School of Public Health found that physical activity seems to have a direct effect on the brain itself. This survey of more than 18,000 women showed that exercise promotes the production of chemicals in the brain, called *nerve growth factors,* that improve the brain cells' survival and growth.

A majority of women with IBS also have symptoms of PMS. Research shows that exercise is helpful to reduce or eliminate the symptoms of PMS because it reduces stress and tension, acts as a mood elevator, provides a sense of well-being, and improves blood circulation by increasing the natural production of endorphins.

Reducing health risks

It's never too late to start exercising. Studies show that even small improvements in physical fitness can significantly improve health and even lower the risk of death.

The exercise program you begin now for IBS will not only increase your well-being and productivity but will give you an edge on many other diseases. For example, exercise decreases the risk of the following:

- Arthritis
- Breast and colon cancer
- Diabetes
- Diverticulosis
- Heart attack
- High blood pressure
- High cholesterol
- Indigestion
- Kidney disease
- Minor illness from colds and flus
- Obesity
- Osteoporosis
- Premature death
- Stroke
- Ulcers

And if your friends worry about coming down with IBS, you may mention to them that exercise can decrease the risk of developing it as well.

The net result for people with IBS who take the time to exercise is an overall improvement in physical strength, energy, and endurance, which banishes fatigue and muscle tension. Stress reduction results in less anxiety, irritability, and depression. Boosting the immune system results in greater resistance to disease. There are even more benefits for IBS when you use special exercises targeting the lymph glands and the hormones. We get to these exercises later in the chapter, in the section "Loosening Up Your Lymph System."

Maintaining your muscles

The body is incredibly adaptable, but if you don't move your muscles for about three weeks, you lose them. Have you ever injured one of your limbs? If so, you probably remember that it didn't take long for your muscles to turn to flab. Unless you exercise, your muscles think you don't care, and they go on strike.

The good news is that when you start to exercise, it takes only about three weeks to see a noticeable increase in strength, muscle bulk, and stamina. A moderate exercise program involves spending 30 minutes a day or an hour four times a week walking, swimming, running, or jumping.

Focusing on psychological fitness

There is no question that having IBS is stressful. If we can't convince you to exercise for any other reason, you should make exercise an important part of your overall wellness program in order to reduce stress. A brisk walk with a positive attitude lifts your endorphins and your mood. A morning walk can improve your mental concentration and creativity and make work easier.

Any type of exercise can reduce anxiety and depression. The calming, meditative postures of yoga, where you take deep refreshing breaths and become centered and grounded, are a balm to what ails us. In some studies, exercise outshines psychotherapy and antidepressive medication in its ability to relieve mild to moderate depression.

Another psychological benefit to exercise is its ability to eliminate insomnia and sleep disturbance. However, it's best to not do heavy exercise at night — save some yoga postures for your bedtime routine.

Relieving pain

People with IBS have three common symptoms — constipation, diarrhea, and pain. The Mayo Clinic says that people with the following conditions, which are characterized by chronic pain, can benefit from regular exercise:

✔ Arthritis

✔ Back pain

✔ Endometriosis

✔ Fibromyalgia

✔ IBS

A common misconception is that exercise increases pain, and when you have pain you should stop all physical activity. Researchers at the Mayo Clinic say the exact opposite is true. Lack of movement leads to deconditioning. (The old "Use it or lose it" adage comes to mind.) Deconditioning, in turn, can lead to even more pain. Being inactive leads to lost muscle tone and strength and less efficient heart action. What can follow are high blood pressure, high cholesterol, and diabetes. Your sleep suffers, and you are subject to more fatigue, stress, and anxiety. Just reading about this decline is tiring!

Exercise releases chemicals called endorphins that block pain signals from reaching your brain. The Mayo Clinic doctors tell us that endorphins are the body's natural pain-relieving chemicals that in many cases are more powerful than morphine! It's pretty difficult to get morphine, yet you have a ready-made supply of endorphins just waiting to be released. We encourage you to do the exercise rather than find a dealer!

Taking the First Steps

IBS is a complex condition. As we discuss in Chapter 10, the type of diet you should follow depends in part on the type of IBS you have. The same is true with exercise, but mostly in the location you choose. People with IBS-diarrhea should be sure to start their exercise programs close to home. People with IBS-constipation, on the other hand, can go on that long-distance run with impunity.

Checking your attitude

The first step in starting an exercise program is getting the right attitude. We live in an instant gratification society, and exercise does not always give us immediate results. In some cases, it can actually make us feel a little bit worse when we first start an exercise program. Plus, exercise takes time away from living our lives.

You can easily reframe exercise as a mini-vacation from your work and daily chores. And you can remind yourself that a bit of muscle ache is, in this case, a good thing.

Getting motivated

Maybe you've never been a regular exerciser. Or maybe you exercised regularly in the past but have experienced some major stress, time constraints, or physical pain that led you to stop exercising, and you're having trouble getting back on track.

The more you exercise, the more the benefits build. But only your will power and effort can get you off the starting block. We want our exercise program to give you the incentive to begin your exercise adventure. Here's how to make it work for you:

- **Check with your doctor to make sure there are no reasons that you shouldn't start an exercise program.** Most doctors say that only people with heart pain should limit their exercise. But it's best to be on the safe side and get your doctor's okay regardless.

- **Identify your major symptom(s) and focus on the exercises for that symptom(s).** In this chapter, we specify exercises for IBS-constipation, IBS-diarrhea, and pain.

- **Set a long-range goal.** For example, give yourself six months to reach a goal of exercising for 30 minutes each day.

- **Set a short-range goal.** A short-range goal can be to simply do 5 minutes of exercise today. Take one day at a time.

- **Take baby steps when you start your exercise program.** Overdoing it at the beginning can set you up for defeat.

- **Vary your activities.** Do aerobics, strength training, and stretching. Walk one day, and do yoga the next.

- **Exercise with friends or take your dog on a walk.** Company, even of the canine variety, can help you stay engaged and pass the time more quickly.

- **Develop a traveling exercise plan.** Take a DVD of your favorite exercises when you go on the road.

- **Keep an exercise diary.** Tracking your progress can be very helpful. Unless you write it down, in three months, you won't remember that you couldn't even exercise for 5 minutes when you began. (After all, now you're doing 45 minutes with no problem!)

- **Pat yourself on the back.**

Researchers found that a group of people who suffered from symptoms of IBS experienced a significant decrease in constipation, abdominal pain, and gas after they began a running program. If nothing else motivates you, focus on getting rid of those symptoms!

Loosening Up Your Lymph System

A properly working lymph system is essential for overcoming IBS and a key factor when considering what type of exercise to do. In Chapter 3, we mention the importance of the lymph. We explain that it's the body's main mechanism for clearing waste products from all its cells. In this section, we describe how important it is to move lymph and how exercise makes that happen.

Lymph vessels (which are separate from blood vessels) travel through every square inch of the body. The lymph system pulls toxins and debris into its channels and eventually dumps them into the bloodstream at an area near the neck called the *thoracic duct*. After the toxins reach the blood, they are filtered by the spleen. Figure 11-1 gives you some idea of the complexity of the lymph system.

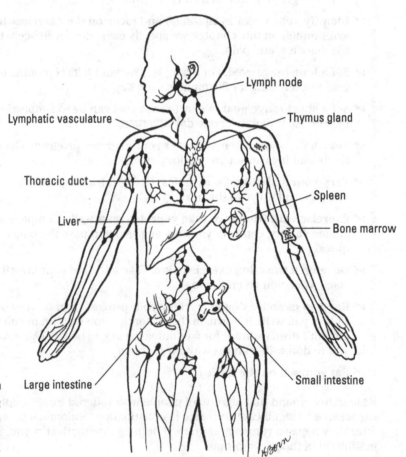

Lymph node

Thymus gland

Lymphatic vasculature

Thoracic duct

Spleen

Liver

Bone marrow

Large intestine

Small intestine

Figure 11-1:
The
lymphatic
system.

Pumping the gunk with muscles

The lymph system depends entirely on exercise to get its work done. Who knew?! Muscles are the pump that makes lymph fluid move. Muscles squeeze the lymph vessels and push lymph fluid from every part of the body to one dumping area and then into the bloodstream.

In Chapter 4, we talk about the many triggers for IBS that can produce yeast, bacteria, and food toxins in the gut. The lymph system works to remove those toxins every minute of every day. And exercise makes the lymph move and helps clear up symptoms of IBS.

If you do not exercise, the lymph system can get sluggish and cause swelling in your body. Swollen ankles, cellulite, and inflammation are the result. Just think of the last time you took a long flight and didn't move for hours. Chances are that your feet became a bit swollen because they weren't moving the lymph fluid. But when you exercise, you move all the toxins and debris from your cells and keep fluid where it belongs — either in the cells or in the bloodstream, not pooling around your ankles.

Any and all exercise is important for general health, and you can pick up any book on health and learn the basics. However, we want to first focus on lymph exercises, which you may not have heard too much about.

Bouncing your lymph system

Bouncing on a trampoline is a vigorous sport. Soaring high in the air, twirling, and diving on a flexible canvas is something that we associate with the circus. But mini-trampolines called *rebounders* have been used for decades for exercise. They provide the same benefits of regular exercise but with the extra enhancement of massaging the lymph circulation.

Research on rebounding is rife with stories about the benefits to the lymphatic system. People who advocate rebounding talk about the acceleration, deceleration, and forces of gravity that pull gently on the body as you glide up and down on your rebounder. This type of exercise acts like a mini external massage and gives your lymphatic circulation enough of a squeeze to make toxins move.

Rebounders can be your best friend if you are housebound with IBS. And, by following a rebounding exercise program and our diet and supplement suggestions in Chapters 9 and 10, you could soon be doing your exercise at the local gym without worrying about your symptoms.

Rebounding for IBS-diarrhea

Simply walking on the trampoline is enough to gently massage your lymph system and increase your circulation. Moving toxins out of the gut and into the lymph system, and pushing gas out of trapped pockets, can help alleviate symptoms of gas and bloating associated with IBS-diarrhea. Some of these benefits can be obtained with a good brisk walk, but they are enhanced with rebounding.

You can improve your workout by raising your knees in an exaggerated fashion, as if you were marching. This action massages the area of the groin, where there is an abundance of lymph tissue.

Rebounding for IBS-constipation

To move constipation along, you need a more vigorous workout. Jumping on the spot, skipping, and dancing are all possible on the mini-trampoline. Just put on your favorite music and bounce. Begin with a few minutes a day, and work up to 20 minutes four or five times a day.

Rebounding for pain

You don't necessarily want to do this type of exercise in the midst of pain. We recommend other exercises for times of acute pain, such as specific yoga postures. However, regular jumping and dancing on the rebounder can not only give you a lymph massage but also increase the level of pain-relieving endorphins coursing through your blood and, therefore, decrease your pain.

T-Tapping your lymph

Teresa Tapp is a physical trainer and exercise physiologist who has designed a unique form of exercise. For the past 20 years, Teresa has been researching her program and providing scientific support for its many benefits, including its effects on the lymph system. The best part of the program is that you can do it by following detailed instructions on a video or DVD in the privacy and comfort of your home (see www.t-tapp.com). The exercises are very simple and can be learned in a few minutes. The exercises provide four types of workouts all in one: aerobic, strength training, stretching, and lymph movement.

Teresa created the T-Tapp system to rebuild primary body functions, such as

- **Assimilation:** Enhancing digestion
- **Digestion:** Breaking down food thoroughly into its nutrient components
- **Elimination:** Balancing bowel function so it's neither too fast or too slow
- **Lymphatic flow:** Increasing the removal of waste
- **Neurokinetic flow:** Enhancing the nerve-to-muscle communication

She has also proven that the special sequence of her T-Tapp movements also stimulates the release of the following substances involved in a properly working gastrointestinal tract:

- ✔ Biochemical factors
- ✔ Hormones
- ✔ Neurotransmitters

One exercise that Teresa is graciously allowing us to share with you is Hoe Downs. This exercise moves lymph in the groin area — an area extremely rich in lymphatic tissue that we rarely target for exercise. If we did exercise the groin more, we would cut the incidence of IBS and hip arthritis.

Hoe Downs don't look that pretty, but they sure do the job. And they can also lower stress levels. Teresa worked for many years as a trainer for runway models, and she says that many of the top models still do their Hoe Downs before they step out before the cameras. Hoe Downs can be done anywhere.

Here are the steps to take:

1. **Hold your arms straight out to the side, then bend them at the elbows.**

2. **Tap your right toes to the floor on the right side with your knee pointed to the right.** At a fast pace, lift your knee four times as you tap your foot and swing your right arm across your chest and leave it there for the count.

3. **With your knee pointed forward, raise and lower it four times and swing your arm back out to the side, leaving it there for the count.**

4. **Repeat the exercise on the left side.** Then do the sequence on both sides all over again.

This exercise may be difficult for you to visualize, so Teresa invites you to go to her Web site, www.T-Tapp.com, and click on a free video that demonstrates Hoe Downs.

Jocelyn had IBS with constipation for years and was nearing the end of her tolerance of constantly feeling terrible. She was also feeling depressed much of the time and was not motivated to do any exercise. Her friend Kay came to visit, bringing a DVD of the basic T-Tapp program to share with Jocelyn. Kay had been doing the workout for just three weeks and was already feeling a change in her body. She offered to lend the DVD to Jocelyn for a week to try it out. Jocelyn followed the instructional video and started doing the basic workout. Within four days, she had a fantastic bowel movement and began feeling like the toxins were finally leaving her body. She ordered the DVDs for herself.

Loving Yoga

Yoga is one of the best forms of exercise for IBS. However, to say yoga is just an exercise does it an injustice. It is a practice that incorporates yoga postures and meditation to help a person come to a more peaceful state. Now that sounds like something that would benefit all of us!

We spoke with Delia Quigley, a yoga instructor, yoga teacher trainer, and author of *Empowering Your Life with Meditation* (Penguin Group), about the benefits of yoga for IBS. Delia said that postures that compress the abdomen and postures that stretch the abdomen are the ones that work best. Think of it this way — when a baby has colic or abdominal cramps, she curls her legs up and goes into the fetal position, probably to press out the gas and try to release the tension. It's the same with adult tummy pain. Actually, Delia told us that one of the main IBS tummy tamers, which we present here, is called Happy Baby!

In the following sections, we present several yoga postures for IBS and describe how to do them.

Happy Baby

Figure 11-2 shows how to do the Happy Baby posture, which has the following steps:

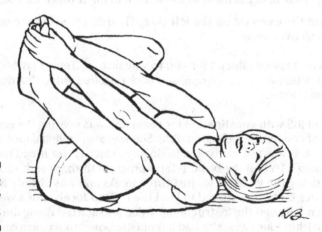

Figure 11-2:
Happy
Baby.

1. Lie on your back on a mat.

2. Put your feet in the air.

3. Bend your knees and grab your big toes with your fingers.

4. Pull your knees into your abdomen.

5. From that position, rock back and forth or side to side.

Ankles crossed, knees to chest

Figure 11-3 shows a posture in which you cross your ankles and pull your knees to the chest. Here are the steps:

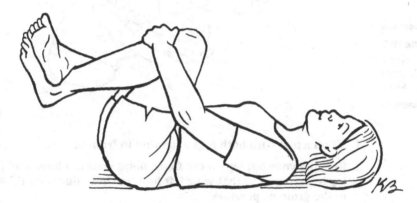

Figure 11-3:
Ankles crossed, knees to chest.

1. Lie on your back on a mat.

2. Pull your knees into your chest.

3. Cross your ankles

4. Wrap your arms around your knees and take deep breaths as you compress your abdomen.

One-legged forward bend

Figure 11-4 shows a great forward stretch that can ease pressure in your abdomen. Here's how to do it:

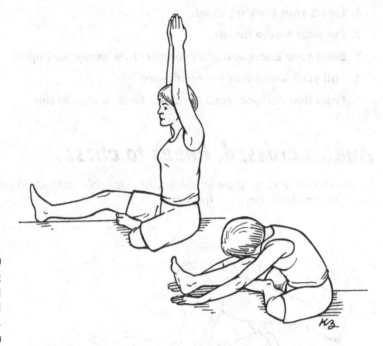

Figure 11-4:
One-legged
forward
bend.

1. Sit on a mat with both legs extended in front of you.

2. Keeping your left leg on the floor, bend your left knee and pull your leg toward you so that your left foot touches your right thigh as close to the groin as possible.

3. Bend forward in that position over your right leg.

4. Take deep breaths as you bend further and both stretch and compress your abdomen.

5. Repeat the sequence on the other side.

Supine twist

Figure 11-5 shows a great stretch that can help ease tension in your abdomen and relieve gas.

1. Lie on your back on a mat.

2. Cross your left leg over your right leg and rest it on the mat to the right of your body, so that you are lying on your hip.

3. Look to your left side and twist your upper body to the left.

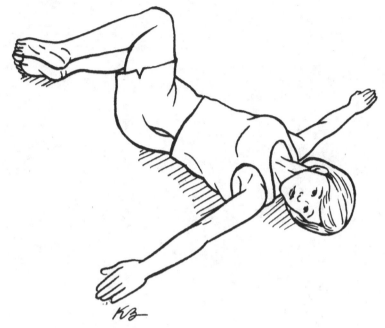

Figure 11-5:
Supine
twist.

4. **Take deep breaths as you stretch your abdomen.**

5. **Repeat the sequence on the other side.**

Exercising Choices

While we think rebounding, T-Tapp, and yoga provide the aerobic, strength training, and stretching exercise you need for IBS, there are many other exercise choices available to you. Whatever activity you decide to try, whether bicycling, jumping rope, swimming, or shoveling snow, you're bound to see benefits to your overall health.

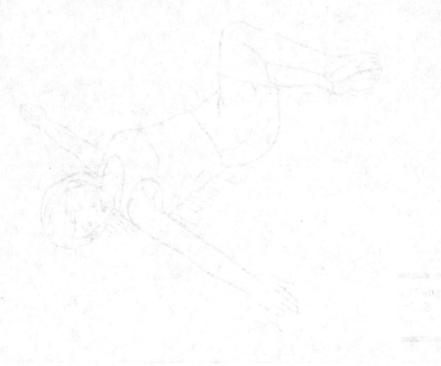

Chapter 12

Treating Stress and Symptoms with Caring Therapies

In This Chapter

▶ Achieving balance with acupuncture

▶ Tapping away symptoms with EFT

▶ Benefiting from the relaxation response

▶ Reducing stress and pain in other ways

*T*hroughout this book, we discuss the fact that stress and IBS have an intimate connection. As we say in Chapter 2, stress does not *cause* IBS. However, stress can trigger IBS episodes, and IBS episodes can increase your stress level. The cycle is a dangerous one, and we want to show you how you can break it.

You may have heard about some of the stress-reducing and pain-reducing therapies we discuss in this chapter, but maybe you don't know whether to try them. And maybe we're going to introduce you to some therapies whose names are completely unfamiliar. We hope you'll keep an open mind and consider how each therapy could become part of your routine as you piece together a treatment plan for reducing your IBS symptoms.

Some of the therapies we discuss in this chapter, like the Emotional Freedom Techniques, meditation, and deep breathing, are types of self-care that you can do either on your own or with a trained practitioner. Others — acupuncture, massage, and hypnotherapy — are administered by a qualified therapist. Each holds the potential to help you better alleviate stress so you can give both your body and your mind a break.

Pinning Down IBS with Acupuncture

Acupuncture has been in use for about 5,000 years. Most people are aware that acupuncture began in China, but you may not know that it wasn't until

1994 that acupuncture needles were reclassified by the U.S. Food and Drug Administration from an experimental device to a standard medical device to be used by a qualified practitioner.

In the West, we tend to think of acupuncture as a stand-alone therapy. In China, however, it is part of a larger system of healthcare called *Oriental medicine,* which includes diet therapy, herbal medicine, medical massage (Tui Na), exercise (Tai Chi and Qi Gong), and moxabustion (which we describe in the next section). A Chinese medicine practitioner in the West is usually trained in acupuncture, moxabustion, and herbal medicine. Medical doctors may take acupuncture courses but are usually not trained in moxabustion or herbal medicine.

An effective Chinese medicine practitioner is one who is skilled at reading your pulses. By holding your wrist and putting several fingers along the pulse, a good practitioner can read all the nuances of your body; identify where the imbalance lies; and use acupuncture needles, moxabustion, and herbal medicine to correct that imbalance.

Using heat to heal

Moxabustion involves burning a small cone of the herb Artemesia vulgarus near an acupuncture point. In the past, cones of herbs were placed on acupuncture points, and the herbs were ignited. When they burned near the skin, they were immediately swept off. These days, large sticks of pressed herbs are lit, held near the skin, and moved away if the skin becomes too hot. Moxabustion is especially suited to treating the pain of IBS because the warmth seems to relax intestinal spasms by activating certain acupuncture points.

Heat from a hot water bottle or heating pad can also be an effective way to turn off pain. Some people curl up with a hot water bottle wrapped in a soft towel tucked into the abdomen. The pressure from the bottle and the heat combine to do the trick.

Stimulating acupuncture points

Acupuncture treatment involves puncturing the skin with extremely thin needles that go into the underlying tissues at specific points. These acupuncture points can be found by practitioners with very sensitive fingers, as well as by using electrical measuring devices. The points lie along lines called *meridians,* which carry a stream of life force called *Qi* (pronounced "chi"). There are 14 principal meridians and 361 basic acupuncture points represented on the surface of the body. Each meridian originates from or flows to a particular organ.

Sir William Osler, the founder of the practice of internal medicine, commented on the use of acupuncture for back pain in his *Principles and Practice of Medicine* in 1892. However, very little acupuncture was performed in the United States apart from Chinese immigrant communities until 1970, when the United States recognized The People's Republic of China. The media was dazzled by the use of acupuncture anesthesia for a journalist's appendectomy, and this story immediately catapulted acupuncture into the spotlight.

Achieving balance

Acupuncture, like herbal treatment, is very individualized. However, in IBS, what the practitioner is looking for is an imbalance in various meridians, mainly the stomach, large intestine, spleen, kidney, and liver. These meridians can be overactive or underactive, suffering from dampness, heat, or stagnation. Inserting needles at the appropriate acupuncture points can help promote the flow of Qi and regain balance in the meridians.

Chinese medicine is a fascinating subject and looks at the totality of the individual condition. In China, traditionally practitioners had to focus on curing their patients because they would be paid only when their patients were well; if a patient continued to be ill, the practitioner received no pay. (That would certainly throw a monkey wrench in our present healthcare system, where doctors get paid only when you are sick!)

Finding a practitioner

The American Association of Oriental Medicine (AAOM) is the oldest organization representing individual practitioners of acupuncture and Oriental Medicine in the United States. The phone number for patient referrals is 1-888-500-7999, or you can visit www.aaom.org/aboutaaom.html.

The American Academy of Medicine Acupuncture (AAMA) was founded in 1987 and is the only national professional society of North American physicians who have incorporated acupuncture into their medical practices. The phone number for patient referrals is 1-800-521-2262, or you can visit www.medicalacupuncture.org. The AAMA often handles more than 1,000 referral requests a month.

Emotional Freedom Techniques (EFT)

In this section, we continue the discussion of meridians and acupuncture points. EFT is a form of emotional acupuncture that doesn't use needles. EFT is part of a new class of treatment in the field of energy psychology. It was founded by Gary Craig, a Stanford engineer who based his work on Einstein's statement that all things (including our bodies) are made of energy. By tapping with your fingers on specific acupuncture points on the body's energy meridians, you can release blocks in your energy system that may be contributing to symptoms of IBS.

We talk a lot in this book about the fact that researchers haven't yet pinpointed a specific cause of IBS. But according to Craig, the cause of any physical illness is one of two things: a disruption in the body's energy system, or unresolved emotional trauma. Therefore, EFT helps resolve emotional issues and disruptions in the body's energy system.

In this section, we provide a shortened version of EFT. We encourage you to visit the Emotional Freedom Techniques Web site (www.emofree.com), where Craig has made the EFT Training Manual available as a free download. By reading the manual, you can increase your efficiency with EFT and improve your success with relieving your IBS symptoms. The description we provide here gives you great information to help relieve your IBS symptoms, but it is not meant to be a substitute for learning the technique from the EFT Training Manual, training videos, or a qualified instructor.

Blocking energy

Many people suffering with IBS have been told that it is all in their heads, caused by some kind of mental issue. We emphasize throughout this book that IBS is real; it is not in your head. However, we also acknowledge that stress, including extreme stress or trauma, can trigger IBS symptoms (see Chapter 4).

EFT explores the possibility that stressful, traumatic events or negative thoughts create disruptions or blocks in the body's energy system. These energy blocks, in turn, cause physical symptoms, including those of IBS.

EFT was designed to be accessible to everybody. To do EFT, you specify the problem that is causing you discomfort, you rate your level of discomfort, and then you tap on specific acupuncture points while tuning into your problem.

Performing EFT

There are three parts to EFT: the setup, the tapping sequence, and checking in. We discuss each in the following sections.

The setup

Choose the problem that you want to work on. The problem may be general like *I have IBS* or more specific like *I'm afraid of having an accident.* Then rate how much intensity or discomfort this problem is causing you right now. Use a scale of 0 (no discomfort) to 10 (very intense discomfort). It may help to make a note in your journal of the problem you are working on and its intensity.

Insert your identified problem into this affirmation statement:

> *Even though I have this **insert problem**, I deeply and completely accept myself.*

The affirmation statement is the same for any problem that you choose to work on. You just insert your problem in the blank space.

While continuously tapping with two or three fingers on the Karate Chop (KC) point on the fleshy part on the side of either hand (see Figure 12-1), repeat your affirmation statement three times, preferably out loud.

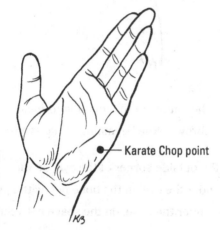

— Karate Chop point

Figure 12-1:
The Karate
Chop point.

When you have repeated the affirmation statement three times, continue to tune into the problem by repeating a reminder phrase that briefly describes your problem. We offer examples of reminder phrases in the tables later in this section.

The tapping sequence

Following is a description of the EFT tapping points as they progress down either side of the body. Each point is illustrated in Figure 12-2:

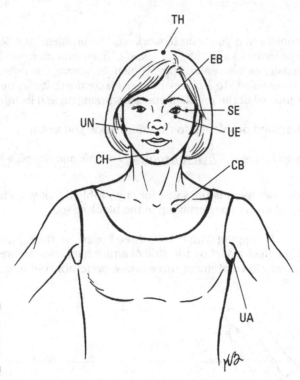

Figure 12-2:
EFT tapping
points.

- TH = Top of the Head — the middle of the top of your head
- EB = Beginning of the Eyebrow — the beginning of the eyebrow near your nose
- SE = Side of the Eye — the outside corner of the eye, on the bone
- UE = Under the Eye — under the eye on the bone below the pupil
- UN = Under the Nose — under the nose, on the space between the nose and top lip
- CH = Chin — halfway between your bottom lip and the tip of your chin
- CB = Collarbone — from the U-shaped notch, down 1 inch and to the right or left
- UA = Under the Arm — about 4 inches below the armpit

While tapping these acupuncture points six or seven times each, repeat a reminder phrase that keeps you tuned into the problem you are working on. Tapping on these points corrects the energy imbalance in your meridian system that is associated with the problem you're tuning into.

Checking in

After a round of tapping, check back in to the problem you are working on and rate the level of intensity that you are feeling after one round of tapping. Use the same scale of 0 (no discomfort) to 10 (very intense discomfort).

Perhaps your intensity has gone from an 8 to a 3 with your first round of tapping. If you still feel discomfort, you can repeat the setup and tapping sequence, but revise your affirmation statement to reflect that you are still working on the same problem. For example, you may say

> *Even though I still have some of **this problem**, I deeply and completely accept myself.*

Your reminder phrase would be *this remaining problem*.

Continue tapping on the same problem that you started with, rating your level of intensity with each round of tapping until you feel like you have dissolved the problem.

Christine Wheeler, one of the authors of this book, is also an EFT practitioner. She has successfully used EFT to treat her own IBS symptoms, *(Even though dad had IBS and I probably "caught it" from him, I deeply and completely accept myself)* and worked with hundreds of clients, helping them to alleviate emotional traumas and symptoms associated with physical illnesses like IBS and allergies, as well as terminal diseases. For more tips on using EFT for IBS, visit her Web site at www.christinewheeler.com.

Identifying IBS problems to work on

Because IBS is a condition with as many symptoms as there are sufferers, it is important to practice making your EFT affirmation statements unique to your own situation. We have put together tables to help you identify problems and develop affirmation statements and reminder phrases.

Dr. Carol Look is an expert EFT practitioner and trainer and a contributing editor to Gary Craig's EFT Web site support list. We thank Carol for her contribution to these tables. We invite you to use the phrases that mean the most to you or invent your own. Notice that sometimes there are many ways to approach the same problem.

In Table 12-1, we present statements and phrases related to IBS-diarrhea symptoms.

Table 12-1	EFT for Diarrhea	
The Problem	*The Setup Phrase*	*The Reminder Phrase*
Unable to control bowels	Even though I can't control my bowels, I deeply and completely accept myself.	Can't control bowels
Can't hold any longer	Even though I can't hold any longer, I deeply and completely accept myself.	Can't hold on
Everything goes right through me	Even though everything goes right through me, I deeply and completely accept myself.	Everything goes right through me
Diarrhea reminds me of having a bad flu when I was a kid	Even though I remember the diarrhea I had as a kid, I deeply and completely accept myself.	Had diarrhea as a kid

In 1992, Ingrid learned EFT with Gary Craig after suffering from IBS with constipation all of her adult life. She would take a laxative every night to ensure that she had some kind of bowel movement in the morning, but without the laxative, nothing happened. Ingrid's day-to-day abdominal discomfort was rated at an average of 7 before she started doing EFT. She did tapping 8 to 11 times every day for about three weeks, and she excitedly reported that she had a bowel movement in the middle of the afternoon for the first time in years! Ingrid said, "It's heaven . . . I wish that everybody was constipated so that they could tap and realize that this stuff (EFT) works." We talked to Ingrid in 2005, and she indicated that she had always carried her stress in her gut. Despite going through very stressful times since learning EFT, she has never developed IBS symptoms again.

In Table 12-2, we list affirmation statements and reminder phrases related to IBS-constipation.

Table 12-2	EFT for Constipation	
The Problem	*The Setup Phrase*	*The Reminder Phrase*
Can't have a bowel movement	Even though my body refuses to let go, I deeply and completely accept myself.	Body refuses to let go
Can't have a bowel movement	Even though I need to be in control, I deeply and completely accept myself.	Need to be in control

The Problem	The Setup Phrase	The Reminder Phrase
Can't have a bowel movement	Even though it's not safe to let go, I deeply and completely accept myself.	It's not safe to let go
Can't have a bowel movement	Even though I am full of it, I deeply and completely accept myself.	I'm full of it

Table 12-3 shows statements and reminder phrases to consider if you suffer from abdominal pain and cramping.

Table 12-3	EFT for Abdominal Pain and Cramping	
The Problem	**The Setup Phrase**	**The Reminder Phrase**
Unbearable pain	Even though this pain is unbearable, I deeply and completely accept myself.	Unbearable pain
Pain is affecting my life	Even though this pain is cramping my style, I deeply and completely accept myself.	Cramping my style
Pain is frightening	Even though this pain is scary, I deeply and completely accept myself.	Pain is scary
Can't have a bowel movement	Even though I can't let go of this stuff in my bowels, I deeply and completely accept myself	It's not safe to let go

While some people enjoy almost immediate relief by using EFT, a key to success with EFT is persistence. After you get used to the EFT protocol, it is easy to practice this technique almost anywhere. We encourage you to tap on your symptoms several times a day if you want to achieve the best results.

If you are using a particular setup phrase and your symptoms aren't changing, alter your phrasing and keep tapping. For example, you may be tapping on *this gas pain,* but try being more specific like *this horrible gas pain that feels like it's going to explode inside me.* Table 12-4 offers other suggestions for phrases to use if gas and bloating are your issues.

Table 12-4	EFT for Gas and Bloating	
The Problem	*The Setup Phrase*	*The Reminder Phrase*
Full of gas	Even though I am full of hot air, I deeply and completely accept myself.	Full of hot air
Embarrassed about gas	Even though the noise and smell of gas is embarrassing, I deeply and completely accept myself.	Gas is embarrassing
Stomach is swollen	Even though I am too big to wear my clothes because of my bloating, I deeply and completely accept myself.	My clothes don't fit
Stomach is swollen	Even though I am full of something that is hurting me, I deeply and completely accept myself.	Full of something painful

For many people with IBS, symptoms change from day to day. Some days are defined by diarrhea, and others are plagued by constipation. Table 12-5 offers EFT phrases if this describes your situation.

Table 12-5	EFT for Alternating Diarrhea and Constipation	
The Problem	*The Setup Phrase*	*The Reminder Phrase*
Alternating diarrhea and constipation	Even though my body can't decide what to do, I deeply and completely accept myself.	My body is confused
Alternating diarrhea and constipation	Even though my IBS symptoms remind me of my confusing life, I deeply and completely accept myself.	IBS reminds me of my life
Can't find any relief	Even though I get no relief no matter what, I deeply and completely accept myself.	I get no relief from this

Finding an EFT practitioner

EFT was developed to be accessible to lay people as well as professionals, so you can use it on your own. However, some people prefer to have the support and expertise of an experienced EFT practitioner, at least at the beginning. EFT can even be demonstrated by telephone.

Gary Craig's Web site, www.emofree.com, provides a place for practitioners from all over the world to list their services. The practitioners listed are not endorsed by Craig.

Meditating for IBS

Meditation conjures up images of people sitting in impossibly contorted positions for interminable lengths of time. You can certainly do that — don't let us stop you — but there are many ways to relax that don't turn you into a pretzel.

One of the best-known ways of achieving a relaxed state was described in 1975 by Dr. Herbert Benson, a professor at Harvard Medical School. This physiological state of relaxation is called the *relaxation response,* and it is also the title of a book Dr. Benson wrote, which was written in 1975 and updated in 2000. This book and another nine that he has written about the relaxation response have sold over 4 million copies. Dr. Benson also founded the Mind/Body Medical Institute, a behavioral medicine research and treatment center in Boston.

Eliciting the relaxation response

Dr. Benson tells us that inducing the relaxation response is not difficult. There are only two essential steps:

- ✔ Repetition of a word, sound, phrase, prayer, or muscular activity
- ✔ Passive disregard of everyday thoughts that inevitably come to mind and the return to your repetition

The relaxation response can also be initiated with the use of imagery, progressive muscle relaxation, meditation, repetitive physical exercises, and breath focus.

The Mind/Body Medical Institute teaches the following process and was kind enough to allow us to reprint the method for you:

- ✔ Pick a focus word, short phrase, or prayer that is firmly rooted in your belief system, such as "one," "peace," "The Lord is my shepherd," "Hail Mary full of grace," or "shalom."

- ✔ Sit quietly in a comfortable position.

- ✔ Close your eyes.

- ✔ Relax your muscles, progressing from your feet to your calves, thighs, abdomen, shoulders, head, and neck.

- ✔ Breathe slowly and naturally, and as you do, say your focus word, sound, phrase, or prayer silently to yourself as you exhale.

- ✔ Assume a passive attitude. Don't worry about how well you're doing. When other thoughts come to mind, simply say to yourself, "Oh well," and gently return to your repetition.

- ✔ Continue for 10 to 20 minutes.

- ✔ Do not stand immediately. Continue sitting quietly for a minute or so, allowing other thoughts to return. Then open your eyes and sit for another minute before rising.

- ✔ Practice the technique once or twice daily. Good times to do so are before breakfast and before dinner.

Relaxing away IBS

The relaxation response was used in a 2001 study on IBS at the State University of New York (SUNY). Adults with IBS were divided into two groups. One was assigned to a six-week treatment program and asked to practice the relaxation response twice a day. The other group was asked to just monitor their symptoms. After the six-week period, participants using the relaxation response reported significant improvements in symptoms of diarrhea, belching, bloating, and flatulence.

Changing Your Behavior

Behavioral therapy encompasses a number of therapeutic modalities, such as relaxation therapy to reduce stress, biofeedback regulation of bowel habits, hypnotherapy aimed at controlling intestinal muscle contractions, cognitive therapy, and psychotherapy.

Behavioral approaches for treating IBS were analyzed by the American College of Gastroenterology Task Force that we mention in Chapter 8. The Task Force evaluated 16 studies involving behavioral therapies. Eleven studies showed that IBS symptoms were significantly improved in patients who received such treatments.

In the following sections, we introduce just a few behavioral therapies you may want to consider as you work to improve your IBS symptoms.

Believing in biofeedback

Biofeedback is a body-awareness technique that allows clients to learn how to feel difficult physiologic states in their muscles and nervous systems. For example, you can actually learn to become aware of your blood pressure changing. A change in blood pressure is experienced as a tone in the biofeedback machine, and you feel what is happening in your body when the tone is present.

Biofeedback is completely painless. You are hooked up to a monitor by a headband or a wristband, and you sit comfortably beside a computer with a video screen that displays body activity and/or you hear a tone related to body function. A trained therapist, who may be a doctor, nurse, or physical or occupational therapist, gives guidance on how to relax in order to change an abnormal response. It could be as simple as counting your breaths, breathing deeply, or repeating a word or phrase.

You can learn how to gain control over the function of your gastrointestinal tract through this method. In most cases, it's a matter of retraining your bowel to work normally. Biofeedback has proven useful in treating IBS, as well as tension and migraine headaches, teeth grinding, and muscle tension. After biofeedback training, you are able to relax your GI tract in stressful situations by remembering what you learned in your sessions.

Biofeedback has the advantages of being noninvasive, having no side effects, and putting you in control. The average number of treatments for IBS is six to eight held over a three-month period. Research on biofeedback for IBS at the National Institutes of Health shows about 75 to 80 percent reduction in symptoms of IBS.

Considering Transactional Analysis

Transactional Analysis (TA) is said to be one of the easiest therapies to understand in modern psychology. TA was originally developed by Eric Berne, who pointed out that we are all comprised of three separate personalities: the Parent, the Child, and the Adult.

Berne found that these three ego states describe how and why people behave the way they do. It appears that each ego state has its own distinct personality, body language, facial expressions, gestures, posture, and vocabulary that make it easy to identify if you know what to look for.

Dividing up your personality

We probably have a bit of all three ego states expressing themselves at any moment in time. Following is a short description of each state and how you are thrown off balance if you go too heavily into your Parent or Child state.

The Parent

This ego state is our ingrained voice of authority. It records all the conditioning, learning, and attitudes we absorb from parents and other adult authorities while we are growing up. These include all the *shoulds* and *musts* that rule our lives:

- Be nice.
- Don't interrupt.
- Don't upset anyone.
- Don't speak up.

Our own personal tape recorder stores millions of such messages. According to TA therapists, virtually all internal stress is Parent-related.

When it comes to IBS, the Parent messages can burn your ears!

- It's disgusting to fart in public.
- What the heck are you doing in the bathroom so much?
- There's nothing wrong with you.
- Stop complaining.
- Don't mess up.
- If you can't hold it in, you're a wimp.
- I'm not stopping the car for anything.

The Child

This ego state expresses the sensations and feelings that we have related to external events and people.

Jut Meininger, who wrote *Success Through Transactional Analysis* (Signet), has separated Berne's Child ego state into two components: the *Adapted Child* and the *Natural Child*. Fear, anger, despair, and moodiness are emotions associated with our Adapted Child. The Natural Child is spontaneous, intuitive, and creative.

The Adapted Child is the storage place for feelings we were conditioned to feel when we were very young, as well as early behavior we engaged in when we adapted to living with our mothers and fathers. Our Natural Child expresses the unfettered feelings and behavior we were born with.

Meininger explains that you can pair off the Adapted Child with the Parent, because they develop simultaneously when we're young and usually operate in tandem. You can pair the Natural Child with the Adult, because they often operate in tandem.

The Adult

Our Adult ego state is where we take in data and decide the best way to react to that information. Berne found that, surprisingly enough, our Adult begins to form at the tender age of 10 months (or even sooner). Its function is to process and compare data. Things usually work best for us if our Natural Child is able to use our Adult to gather enough data to enable our Natural Child to get what it wants.

Minding the body connection

The mind–body connection is very important in IBS. Jut Meininger told us that we all store our negative Adapted Child feelings somewhere in our organs. That's where reprimands from parents and teachers, taunts from other kids, and abuse coming from any direction are tucked away.

Meininger referred us to Louise Hay's work in *Heal Your Body* (Hay House). Hay says that people who are taught as children to be unforgiving and not give up their pasts are inclined to be constipated. The Parent message is, "Don't screw up or make a mistake because you won't be forgiven." This puts a person in a constant state of tension and fear. This tightening happens physically as well as psychologically, and the intestines just won't let go.

Hay also says that people who are afraid of rejection and learn that behavior as children are inclined to have diarrhea. The Parent messages that can induce fear of rejection are very wide-ranging. They may include

✔ Don't be yourself. Be the way I want you to be.

✔ Don't feel what you feel. Feel what I tell you to feel.

When we say that IBS makes people anxious or embarrassed and limits their social interaction, in TA language Meininger says that "things outside ourselves don't cause us to feel certain feelings." What actually happens is that "we cause ourselves to feel these feelings when we replay our own negative Adapted Child feeling tapes."

Thus, we cause ourselves to feel anxious or embarrassed by repeating various self-defeating Parent messages in our own heads. Some of those messages can be

✔ You look foolish.

✔ You're making a scene.

✔ You just farted.

If we learn to give up the Parent messages we keep repeating to ourselves over and over again in our heads, we can then give up the corresponding negative Adapted Child feelings that we associate with these messages. For example, stop telling yourself that you look foolish, and you will give up feeling embarrassed.

Practicing TA

Including *Success Through Transactional Analysis,* there are several good books on TA that can help you understand how your ego states may get in the way of your health. We list some for you in Chapter 21. TA, however, is way more effective if you have a few sessions with a TA practitioner.

The way TA sessions work is by creating a contract between the counselor and the client to solve here and now problems. The focus is on creating workable problem-solving behaviors and showing a client how her Parent and Child ego states may be interrupting her Adult.

Sometimes just knowing that it's your Adapted Child who is worried, embarrassed, and freaked out — not your Adult — is enough for you to get over a particular embarrassing time in your life.

We can't provide enough information in this book for you to do TA on your own, but we encourage you to go to the International Transactional Analysis Association's Web site at www.itaa-net.org. This association has members in 56 countries. You can check the Web site for more information on TA and to help you locate a practitioner in your area.

Hypnotizing the pain

People all over the world and from the beginning of time have achieved trancelike states in religious and healing rituals by means of rhythmic chanting, monotonous drum beats, and staring at fixed points. The term *hypnosis* was not coined until 1842, but snake charmers, yogis, and fakirs have induced trancelike states for centuries to perform astounding physical feats — tests of strength and the ability to conquer pain.

Even though hypnosis is one of the oldest remedies used to battle physical diseases and mental disorders, it is not widely practiced by allopathic doctors so it is not frequently mentioned in the treatment of IBS. However, one study showed that more than 70 percent of family doctors thought that *hypnotherapy* (the use of hypnosis in the treatment of illness) may have a role to play in the management of patients with IBS.

The American Medical Association officially recognized hypnotherapy as a medical modality in 1958. Hypnotherapy as a treatment for IBS has been validated by the international expert groups that produced the Rome II Diagnostic Criteria for IBS (see Chapter 2) and the British Society of Gastroenterology.

Directing the gut

Gut directed hypnotherapy (GDH) was developed specifically for IBS patients in 1984 by Dr. P.J. Whorwell at the University Hospital of South Manchester. It boasts a success rate of 80 percent for symptoms of abdominal pain, bloating, diarrhea, and/or constipation.

An effective GDH treatment program can vary from 6 to 12 sessions that take place every week. Here's what to expect: The first session focuses on taking your history and outlining the treatment plan. From then on, each session is recorded on tape, and the client listens to the tape every day until the next session.

In Chapter 21, we list two hypnotherapy resources to check out. Individual hypnotherapy practitioners may know about GDH and treating IBS; be sure to ask about it when you phone to make an appointment.

Reviewing the research

We found study after study that shows hypnosis — even self-hypnosis — is a scientifically proven tool used in modifying gastrointestinal functions, such as mucus production, intestinal movement, and intestinal sensitivity, and how the brain perceives GI symptoms.

Hypnosis acts on the physical level; it doesn't just erase your bowel from your mind. But it also functions on the psychological level, and suggestions can be given to help with symptoms of anxiety and tension.

Researchers sometimes do very strange things in the name of science. In one study, a balloon was blown up in the rectum of each IBS patient. (Okay, get the image of a big birthday balloon out of your mind — this was a tiny balloon.) Before hypnosis, this experiment produced very uncomfortable sensations, triggering IBS episodes of pain and rectal urgency. Under hypnosis, most patients were not affected by the balloon but experienced normal rectal sensations.

In the 1980s, several studies on IBS patients showed remarkable results using hypnotherapy. In one study, 40-minute sessions of hypnotherapy held on 4 different occasions were performed over 7 weeks on 33 patients. Twenty patients improved, and 11 of them had almost complete relief of their symptoms. The patients were followed for three months and did not relapse. The same investigators on that trial reported that hypnotherapy in small groups of eight patients is as effective as individual therapy.

The results of a comparison trial of hypnotherapy, psychotherapy, and placebo in a group of patients with severe IBS were very interesting. The group given psychotherapy showed a small but significant improvement in abdominal pain, abdominal distension, and general well-being but not in the number of times they went to the bathroom. The hypnotherapy patients showed a dramatic improvement in all aspects of the condition with no relapses in the three-month follow-up period.

In 2005, a review paper reported an accumulated 644 patients who took part in 14 published studies on hypnotherapy. The results showed that hypnosis consistently produces significant results and improves the defining symptoms of IBS in the majority of patients, as well as positively affecting quality of life, anxiety, and depression. In one study, patients who were followed for five years maintained their wellness.

Hypnotizing yourself

Studies show that hypnosis can reduce dependence on medication and decrease doctors' visits, which amounts to economic savings. But hypnosis administered by a professional obviously involves consultation costs. Self-hypnosis tapes are an affordable option you may want to consider.

One study compared a group of patients who received hypnotherapy and a group who listened to a hypnotherapy audiotape. The results were not surprising. There was an improvement in symptoms in the group that listened to the audiotape but more improvement in the ones who received a hypnotherapy session. The researchers concluded that the ease and economy of the audiotape makes it a useful treatment option, and people who do not improve sufficiently with the audiotape could then opt for hypnotherapy.

Finding a hypnotherapist

If someone is going to be giving your brain suggestions, you want to make sure that person knows what he's doing. Anyone can train to be a hypnotherapist, so you may want to consider going to someone who is also a trained psychologist or psychiatrist with a medical background — ideally, someone who knows about IBS.

We provide information about two hypnotherapy resources in Chapter 21. And remember, you are looking for someone to do therapy, not parlor tricks. You want someone who practices hypnotherapy and not just hypnosis.

Part IV
Living and Working with IBS

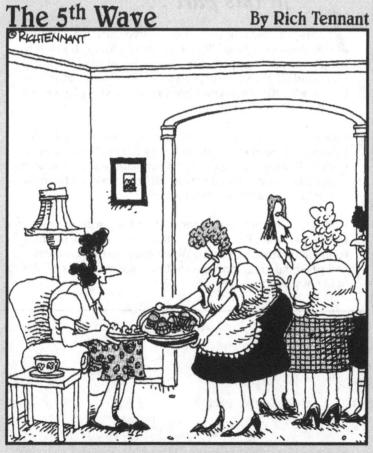

The 5th Wave   By Rich Tennant

"Oh, no thank you Bernice. My doctor's told me to avoid foods containing too much lactose, gluten, or hand grenades."

In this part . . .

In this part, we talk about how to live with this chronic condition every day. We recognize the frustration felt by people who are trapped in the house because of IBS symptoms, and we give you ways to cope. We also address how to deal with IBS when you have to go to a workplace every day despite your symptoms.

Children with IBS are a special concern; perhaps if we can lighten their load early on, they may not continue to experience IBS when they grow up. We explain how to deal with the emotional strain of a chronic illness, which is the most important factor for helping children.

Finally, to continue to deal most effectively with your IBS symptoms, you need to know what's on the horizon in terms of treatment options. We discuss current research and potential breakthroughs that may improve your quality of life in years to come.

Chapter 13

Getting Out of the House: Living with IBS

- -

- -

*H*eather Van Vorous, author of *The First Year: IBS* (Marlowe & Company), wrote that she had IBS for 20 years before she met anyone else who had the condition. When she realized that up to 20 percent of the population suffers from IBS symptoms, she understood that most people were in the closet. Since writing about IBS, Heather has been swamped with letters and e-mails from sufferers who confirm that they suffer in silence.

Living with IBS can be a real challenge. Learning how to manage the symptoms is a difficult task that we want to make much easier for you. We acknowledge that your spontaneity factor may be cut down several notches when you know that your symptoms can rear up at any time. (Boom! There goes the dinner party or trip to the zoo.) You have to be a quick change artist because your plans are always changing.

IBS is one of the most unpredictable medical conditions. You may wake up in the morning and greet the dawn with a smile, and within an hour you're in agony with abdominal cramps and an urgency to go to the bathroom. Or bloating can occur just because you go from a horizontal position in bed to a vertical position walking around your home.

We hope that with the information in Part III of this book about supplements, diet, exercise, and therapies, you will feel more confident about your ability to manage your condition and live a more normal life. However, we know that many people with IBS are afraid to stray far from a restroom, which decidedly curtails outside activities.

The intent of this chapter is to give you more tools and the extra boost of confidence that will get you out of the house.

Taking responsibility for your life is the first step to learning how to cope with your condition. When you lift your head up and look around at all the available options, you are empowered to improve your quality of life and cancel out any notion that you are a victim of your illness. It also means that you are not a passive patient but an active participant in your healthcare.

Taking Steps Toward Better Health

In other chapters, we discuss the following essential facets of taking responsibility of your illness:

- ✔ **Good nutrition:** As we discuss in detail in Chapter 10, diet is crucial for managing IBS. With most chronic illnesses, you just have to avoid foods contaminated with food additives, preservatives, pesticides, and herbicides. With IBS, you have to also pay attention to food allergy, food intolerance, and food sensitivity (see Chapters 4 and 17).

- ✔ **Exercise:** Mind, body, and spirit are all revved up when you get your blood circulating. Mood-elevating hormones are stimulated by exercise, your heart responds to regular activity, and exercise builds strong muscles, which help with weight loss. Plus, exercise boosts your confidence, helps abolish insomnia, and creates strong bones that help your posture. See Chapter 11 for how to start an exercise program.

- ✔ **Spirit:** Yoga, meditation, the relaxation response, and deep breathing are all necessary timeouts for our physical, mental, and emotional health. See Chapter 12 for information about all these techniques.

- ✔ **Research:** This may be the first book you have read on IBS, but it shouldn't be your only resource. In Chapter 16, we discuss how you can keep up-to-date on information about IBS, and in Chapter 21, we give you Web sites and books you can go to for more information.

In this chapter, we add to this list of ways to help your situation. But first, we want to acknowledge the impact that IBS may be having on you right now, so you realize you are not alone.

Surveying the Effects of IBS

In 2003, the International Foundation for Functional Gastrointestinal Disorders (IFFGD) commissioned a nationwide survey of IBS patients in the United States. The IFFGD found that many patients live with the condition for years in isolation, trapped in the house. And those people who try to find out what's wrong with them often see many doctors before being correctly diagnosed. The survey also found that its participants had tried an accumulated 300 different types of prescription and over-the-counter medications in searching for relief.

Here are some results of the survey that show the impact IBS can have:

- ✔ Nearly half of the survey participants reported suffering five or more years with symptoms before a diagnosis of IBS was made.

- ✔ Nearly 45 percent of participants reported severe symptoms, with another 40 percent having moderate pain.

- ✔ Participants described IBS symptoms as seriously impacting their daily lives; more than 25 percent said they missed work or school due to their condition.

- ✔ Of the survey participants, 71 percent reported two or more episodes of IBS per week, and nearly half reported daily events.

Counting the Costs

The frantic trips to the washroom that result from IBS can disrupt your home, work, and social life. The financial cost can be substantial, and the emotional cost includes a huge deficit in confidence that only adds to your burden.

Medscape's clinical update on the "Diagnosis, Pathophysiology, and Treatment of Irritable Bowel Syndrome" (www.medscape.com/viewprogram/2749) lists the following costs of IBS:

- ✔ **The direct costs of medical care:** This includes office visits, emergency room visits, procedures, testing, medications, and hospitalizations. An estimated 3.5 million doctors' visits are made every year for IBS, making up one quarter of a gastrointestinal specialist's practice. (But keep in mind that only 10 to 25 percent of people with IBS symptoms seek medical care. And other sources say that up to 50 percent of people who make appointments with a GI specialist have symptoms of IBS.)

  Some bean counters have tallied that people with IBS have medical expenses that are more than 30 percent higher than those of people without IBS.

- ✔ **Indirect costs to society from lost productivity:** These costs result from absence from school, work, and other activities. The 75 to 90 percent of people with IBS symptoms who *don't* go to doctors often stay home from work when symptoms flare, or they can't produce at full capacity even if they make it to work.

> ✔ Intangible costs reflecting human suffering
>
> ✔ Intangible costs suffered by your family and social circle

As we mention in Chapter 5, several conditions are associated with IBS. Women with IBS seem to be more susceptible to chronic pelvic pain, painful intercourse, bladder symptoms, and migraine headaches. Therefore, more than bowel symptoms are driving the financial, emotional, and social costs of IBS.

Financing IBS

The annual office visit bill for patients with IBS is in excess of $8 billion. When you add to the doctors' visits the outpatient, inpatient, and diagnostic testing, the estimated total costs in the United States for IBS medical care are around $30 billion per year. (We're told that figure excludes prescription and nonprescription drugs.)

Obviously, absence from work and school adds to the costs of having IBS. And another price tag to consider is the amount of money people spend on changing their diets, taking supplements, and seeking noninsured services for IBS therapies, such as those we talk about in Chapter 12. The sidebar "Paying for alternatives" offers some insight into what that price tag may be.

Here's an interesting statistic: For people who have gastroesophageal reflux disease (GERD), drug costs are estimated to account for 63 percent of their total direct medical costs. However, only 6 percent of the direct medical costs for IBS are attributed to medication. Why? Because, as we discuss in Chapter 8, there are so few workable drugs for IBS.

Paying for alternatives

When we consider the medical expenses associated with having IBS, we should recognize that those expenses include payments for services that fall outside the scope of Western (allopathic) medicine. Many people seek help from traditional or naturopathic medical professionals — those who emphasize using diet, exercise, meditation, Chinese medicine, and other tools for improving your health.

Dr. David Eisenberg tabulated that people in the United States made 629 million visits to nonallopathic medicine practitioners in 1997. This number exceeded the total visits to all U.S. primary care physicians that same year.

People spent an estimated $21.2 billion in 1997 to get services from traditional or naturopathic medical professionals. At least $12.2 billion of that amount was paid for out-of-pocket. This figure exceeds the out-of-pocket expenditures for all U.S. hospitalizations that same year.

On the other hand, only 21 percent of the total direct costs of GERD care are consumed through hospital admissions. In contrast, 63 percent of IBS-related direct costs are attributed to hospital admissions for acute care and for in-hospital tests for evaluation and diagnosis.

Considering the emotional cost

IBS is associated with some very strong emotions, including anger, anxiety, depression, loss of self-esteem, shame, fear, self-blame, and guilt. Perhaps the biggest cost of IBS is the loss of confidence.

When you have daily pain and either constipation or diarrhea, you are always aware of your condition. But because of embarrassment, you may not share your concerns with others. It's like there's a little devil with a pitch fork tormenting you all the time — not just sitting on your shoulder but actively poking your intestines — and you can't tell anyone!

Fearing public places

Perhaps you developed your IBS symptoms after an infection, but you periodically suffer from all the symptoms for no apparent reason. (In other words, you can't associate the symptoms with eating specific foods or experiencing some other specific trigger, so your symptoms are unpredictable.) If you have a severe attack of pain when you are out, that's one thing: You limp home and try to recover. But if you suffer the horrors of bowel leakage in public, you are going to think twice about going out again. The old adage "Once bitten, twice shy" has IBS written all over it. We talk more about losing bowel control in public in the upcoming section "Analyzing the social cost."

Agoraphobia means the fear of open places. An agoraphobic is a person who is afraid to go outside. That designation is usually given to someone who gets anxiety attacks or panic attacks in public, usually for no apparent reason.

Many people with IBS are afraid to go outside, but the reasons are very apparent. They get panicky in public places, terrified that they won't find a restroom or get to it before they have an accident. They are also afraid of passing gas in public, in case something else comes out along with it.

Fear begins in the mind as a concern, then becomes a worry, and can shift into a full-blown panic attack. For some people, the panic sets up a rumbling in the stomach. (As we explain in Chapter 3, there's an intimate connection between the mind and the gut, which is home to more neurotransmitters than your brain.) In people with IBS-constipation, fear can cause spasms and pain. In IBS-diarrhea, fear can mean a frantic trip to the bathroom.

Fearing food

Another fear common to people who have IBS is eating. For people without IBS, this sounds bizarre. Eating is the most natural (and necessary) thing in the world. But people with IBS have an incredible burden: They are afraid to eat because just eating a meal can trigger a bout of symptoms.

Fearing the future

Fear of never finding a solution to your problem may prevent you from living life to the fullest. Here are some things that many IBS sufferers have come to believe about the condition:

- IBS is impossible to treat.
- Having IBS means that I am doomed to a life of misery.
- There is no cure for IBS.
- I will never eat a normal meal again.
- No one will love me because of this condition.
- My body is betraying me and rebelling.
- I will never have a normal bowel movement.
- My friends and family think I am a pain in the ass — literally.
- IBS controls my life.
- Nobody believes that I am ill.

These are serious and genuine complaints. While there may be some truth to these concerns, we believe that there are many ways to take this condition by the scruff of its neck and shake out some very workable solutions. In the next section, we offer suggestions that can help you do just that.

Tackling Social Situations

"Where's the bathroom?" is not a great pickup line. But if you're on a date and you have IBS, that question is probably on your mind constantly. (If your date thinks that he is the total focus of your attention, he is sadly mistaken!)

In this section, we discuss some topics that you may not feel comfortable talking about with anyone — unpleasant stuff like fecal incontinence and nasty odors. We hope the information we provide here will help you realize not only that you aren't the only person in the world worried about such things, but also that there are steps you can take to minimize the impact these problems have on your ability to get out and socialize.

Experiencing fecal incontinence

One of the most feared events in the world of IBS sufferers is fecal incontinence. In Chapter 2, we note that there's a word to describe what happens when you pass gas and lose some bowel contents at the same time: *sharting*.

This is not a symptom that you want to share with *anyone*. Face it: If you told people that you had these kinds of accidents, you'd fear that image would be on their minds anytime they saw you or even thought of you. It's just too unbearable to imagine. After the age of 3 or 4, society expects that stool goes in the toilet. So there is a great stigma to fecal incontinence.

We aren't going to try to convince you that you should tell everyone that you have this problem. However, you should tell your doctor, who is sworn to secrecy and will absolutely not laugh at your troubles.

In one large study, researchers interviewed patients in the waiting room of family doctors and GI specialists about fecal incontinence. Anonymously, about 18 percent of the patients admitted they were bothered by fecal incontinence. However, only 25 percent of them had ever discussed the problem with their family doctor, and only 50 percent had ever discussed it with a gastroenterologist. And these were people sitting in the doctor's office at the time! Please, do yourself a favor, and find the courage to talk to your doctor.

You may think that only people with diarrhea would be affected by fecal incontinence. The pressure of liquid stool building up in the rectum and wanting release is sometimes too much to hold back. When a bubble of gas sneaks toward the anal opening and tries to squeeze out, sometimes more than a bubble of gas escapes.

But severe constipation can also lead to bowel incontinence. A large amount of stool can fill up the rectum, and because it is so hard and solid it can't pass through the anal opening. This condition is called *impaction*. The impaction can weaken the anal muscles, allowing liquid stool to ooze around the impaction and leak out. Occasionally, impaction can cause the stool to harden like a stone, forming a *fecalith* that must be removed by forceps or surgery. If you have such a blockage, diarrhea is the only way stool can pass around it.

Using perineal pads

You may find that wearing a small panty liner called a *perineal pad* (the kind that women use for the light days of their periods) is all you need to boost your confidence. For you men out there, these pads have an adhesive strip that attaches them to your underwear. They have absorbent material on one side and plastic on the other to prevent moisture from reaching your underwear. They are small and convenient to carry, even in your pants pocket. If your problem is the loss of a little bowel content when you pass gas, this type of liner should be enough to prevent staining or embarrassment.

Considering diapers

But perineal pads may not provide enough coverage for everyone who suffers from fecal incontinence. Before we discuss the diaper option, we want to mention another option that you *shouldn't* try.

Believe it or not, some people resort to inserting a tampon in the anus, or blocking the anus with a roll of gauze, to prevent bowel leakage when going out in public. We don't recommend this drastic measure because it can dry up normal anal mucus secretions that keep the lining of the anus healthy.

Okay, with that out of the way, let's talk diapers. Some people are forced to use adult diapers to deal with the unexpected if they want to have a social life. You may lament that those bulges won't do wonders for your hot new outfit. But if you want to get back to living a more normal life, you have to be willing to adapt.

When you think of adult diapers, you may associate them with elderly folks who suffer from urinary incontinence. But younger people with IBS, an inflammatory bowel disease (Crohn's or ulcerative colitis), or bowel cancer wear them as well. Tell yourself over and over that diapers aren't just for babies (no matter what your mother used to say!). They are an invaluable resource for people who need them.

Many of the diapers available are designed for people who are bedridden. But if you keep looking, you can find one that suits your needs. Look for products called *adult briefs* — they come in various weights and sizes for light incontinence to heavy incontinence.

The Internet makes it especially easy to research, window shop, and order these products in privacy. Calling a manufacturer directly can also help you find the best product for you. In fact, most department stores don't carry the best brands. Some brand names of products used for fecal incontinence include Molicare, Abena, Tranquility, Tena, and Select.

Many adult briefs have absorbent material that neutralizes odor, as well as anti-leak cuffs. And of course, they are all disposable. You probably aren't looking for a product with a large capacity or one that's made for overnight use. You mainly need something to wear at work or on social outings to feel safe. (Chances are you may not even need them, but they definitely act as a security blanket for your rear end.)

Here are some tips for getting the best use out of these disposable garments:

✔ Change briefs as soon as possible after use.
✔ Practice good skincare habits. Wash with mild soap and water or the adult version of baby wipes (called, appropriately enough, *adult wipes*), which are available at pharmacies, online at pharmacy sites, or at Assisted Living Store, Inc. (www.assistedlivingstore.com).

> ✔ Use a skin cream that acts as a barrier to irritating fecal matter. The best ones contain zinc oxide (an ingredient used in babies' diaper cream), which is also healing for damaged skin.

If you prefer, instead of diapers you can wear washable plastic pants over your cotton underwear. (You don't want to use plastic pants directly next to the skin.) To cut down on the rustle and squeaking when you walk, wear another pair of cotton panties over the plastic pants.

Using fiber and diet to combat fecal incontinence

Most programs for fecal incontinence focus on two ways to treat this condition: solidify the stool and slow the gut. These solutions assume that your problem is incontinence due to diarrhea. Taking fiber is the most common way to firm up your stool. We discuss the benefits of fiber in Chapters 8 and 10. The key to success with fiber is to introduce it very slowly so your intestines get used to it; if you take too much, you could cause gas, bloating, and irritation.

As we note earlier, incontinence can also occur due to fecal impaction. If that's your situation, treatment with fiber, fluids, and mild laxatives, as well as identifying the triggers for constipation, can help you overcome the problem.

Identifying your food triggers and eliminating them can often reduce your IBS symptoms, including severe ones like fecal incontinence. Chapter 10 walks you through an avoidance and challenge diet that can help you figure out what your food triggers are.

Fasting is not a long-term solution for fecal incontinence, but it may help you get through a specific event. It works because food consumption triggers contractions throughout the GI tract. In IBS, these contractions often create the need to defecate. If you have poor bowel control, urgency and incontinence may result.

Eating a large meal, especially one full of fatty foods, can stimulate GI secretions that increase your bowel motility. So especially when you're in public, keep those portions light.

Taking medications for fecal incontinence

Using a medication before going out is one way to cope with the physical and emotional reality of IBS accidents.

Imodium

Imodium (which we discuss in Chapter 8) is useful for treating fecal incontinence because, in addition to slowing down your gut, it actually tightens the anal sphincter. It generally works best at night, but you may find it helps during the day as well. You have to try it to know for sure. You don't want to use it if you are prone to constipation, but otherwise it is safe to use to prevent episodes of fecal incontinence.

Take Imodium 30 minutes before meals if you often have diarrhea and/or incontinence immediately following meals. If you have early morning urgency, watery stool, and incontinence, a tablet or two at bedtime may help.

Questran

Questran (see Chapter 8) is a resin that binds bile acids. This drug was actually designed to lower cholesterol, but it also has a binding effect in the bowels. If you've had your gallbladder removed, resulting in watery stool after a meal, you may find this medication useful. However, gassiness and bloating are possible side effects.

Amitryptyline

Amitryptyline in high doses is used as an antidepressant. Lower doses are used in chronic fatigue syndrome and fibromyalgia for treating sleep disorders or helping decrease chronic pain. However, the drug does have a constipating effect, and some doctors use it to treat fecal incontinence when fiber and Imodium don't work.

Covering up odors

Chlorophyll capsules are used to control body odors. One widely available chlorophyll product is called *Nullo Internal Deodorant Tablets*. It was developed for people with colostomies, ileostomies, and fecal incontinence. One to two tablets are taken by mouth, or a tablet or two can be put in an empty pouch. (We were interested to learn that Nullo is used by hunters to disguise their scents from animals!) The only drawback appears to be that chlorophyll coming out the other end will stain your panties green.

For people whose main trouble is flatulence, two innovative companies are producing products to help control those odors. At www.GasbGon.com, you can find a flatulence filter seat cushion with replaceable carbon filters, which supposedly absorbs both the sound and the odor. And at www.flat-d.com, you can find charcoal pads that are worn in undergarments, which supposedly eliminate the odor of flatulence. We haven't investigated the effectiveness of these products, but we like the idea that companies are creating products that may comfort people who are embarrassed, not entertained, by flatulence.

Preparing to go out

Some simple steps can go a long way in helping you cope with distressing IBS symptoms. To prepare for an outing, use the following tips as a guide:

- Make a point of using the toilet before leaving the house.

- If you are in a bad cycle of symptoms, wear a perineal pad or adult briefs.

✔ Carry adult wipes and a change of underwear.

✔ Make a mental list of public restrooms.

Keeping a diary of episodes of incontinence can help you sort out what could be causing the problem in the first place. Take special note of

✔ When it occurs

✔ Possible triggers, such as stress, food, or fluid

✔ Associated symptoms of pain, gas, and bloating

Trying EFT to Overcome Anxiety

In Chapter 12, we introduce the Emotional Freedom Techniques (EFT), which can help reduce anxiety and fear — including the anxiety and fear of leaving the house. Take a few moments and think about the things that bother you most about going out. What you're doing is defining the problem.

To make EFT work for you, it's important that you do it the same way every time. The only thing that changes is the problem you're tackling. To try EFT for overcoming your fears of leaving the house, refer to Chapter 12 to see how to do the tapping sequence, and create statements that describe how you are feeling when you think about going out in public.

Connecting with Others

Connecting with other people is one of the most important steps you can take when dealing with IBS. Keeping this condition a secret from your friends and family can lead to all kinds of tension and misunderstanding. Being alone with your illness in your house is one thing, but being alone with it in your mind is even worse.

Supporting someone with IBS

This section is one to share — with anyone you want to have a better understanding of how to help you.

Following are some things you should definitely do:

✔ Listen, listen, and listen more

✔ Commiserate

✔ Believe what this person is saying

✔ Offer help with chores, projects, and errands

✔ Keep this person's IBS a secret if that's what he or she desires

And here are some things you shouldn't do:

✔ Try to give advice

✔ Tell horror stories about your own (or others') bowel conditions

✔ Act bored or restless when you're being asked to listen

✔ Give this person more work to do

✔ Make jokes — unless the person with IBS initiates them

Communicating with your partner

We assume that your partner knows about your illness (it can be difficult to hide), but he may not understand fully what it costs you physically and emotionally. You may hear an edge in his voice when you have gone to the bathroom six times and he is still waiting his turn. That's to be expected. But it also means that you need to take time periodically to have the *IBS Talk*.

The IBS Talk reminds your partner what IBS is all about, how it affects your body, and the kind of support you need to keep your life together. It's just a reminder about the nature of your illness. Your partner may have forgotten some of these things — lucky him. But it's with you every day, and you can't forget. If you sense that his impatience is overriding his sensitivity to your issues, just say, "It's time for the IBS Talk." Even that one sentence may shift the mood and serve as the necessary reminder.

The IBS Talk doesn't give you the right to run the relationship based on your illness, however. You must be careful not to use your IBS to get your way, no matter how tempting. Playing games like that is not a good relationship-builder, and crying wolf about your IBS will get you in trouble — when you have a serious bout of IBS and really need support, you may not get it.

Key to the success of the IBS Talk is to be able to express what is going on without your partner trying to fix the situation. Most people, when faced with a problem, want to fix it. They just have to be reminded every so often that you need them to listen — you aren't looking for a quick fix.

Having sex

IBS is not a sexy illness. Intercourse can be painful even when you aren't having an attack. And if you *are* having an attack — forget it:

- ✔ In the middle of a painful abdominal spasm, sex is the last thing on your mind.

- ✔ If you are having frequent diarrhea, you are absolutely not going to put yourself in the reclining position only to have to interrupt the proceedings to hop into the bathroom.

- ✔ Intercourse when you have constipation can also be extremely painful — you don't want someone lying on you, and you don't want any pressure on your swollen intestines.

The IBS Talk that we describe in the previous section is really helpful to have when your partner wants to have sex and you — your body, your mind, and your intestines — are absolutely not interested. Your partner has to know that when your pain sensitivity is sky-high, all the romance and sexual tension in the world can't overcome pain. If he doesn't want his feelings hurt, he has to know when to back off and wait for a more appropriate time.

If your partner is feeling rejected in the bedroom because you are in the bathroom, be sensitive to those feelings. We recognize that it can be a long road from sick to sexy, but when you are feeling well, think about initiating sex. Don't use your IBS symptoms as an excuse to avoid intimacy. (One person told us that her IBS is to her what a headache was to her mother.)

Telling your friends

A big *faux pas* in a relationship is when your partner blurts out to mutual friends that you have IBS without asking your permission. That is usually a major breech of trust. Be blunt with your partner about what you consider private and what you consider public information.

If your friends need to know that you have symptoms because you are going out or traveling by car together, you need to make a decision. If these are close friends who you see often, you don't want to have to tell white lies all the time to avoid the topic. Plus, you may find that if you clue them in, you can get the support from them that you really need. However, if you're going out with people you rarely see and don't know very well, you always have the option of simply saying that you have food poisoning. It's your call.

Nearly one in five people suffers from IBS, so when you tell your friends about it, you may find that you aren't alone in your suffering. While we were writing this book, most people we talked to knew at least one other person who had IBS.

Taking baby steps

If, after reading this chapter, you still aren't convinced that it's safe to leave the house, we have a few more suggestions to get you back on the path to being a social person:

- **Have at-home dates with your partner:** If you feel trapped in the house, your partner may feel that way too. To avoid letting that situation turn into a source of resentment, schedule fun activities that the two of you can do at home. Set up movie nights, play games, or find a hobby that the two of you can pursue from the comfort of home.

- **Invite people to your house:** As long as you know that your own bathroom is just up the stairs or around the corner, you should feel confident enough to ask friends to your house. If throwing a party for 30 people seems like too much, start small: Pick two or three people you know and trust, and ask them to come for dinner. When you see that it's possible to enjoy yourself this way, you can gradually work your way up to hosting bigger events.

- **Take short trips to public places:** Even as you work on improving your social life at home, don't stop making the effort to get out of the house. If the thought of trying to sit through a movie gives you shivers, plan much shorter outings to start with. Ask your partner to make a quick trip to the mall with you, or spend 15 minutes walking in the park. When you discover that you can survive, and even enjoy, these shorter outings, you can gradually increase the amount of time you spend in public. With each success, you should find it easier to walk out the door the next time.

Making Web connections

Another way to socialize from home is to connect with people electronically. Online support groups exist for almost every condition or disease you can imagine. In an age where you can barely get a nod from your next door neighbor, if you send out an appeal to an online support group, you could get a dozen replies (and hundreds of people may read your message). Those replies in turn help others who have similar concerns. It seems to be a win–win situation.

In surveys of people with certain diseases (including cystic fibrosis, diabetes, and amyotrophic lateral sclerosis), results show that those who participate in online support groups fare better physically and emotionally than those who don't. And finding a support group is easy: Just use the key words "IBS support group," and you may be amazed at what pops up.

Most moderated online support groups prohibit promoting businesses, but some participants may encourage you to take specific products to help your IBS symptoms. Be sure to look at the signature line of the person offering advice. If the signature line includes a Web site, check that site to see if the product being recommended to you is promoted there. Be cautious of advice coming from someone who may benefit financially from it.

Joining a mailing list server

When Ginny finally got a diagnosis of IBS after several years of suffering, she went online to collect as much information as possible on her condition. She joined some mailing list servers and chat rooms and began sharing information and tips with other people with IBS. Before long, she noticed postings from Kevin that she thought were kind, caring, and funny. Little did she know that Kevin was noticing her postings as well. Soon, they started to correspond on their own, and they discovered that they lived within five miles of each other!

A *mailing list server* (such as LISTSERV) is the name given to the software for e-mail list applications. The way it works is simple: People join a list, and when they want the rest of the group to receive a message, the list server sends the message to all the members of the list.

The list server has two basic functions:

- ✔ It can send out announcements from the list server owner or moderator.
- ✔ It can send out a post to all members signed up for particular discussion group.

Distinguishing moderated from unmoderated lists

Many discussion groups are moderated, which means someone reads all the postings. The moderators are not checking for spelling mistakes but to make sure the message is appropriate for the list. Censoring can and does happen, but supposedly only to eliminate e-mails that don't meet a list's posted standards or that contain advertising or foul language. Most lists archive their posts so you can read messages from years of postings.

An unmoderated list is wide open. Members can post anything and everything they want. It's up to the reader to delete messages he doesn't like. Messages on unmoderated lists move very quickly because they don't end up in the moderator's e-mail inbox begging to be sent on.

The problems with unmoderated lists are many and varied:

✔ Unfocused conversations occur, which are better held in an online chat room.

✔ The conversation can be dominated by someone with time on her hands but nothing important to say.

✔ There is high potential for *flaming* (sending mean-spirited messages).

Following list server etiquette

When you subscribe to a list server, be sure to save the first message you get. It contains important information, including how to unsubscribe. Nothing is worse than tiring of a group, only to keep on receiving its messages every day.

Following are additional tips for participating in a list server:

✔ Write an appropriate, short, and clear subject line.

✔ Think about what you want to say and the group you are addressing, and make your message short and concise.

✔ Be on your best behavior. Think of it this way: Is this a message that you want your children to read?

✔ If you want to save time when reading your messages, just go by the subject line. If it interests you, open it. If not, discard it.

✔ Set up a special e-mail address to collect messages from different list servers.

People with IBS who meet others online tend to have positive experiences. We talk more about online resources for people with IBS in Chapter 16.

Chapter 14

Working with IBS

....

In This Chapter

▶ Recognizing how IBS affects your work life

▶ Taking steps to get through your workday

▶ Discussing your IBS with the people at work

▶ Considering working from home

▶ Using EFT to cope with work stress

....

With up to 20 percent of the population having IBS, that means if there are five people in your office, chances are one of them has IBS. Oops, that's you! Okay, different example: If there are *20* people in the office, 4 of them could have IBS. So chances are that at least some of your fellow employees (and maybe even your boss) may already know about IBS.

IBS affects people during their most productive work years. People who have IBS are almost *four times* more likely to miss work than those who don't. For these reasons, IBS is the second most common reason for not showing up at work (right behind the common cold).

Unfortunately, IBS tends to put a crimp — and sometimes a cramp — in some professions. It makes police work and skyscraper construction more difficult, for example, just because these folks don't have immediate access to a bathroom. Some people leave the workforce altogether because of IBS and must live on disability or a pension.

Our goal in this chapter is to help you consider less drastic options than getting out of the workforce completely. While we start the chapter by looking at some blunt facts about ways that IBS negatively impacts your productivity and your ability to seize certain work opportunities, we don't stop there. We offer suggestions on how to better cope at work, and we encourage you to consider negotiating to work (at least part of the time) at home, if your profession allows.

Facing Facts about IBS on the Job

We're realists, and we know (especially from talking with many, many people during the course of writing this book) that IBS has a definite impact on your work life. In the following sections, we address some of the most common problems that people with IBS face on the job, so you realize you aren't alone.

Producing less work

Don't you sometimes feel that scientists will study anything that moves? A journal called *Alimentary Pharmacology & Therapeutics* reported on one study in which a standardized questionnaire was given to a group of people with IBS to see how they fared at work. This group of 135 IBS patients indicated that they lost an average of about 12 hours per week due to their illness. That means that someone with IBS may be losing about two out of five days of work per week! This would not be good news to an employer, so we can see why some people don't want anyone (especially the boss) to know they have IBS.

Keep in mind that not all of the hours lost result from physical absence from the workplace. Instead, this study took into account lost productivity on the job (due to time spent in the bathroom, for example). This study estimates that an employee with IBS costs the company 50 percent more than someone without IBS.

If you have IBS, the last thing you want to hear is that you're a financial burden on your employer. Most people with IBS already feel that their illness is an imposition to friends and family. But our goal here isn't to make you feel guilty; it's to consider not only how your IBS affects your work, but how your work affects your IBS. Many people we have talked to can trace the onset of their IBS to coincide with a new job, an increased workload, a change in staff or management, or a reduction in job satisfaction. We discuss the connection between work stress and IBS further in the upcoming section "Suffering from stress."

Passing up promotions

It's sad but true that if your new job description involves traveling, entertaining, or (heaven forbid!) golfing with business associates, you may feel compelled to pass up the promotion if you suffer from IBS. We hear stories like this all the time. And this decision is perfectly justifiable for many people who don't have their IBS under control.

But we believe there are better ways to handle the adventures of a new job and the stresses of work itself. We offer some specific tips in this chapter, and we encourage you to look back at previous chapters to realize that you have a wealth of tools at your disposal (including diet, exercise, and stress-reducing techniques) that can help you better handle travel and social events without incident.

Suffering from stress

If misery loves company, you may be reassured to know that lots of people feel high levels of stress on the job. (If you need proof, see the sidebar "Stressing at work.") But you have the added burden of having a condition that not only *creates* more stress for you at work but can actually be *triggered by* that same stress. We discuss stress as a trigger of IBS in Chapter 4. Most articles written about stress these days mention IBS as one of the physical ailments that is most affected by stress at work.

Stressing at work

A ten-year study done in Canada provides a valuable perspective on work-related stress. Called "An Examination of the Implications and Costs of Work-Life Conflict in Canada," this study is available on the Public Health Agency of Canada Web site at www.phac-aspc.gc.ca/dca-dea/publications/duxbury_e.html.

Studies on IBS find that people with this condition are stressed out, missing work days, and unproductive because of their illness. But, not surprisingly, this study found that people with IBS haven't cornered the market on work stress; almost 40 percent of all workers studied experienced a high degree of work-related stress. Considering that people spend on average 70 percent of their lives at work, this is not a feel-good statistic.

Following are some of the findings from the study:

- One-third of Canadian employees report high levels of depressed mood.

- Half of Canadian employees experience high levels of perceived stress.

- One-quarter of Canadian employees feel "burned out" from their jobs.

- The number of Canadian employees who report high levels of work-life conflict and perceived stress is increasing.

- The number of work absences and physician visits is on the rise.

- The number of Canadian employees who report high job satisfaction, life satisfaction, and that they are in good health is decreasing.

- Women report substantially more work-life conflict than men, regardless of job type or dependent care status.

High work-life conflict is associated with

- Decreased wellness in terms of greater perceived stress, depressed mood, and burnout; and poorer physical health

- Reduced job satisfaction and organizational commitment

- Greater use of the medical system

- Increased absence from work

Many psychologists indicate that women seem to be more stressed out at work than men. And, as we note in Chapter 5, women are much more likely than men to suffer from IBS. While factors other than work are certainly at play here (think hormones, for example), this is not a good combination.

Some of the war stories we hear from people coping with IBS at work are nothing short of terrifying. People are denied bathroom privileges by vindictive supervisors, called hypochondriacs by their coworkers, or given more work when they complain to the boss. These examples, which we'd like to believe are exceptions rather than the rule, are symptomatic of an abusive work environment that places profits first and employees last. And they do nothing but heap additional stress on the person in question.

Ironically, a company that punishes workers in the name of profits simply aggravates the problem: It creates more stressed-out workers, whose health suffers further. As the disability payments and healthcare costs add up, we truly believe that companies will be forced to wake up and deal with the stress they're causing. (A glimmer of hope: Some human resources departments in large corporations are beginning to incorporate stress management, exercise, and massage into their workers' daily routines.)

Making Your Workday Bearable

We're optimistic that the information in this book will help you better manage your IBS in the long run so you find yourself not suffering symptoms as much as before. But, again, we're realists. The road to better health can take time, and in this section, we aim to help you cope with work even when your IBS is flaring up.

Starting your day off right

Coping with work actually begins at home. Many people with IBS can have three to four bowel movements before they even leave for work. And diarrhea isn't the only culprit: Pain and spasms because of gas or pain from the pressure of constipation can also interfere with the start of your day. (If you have constipation, you may feel the constant urge to go. In that situation, you know you need to be near a bathroom just in case the next effort produces results.)

A combination of factors can create a morning attack of IBS:

- Your stress hormones get revved up with the activity of standing upright and moving around.
- Whatever you eat for breakfast sends your gut into action.

✔ You may fear having an accident in the car on the way to work. (If you experience diarrhea in the morning, your body may actually be attempting to empty your colon so you *won't* have an accident.)

So how do you avoid any or all of these triggering events?

✔ If you know that the simple act of getting up in the morning triggers IBS symptoms, set your alarm 30 or 60 minutes early. Give yourself enough extra time in the morning to work through those symptoms and still not feel rushed or panicked (which will only make your symptoms worse).

✔ If what you eat seems to cause symptoms, and if you're afraid that those symptoms will make themselves known during your drive to work, we have two pieces of advice:

   • For a long-term solution, use the avoidance and challenge diet we present in Chapter 10 to determine what foods you need to avoid in order to reduce your symptoms. You may find that you need to eliminate milk, toast, or fruit from your breakfast menu, but you should also be able to find safe foods that you can eat every day without triggering symptoms.

   • In the short run, pack your breakfast and take it with you to work. If you're worried about getting diarrhea, better to deal with it in the office than in the car.

Having an accident-free commute

If the drive to work is itself a source of stress because you're afraid of having an accident (*in* the car, not *with* the car), following are some tips to consider:

✔ As we mention in the previous section, pack breakfast and wait until you are at the office (and near a bathroom) before eating.

✔ Give yourself plenty of time to make the drive to work. The last thing you need is to feel a rush of stress brought on by a traffic jam.

✔ Use the Emotional Freedom Techniques (EFT) that we explain in Chapter 12 by tapping with one hand when you are at stoplights. Use phrases that relate to your commute, like "I'm always getting stressed in traffic" or "Getting to work is such a hassle."

✔ If necessary, take medications that will help you to get to work safely. Taking Imodium about 30 minutes before you walk out the door may solve any concerns about diarrhea. This medication, which we describe in Chapter 8, slows down the bowel, and for some people it tightens the anal sphincter during the day as well as at night.

Doing EFT discretely

Maybe you're wondering how to do EFT without raising eyebrows at work. (We explain how to use this technique in Chapter 12.) The best thing to do is to head for the bathroom, which is a great place to get the privacy you want for tapping.

If you can't get away from your desk when you hear and feel the familiar rumblings in your gut, think about what is happening in your body and just tap on random EFT points and the karate chop point. Sometimes just tapping on the points can alleviate some of the discomfort.

If you need to be *really* subtle, you can even sit with your chin in your hand and tap on the point under your lip while you take some deep breaths.

Dealing with an attack at work

Prevention is the best medicine for IBS. We strongly encourage you to follow the advice we offer in other chapters:

- ✔ Consider taking dietary supplements, such as those we discuss in Chapter 9.
- ✔ Eat an IBS-friendly diet, which you can design based on information we provide in Chapter 10.
- ✔ Exercise, even if you don't feel like it! (We get you started in Chapter 11.)
- ✔ Practice stress-reducing techniques, such as the Relaxation Response and EFT, which you can read about in Chapter 12.

But we also realize that you're bound to experience an IBS attack at work sometimes, no matter how hard you work to keep the symptoms at bay. Perhaps it's that tiny sliver of birthday cake that you were *forced* to eat at a staff party or the added stress of an imminent deadline. For whatever reason, if pain and bloating get the best of you or you find yourself going to the bathroom every half hour, we have some tips for coping with an acute situation:

- ✔ Take several deep breaths.
- ✔ If diarrhea is the problem, take an Imodium.
- ✔ If bloating is the problem, take a peppermint capsule.
- ✔ If pain is the problem, take homeopathic Mag phos.
- ✔ Use the self-hypnosis technique that we explain in Chapter 12.
- ✔ Visualize yourself with a healthy bowel relaxing on a tropical beach.
- ✔ Do EFT (see Chapter 12) and use phrases like "The pain is unbearable," "I have severe bloating," "I'm afraid that I'll lose control of my bowels," "I'm afraid to eat anything for lunch," or "I'm stressed about this deadline." See the sidebar "Doing EFT discretely" for suggestions on how to use this technique without drawing attention.

Masking odors at work

When the worst happens, and you have a smelly bowel movement at work that threatens to become the subject of unwanted jokes, there are ways you can minimize the fallout:

✔ Keep a natural bathroom deodorizer in the washroom. One called Natural Magic Citrus Odor Blaster is a room spray that breaks down sulfur bonds from escaping gases.

✔ A product called Just a Drop is a natural concentrated plant extract that you drop into the toilet to remove smells.

Of course, you can always just flush as quickly as possible and trust that the bathroom vents will clear the air.

Talking to Your Boss and Coworkers

If you're a full-time employee, you should have sick days, vacation days, and personal days that you can use to negotiate the time you need off. But before yours are used up, you have to have a plan. If you're taking quite a bit of time off work, you may want to consider having a discussion with your boss about your illness. Together, you may be able to come up with ways that you can keep your IBS from interfering with your productivity and comfort at work.

We certainly understand that some bosses and coworkers are easier to talk with than others. And if you absolutely know that your boss is going to react negatively to what you have to say, we respect your decision to keep your IBS private and cope with the situation in other ways. But we certainly hope that the majority of people reading this page have a slightly better work situation than that. If you can muster the courage to tell the truth, you may find that you get a lot of support — perhaps even from people who have personal experience with what you're going through.

Deciding when to tell

Timing is everything, and one of your biggest decisions relates to when to discuss your IBS with the people in your workplace. Following are some options to consider:

✔ **When you first interview for the job:** If you feel that your condition may interfere with carrying out the duties of a job you're considering, it may be a good idea to let the cat out of the bag early on. First, you want to know what kind of company you are working for. Some companies don't hire people with medical problems, even though that hiring practice is illegal. You want to know up front if a company seems tolerant of people with medical conditions; otherwise, your job may be an uphill battle. Also, if your company has to pay health insurance, it may come out in your application that you have IBS, and you could be chastised for not disclosing your illness.

✔ **When you are running out of allotted sick days:** Don't wait until your sick days or vacation days are gone to tell your boss that you have IBS. The stress of not being able to take a day off will only increase your symptoms.

✔ **When you feel like your work quality is suffering:** You probably don't want to have this discussion when a deadline is looming and everyone is too stressed to think about how to help you. Instead, talk about your condition when things aren't too busy at work and you can take the time to discuss options that can improve your performance on the job.

There are both state and federal laws that prevent employers from discriminating against people with medical conditions. And your condition must be on record if you are fired because of poor performance that you attribute to your illness. Yes, we know, it can sound like a Catch-22.

✔ **When coworkers start to ask you what is wrong:** Despite your best efforts to hide or disguise that you have an illness, your coworkers are likely to be the first to notice your extra breaks, absences, and trips to the bathroom. You may want to tell them about your challenges before they decide that you are just slacking off.

✔ **When your trips to the bathroom become fodder for jokes:** It is embarrassing enough to have to use an office bathroom that may inadequately camouflage sounds and smells. You certainly don't need the added stress of insensitive comments from coworkers who don't know that you have an illness. Telling your coworkers may protect both of you from the embarrassment of nasty bathroom humor.

Deciding what to say

When you make the decision to talk with your boss or coworkers, here are some general ideas you want to get across:

✔ You have a chronic condition that can flare up with no apparent warning. (Having printed material on hand or a note from your doctor to describe IBS can be very helpful.)

✔ You are taking steps to deal with your IBS, such as watching what you eat or taking supplements or medications to reduce the symptoms.

✔ Despite these steps, you still may need to visit the bathroom several times a day, and some days will be more of a challenge than others.

✔ Most importantly, despite these challenges, you remain a hard worker committed to your job.

If your company has a human resources department, you may be in luck. Because IBS is a condition that comes up in articles on work-related stress, you may be able to talk to someone who understands your situation. All it takes is one knowledgeable person in a department, and you have someone to talk to about some basic ground rules regarding you and your IBS. For example,

- ✔ Your condition may make it difficult for you to be on time for work every day.

- ✔ You need to be close to a bathroom.

- ✔ You may have to rush out of a meeting suddenly.

- ✔ You may have really bad days when you need to stay home altogether.

- ✔ You are not the right person to make home visits to clients.

- ✔ In exchange for flexibility at work, you promise to work all your hours.

- ✔ You would love to discuss the possibility of working from a home office, even if it's just part-time. (We discuss this subject in more detail in the next section.)

If you are a hard worker and sincere, telling your boss or HR representative about your condition may have very positive results. For example, it may get you a desk nearer the washroom or lead to you working from home part of the time.

Plus, when you start sharing your IBS story with other people, you may find that they too have physical, emotional, or personal issues that they are dealing with. Opening up may be the first step toward developing better relationships at work, which can ultimately ease some of your stress. But only you can decide when and how to have this type of conversation.

Working from Home

Jamie was a talented Web designer working for a large company. But his unpredictable IBS with constipation caused him regular and sometimes debilitating cramping and abdominal pain, and Jamie sometimes found it impossible to sit at his desk for long periods of time as his job required. When he was in pain, he was not at his most creative. He was having a difficult time meeting client deadlines without taking work home to do in the evenings and on weekends. He was spending 40 hours a week at the office even if he wasn't able to get any work done, and then he was working on projects in his free time.

Jamie was getting overwhelmed and had little downtime to recover from his pain attacks. Finally, he decided to talk to his boss to see if something could be done. Fortunately, Jamie was a valued employee who was well-liked by clients, and his employer was able to make some accommodations for his illness. They negotiated that Jamie could do his design work from home and would be available to meet with clients, which he could often do by phone. From home, Jamie was able to monitor his IBS symptoms more easily and work more when he was feeling well, allowing him time to recuperate when he did have his painful attacks.

As we note in the previous section, one of the things you may want to request when you discuss your IBS with your employer is that you have the flexibility to work from home, even if only part of the time. Obviously, this situation won't work for everyone. If you work in retail sales or any other job that requires your physical presence, you aren't going to get far if you ask to work from home.

But many jobs *can* be done from a home office; all you need is a phone and a computer. Writing, editing, phone sales, medical transcription, public relations, multilevel marketing, selling certain products . . . many possibilities exist. If your current job seems like a good candidate for some at-home work hours, draft a proposal that seems logical and fair for both you and your employer. (You may offer to make yourself available for activities that require your presence in the office, such as staff meetings or client meetings, for example.)

If your current job can't mesh with an at-home situation, you may want to consider whether it's worth the effort to change careers in order to have that option. If starting your own business seems intriguing, go to the U.S. Small Business Association Web site at www.sba.gov for a host of resources that can help.

Getting support at home

Although this chapter is about dealing with IBS in the workplace, we want to remind you that it's a good idea to talk about your IBS with your family and trusted friends as well. They have to know that IBS is a real condition that greatly affects your life. When they understand that fact, they will know why you sometimes take time off work or come home from work sick and irritable.

Knowing you have support at home helps takes some of the stress out of work, and it may give you more confidence to confide in someone you trust at work. For tips on how to talk with your partner or your friends, see Chapter 13.

The downside to working at home is that you don't get out and socialize with other people. As we explain in Chapter 13, that can also be a downside of IBS. Don't let working at home become an excuse to be a complete recluse. Be sure to read our tips in Chapter 13 so you can continue to have a social life, even at times when your IBS is acting up.

Regaining Power in the Workplace

Rosalind Joffe coaches individuals with chronic illness to thrive in the workplace. She has developed a seven-step program for "Regaining Power in the Workplace with Chronic Illness." With her permission, we want to share her program with you. It's not specific for IBS, but it's a commonsense approach to dealing with a long-standing illness at work:

1. **Focus on what you can control.** You may not be able to control the course of your illness, but you can control the direction you take and the choices you make regarding that illness in the workplace. *View your chronic illness as a challenge to meet, not an obstacle in the way.*

2. **Ignore the naysayers.** People will tell you that since work is stressful, rest is the solution for chronic illness. Not true. Unpleasant work, too much work, or work that is too physically demanding can be bad for anyone's health. Not working can be stressful, too. Your chronic illness presents you with more challenges than before, but throwing in the towel is not the only option. *Shape your work environment to meet your needs, and you'll help yourself.*

3. **Come out of the closet.** Chronic illness is nothing to be ashamed of. If your illness impacts your work, keeping it a secret depletes your precious energy and gets in your way. Know your rights under the Americans with Disabilities Act (ADA) and Family Medical Leave Act (FMLA). Maintain your right to privacy. And be judicious with your information. But don't take on the burden of pretending that you don't have a chronic illness. *Be as public as you need to be and as private as you want to be.*

4. **Don't just survive — thrive.** It's easy to feel that survival is enough. And most people won't expect more from you. But chronic illness or not, you weren't born for mediocrity. Raising the bar doesn't mean doing more than you can; it means aiming high and seeking what you need to thrive. *Reach beyond relief; go for the satisfaction.*

5. **Control the message.** Other people on the job expect you to set the tone, and you can influence the way they respond to your illness. Design and control your message: What and how much do you want to say? To whom do you want or need to say it? When and where do you want to talk? *Get out in front of the conversation.*

6. **Don't let your illness define who you are.** Some people might try to paint you as a martyr; others may consider you less worthy of recognition or promotion. Neither extreme works to your advantage; each gets in your way. The message you want to convey is that your chronic illness is simply one of several cards in your deck, just like everybody else. *Having a chronic illness is neither a source of shame nor a source of pride.*

7. **Look for the silver lining.** Although you may not believe it now, work-place success in the face of illness can be transforming. Many of us have found new strength and confidence, qualities we never knew we had, as a result of our illnesses. We use this newfound power to face other life challenges. *It need not all be about the bad news.*

Chapter 15

Helping Children Cope with IBS

. . . .

In This Chapter

▶ Realizing that IBS is different for kids

▶ Dealing with pain

▶ Comforting your kids

▶ Treating symptoms with homeopathy

. . . .

Children are not mini-adults, especially when it comes to IBS. They may have the same symptoms of IBS that adults suffer, but they don't have the coping mechanisms that tend to come with maturity. Here's a partial list of frustrations that children with IBS suffer, which we address in this chapter:

✔ Tummy pains are common in children, which means it's tough for them — and their parents — to know when the problem is IBS.

✔ Stress from an emotional upset or trauma can trigger IBS.

✔ Embarrassment about bodily functions makes it difficult for children to talk about this condition.

✔ At school, children are often not allowed to leave class for any reason. If they leave for an urgent bathroom visit, they may be taunted.

✔ A child may not want anybody at school to know about this condition.

✔ Children don't really have control over what they eat and don't make the association between food and IBS.

✔ No IBS medications are particularly safe for children. When kids do take drugs, they may experience side effects.

Realizing a Tummy Ache Is Something More

Every one of us had tummy upsets and pain when we were kids. Who doesn't remember feeling a mother's soothing hand on his abdomen or a cool cloth on his forehead? But some kids deal with more than the usual tummy ailments that result from picking up a bug at school or eating too many sweets.

Recurrent abdominal pain is the most common pain complaint of childhood. It affects 10 to 15 percent of school children, resulting in absences from school and impaired quality of life. One study showed that one-third to one-half of children with recurrent abdominal pain continue to report abdominal pain and related symptoms (such as IBS) when they are adults.

You may not believe that a child as young as 4 years old can have IBS, but she can. IBS is more common in the late teens and early 20s, but that doesn't mean it can't strike earlier in life.

You must be aware of how quickly a child can dehydrate and become very ill when she loses a lot of fluids with frequent bowel movements. Dry skin, not going to the bathroom to urinate, sunken eyes, and lethargy are common signs of dehydration.

Finding out what's wrong

Before you can cope with IBS in your child, you have to find out what's wrong. But some children don't tell their parents what they're experiencing. What do you do then?

The key is to pay attention. If your child has frequent bouts of abdominal pain and constipation or runs to the bathroom all the time, she may have IBS. If she doesn't talk with you about her symptoms, she's probably either embarrassed or thinks something is deadly wrong and is in denial.

Be observant of your child's behaviors. Then, gently ask what's up and give her all the openings she needs to talk with you. When she finally talks, reassure her of your unconditional love and support, and let her know that you'll help her deal with this problem.

Next, find out all you can about IBS — this book is a great start. Get a proper diagnosis by ruling out other conditions, which we discuss in the next section. Then, work on making lifestyle changes involving diet, exercise, and stress-releasing tools (see Part III of this book). Encourage your entire family to participate in these changes so your child doesn't feel further isolated.

Ruling out other conditions

When abdominal pain, gas, bloating, diarrhea, and/or constipation occur in a very young child, you must rule out the following conditions and diseases that cause digestive upsets:

✔ **Gluten enteropathy (celiac disease):** As we explain in Chapter 2, people with this disease cannot tolerate *gluten,* a protein found in wheat, rye, oats, and barley. Their symptoms may mirror those of IBS. A blood test can help rule this condition in or out, although some doctors insist on performing a small bowel biopsy to identify this condition accurately. (If a small bowel biopsy is required, the procedure will be done under sedation so that your child will not feel the procedure or be traumatized.) If the test results are positive, the treatment is lifelong avoidance of wheat, rye, oats, and barley. Identifying this condition early can curtail a lifetime of disability.

✔ **Lactose intolerance:** Most kids eat dairy products, and most gastroenterologists who investigate gas, bloating, pain, constipation, and/or diarrhea in a young child will test for lactose intolerance with a hydrogen breath test. The test is simple: After drinking a glass of milk laced with extra *lactose* (milk sugar), your child simply breathes into a machine. If the test results are positive, the treatment is to avoid milk products or to take lactase milk enzyme tablets when eating them.

✔ **Inflammatory bowel disease (IBD):** Blood in the stool, along with copious watery stools (more than 10 a day) and a slight fever, is an indication of an IBD — Crohn's disease or ulcerative colitis. We discuss these diseases in Chapter 2.

If your child is having copious watery stools, the situation can be life-threatening because water loss can lead to dehydration and damage to certain organs — namely the kidneys and the heart. An immediate trip to the emergency room is best. After your child is stabilized in the hospital, doctors will want to find out what type of bowel disease he has by using these tests:

- **Blood tests:** These tests indicate if there is an infection or an inflammation in the intestines. An infection is quite possible if the white blood cells are elevated. Evidence of inflammation is found in a blood test called the *sed rate* (or sedimentation rate), which is a measure of inflammatory products in the blood.

- **Endoscopy:** A sigmoidoscopy of the lower intestines can diagnose ulcerations that are a sign of ulcerative colitis. A colonoscopy that travels around the whole intestine may find ulcerations higher up than the sigmoid area. We discuss both tests in Chapter 7.

- **Barium enema:** This test is usually necessary to diagnose Crohn's disease, which can affect the last section of the small intestine as it is attached to the large intestine. (A colonoscopy cannot see into the small intestine.) When barium chalk is introduced through the anus and rectum with an enema, some of the barium goes into the small intestine and outlines ulcerations and scarring that can be seen on an x-ray.

Endoscopies and barium enemas are performed when your child is under sedation and should be done with the utmost sensitivity. You can turn to homeopathic medicine for the fear and anxiety that many children experience with blood tests, hospitalization, and other medical investigations. The best one for fear and panic is Aconite. You find out more about these remedies at the end of this chapter.

Struggling with the pain

Doctors who study IBS in children have found that because they haven't developed adult coping skills, they tend to put up with the pain, which is called *passive coping*. However, they also feel victimized by the pain, which is called *catastrophizing*. Kids sometimes use the following phrases to describe their condition:

✔ There is nothing I can do, so why even bother trying?

✔ Nobody understands.

✔ I just can't talk about this with anyone; it's too embarrassing.

✔ I just can't stand this anymore.

✔ There is something horribly wrong with me.

It's true that adults with IBS often think these very same things and have the same feelings of isolation, but for a child these thoughts are as overwhelming as the condition itself.

Overcoming the Stress of IBS

Adults tend to forget that children's lives can be as stressful as theirs — maybe even more stressful. Here are some examples of the stress on a child who has IBS:

✔ I have to get up early for school even though I couldn't sleep all night because of the pain.

✔ My mother forces me to eat breakfast, which only makes me feel worse.

✔ Some mornings I have to go to the bathroom five times before I can leave the house.

✔ I'm always late for school and spend the first period in detention.

✔ There's no way I'm telling anyone at school what's wrong with me because they will make my life even more miserable.

✔ I sit in agony in class because the teacher won't let anyone leave the room without a note.

✔ I farted once in class. I just couldn't help it — the pain was so bad. Six months later, the creeps in my class still bug me about it.

✔ I'm seriously considering asking my mom if I can be home-schooled. I can't take it any more.

✔ After my grandmother died, I just couldn't stop going to the bathroom.

✔ I think I'll ask my mother if I can go to the doctor myself. There is no way I want anyone else in the room when I have to tell the doctor what's wrong with me.

✔ Every time I'm around my uncle, I feel sick to my stomach. He yells and makes stupid jokes, but my father says I'm being rude because I don't want to be around him.

This list is enough to take your breath away. It's impossible to protect your child from her own sense of embarrassment. It's also nearly impossible to protect her from harsh comments from other kids. But there are many things you *can* do to instill confidence in your child, let her know her feelings are important, and let her know you support her.

In the following bulleted list, we provide specific suggestions for making your child's life a little easier. Using the preceding list, we walk through each item and offer solutions to consider:

✔ **I have to get up early for school even though I couldn't sleep all night because of the pain.** This is a common complaint, and we offer two possible solutions:

• *Diet:* Watch what snacks your child has at night. Offer him applesauce and mashed potatoes, which rate high on the list of soluble fiber foods that soothe the tummy. (We talk about the importance of soluble fiber in Chapter 10.) Ice cream, which is high in fat, sugar, and dairy, is a no-no. Popcorn is also a no-no because it's hard to digest and can irritate the gut, making it one of the worst insoluble fibers.

• *Emotional Freedom Techniques (EFT):* In Chapter 12, we describe EFT and explain how easy it is to use on yourself to reduce stress and IBS symptoms. Take a look at that chapter, and show your child how to do EFT on himself. An example of a setup phrase that he may use would be, "Even though I have a hard time sleeping because of the pain, I'm still a great kid." The reminder phrase would be "Pain keeps me from sleeping."

✔ **My mother forces me to eat breakfast, which only makes me feel worse.** Of course you want your child to eat breakfast, but you must make sure the food you offer doesn't trigger IBS symptoms.

You may find that a breakfast of a soluble fiber food, like cooked oats or barley, along with diluted orange juice or apple juice may be a good choice. You have to experiment to find out what affects your child in good and bad ways. Our advice in Chapter 10 can help.

✔ **Some mornings I have to go to the bathroom five times before I can leave the house.** Frequent bowel movements in the morning are common in IBS. Possible culprits are the food eaten the night before, the worry about getting to school on time, the fear of pain or having to go to the bathroom, or the worry about having an accident.

The first thing to do is make sure your child wakes up early enough to allow for extra bowel movements. If she isn't sleeping well because of pain, waking her early may seem wrong, but giving her an extra 15 minutes or half hour to get ready for school may reduce some stress if she's always worried about being late.

Here are two other possible solutions:

- *Diet:* The dietary advice in the previous two bullet points applies here. Make sure your child is eating soluble fiber foods both at bedtime and for breakfast, and try to discover what foods are particularly good and bad for her symptoms.

- *Emotional Freedom Techniques (EFT):* Your child can use these simple tapping routines in the morning to deal with the fears and worries of having IBS (see Chapter 12). An example of a setup phrase to use in the morning would be "Even though I'm always late for school, I'm still a great kid." The reminder phrase would be "Always late for school."

✔ **I'm always late for school and spend the first period in detention.** This can happen when a child refuses to tell the teacher or principal what is going on. Your child may develop a rough-and-tough attitude to cover up the problem and be identified as a kid with a chip on his shoulder. He may even get in fights and bully other kids so he won't be bullied.

When your child's school performance is being affected by IBS, you need to tell the principal, school nurse, or school counselor. However, before you do, you must have their assurance that the information is strictly confidential.

✔ **There's no way I'm telling anyone at school what's wrong with me because they will make my life even more miserable.** It seems that children have the uncanny ability to ferret out the weaknesses in other children and torture them with that knowledge. There is no use telling your child not to worry about this quirk of human nature. We can't miraculously change people's behavior, but we can offer a suggestion.

When your child expresses this fear, it's time to have a long talk about bullies. You want your child to understand that bullies are bullies because they are hiding weaknesses of their own. They lash out at other kids so no one can spot their weakness. Most kids understand this explanation. Ask your child to describe the bullies in his school. You may be able to figure out pretty easily what is driving their behavior.

✔ **I sit in agony in class because the teacher won't let anyone leave the room without a note.** This is definitely a situation where you want the teacher to know that your child needs access to the washroom on his schedule, not the teacher's. Some teachers find creative ways to acknowledge a child's needs. Rather than informing the whole class that Johnny has to go to the washroom, a teacher may ask him to pick up something from the secretary's office or do some other errand.

✔ **I farted once in class. I just couldn't help it — the pain was so bad. Six months later, the creeps in my class still bug me about it.** If your child shares an embarrassing moment like this with you, consider sharing some of the worst moments in your life — as long as they aren't too risqué. EFT can also help reduce the stress (see Chapter 12).

It's also important to discourage your child from holding in painful gas or bowel movements and to make sure she understands that doing so can lead to long-term bowel problems. This is another situation where it is important to have a conversation with the teacher to ensure that you child is able to leave the classroom when having gas or urgency.

✔ **I'm seriously considering asking my mom if I can be home-schooled. I can't take it any more.** While home-schooling may be an option for a child who is severely ill with IBS, it may cause other problems. It can be an isolating experience; you have to work hard to provide your child with social activities that help develop interaction and communication with other children. A frank discussion with your child about the pros and cons is the only way to handle this question.

✔ **After my grandmother died, I just couldn't stop going to the bathroom.** A tragic event such as a death in the family can trigger an underlying bowel sensitivity. The symptoms of IBS and the grief become inter-meshed and can provide an ongoing source of emotional irritation for a child. Here are some possible solutions:

- *Talking with your child:* As a parent, you should encourage your child to talk about the death of a family member. The whole family can participate in remembering the person who has died by spending time each day or each week talking about the person, looking at photos, and sharing memories. Such shared events can go a long way toward helping a child deal with stress. Psychologists find that the biggest problems seem to occur when families don't talk about the death.

- *Counseling:* Your child may benefit from getting psychological counseling about death, dying, and how to deal with grief. If you don't know how to find a counselor, ask a school counselor for suggestions.

- *Emotional Freedom Techniques (EFT):* EFT (see Chapter 12) can help with underlying feelings of guilt, fear, and loss that your child may be experiencing. An example of a setup phrase may be "Even though I got sick after Grandma died, I'm still a great kid." The reminder phrase would be "I got sick after Grandma died."

✔ **I think I'll ask my mother if I can go to the doctor myself. There is no way I want anyone else in the room when I have to tell the doctor what's wrong with me.** This is a common sentiment expressed by kids with IBS. Ask your child if he does or doesn't want you in the room, and make sure you respect the answer. If he says he would rather be alone with the doctor, don't be insulted. Your child does have a right to privacy, and yes, he is growing up!

✔ **Every time I'm around my uncle, I feel sick to my stomach. He yells and makes stupid jokes, but my father says I'm being rude because I don't want to be around him.** If your child makes a statement similar to this, treat it very seriously. She should not be exposed to verbal abuse, even if it's not directed at her. And in the worst case scenario, your child could be trying to tell you that she is being physically abused.

Never force your child to kiss, hug, or otherwise interact with someone she seems to be afraid of. There are often very good reasons for that fear.

Maintaining Balance at Home

Having a child with IBS, or any other chronic illness, puts a strain on the family and produces interesting family dynamics. We often hear that in families with a sick child, that child seems to get all the attention and the other children feel left out.

Some children may feel that the only way to get attention from parents who are too focused on a sick sibling is by being sick themselves or by acting out. You don't want either of these situations, which add considerable stress. Instead, it's best to use preventive psychology. It really doesn't take much to acknowledge your other children, praise them, take them on special outings, and give them responsibilities that let them know you trust them.

You don't have to ask to know that a child feels neglected, perhaps even abandoned, when you spend extra time with a sibling. The healthy child may find it hard to rationalize that you have to spend more time with the sick child. Instead, he just knows how he feels — and it doesn't feel good. Most children who have sick siblings actually think that their parents don't love them as much. This is the dreaded fear you have to dispel.

Obviously, your child with IBS also has his own emotions about his condition to deal with. He may feel that he is a burden and worry that you don't love him because he's such a handful. That's one reason most children with IBS don't want to share their symptoms with anyone — even their parents.

And as if attending to your children's needs isn't tough enough, you also have to make sure that you and your partner don't get off track. For example, if Mom does most of the caregiving, Dad can feel left out. It's important to guard against this happening. And no, that doesn't mean just telling Dad to grow up! Ideally, it means dividing the caregiving as equally as possible between the two of you.

What else can you do to make sure your family sticks together when you're learning how to cope with IBS in your child? Make lifestyle improvements everyone's goal, leading to a healthier family in general. For example,

- ✔ Eat better by planning and cooking meals together.

- ✔ Exercise as a family, such as by biking, walking, or canoeing.

- ✔ Have weekly meetings (but *not* over dinner, which needs to be stress-free) when you talk about anything that's causing stress or frustration.

- ✔ Learn how to give each other neck rubs.

Using Homeopathy for Your Child's Emotions

Stress and emotions play a key role in triggering IBS symptoms, as we explain in Chapter 4. As an adult, what do you do when you're overwhelmed with stress, depression, or anxiety? You may ask your doctor for a prescription, such as valium or an antidepressant, to help you get back to feeling normal. And when your child experiences those same types of emotional problems, your first thought may be to get a quick fix in the form of a similar prescription.

But such prescriptions are usually not suitable for children. Both their physical systems and their emotional lives are too delicate. (In 2005, the European Medicines Agency recommended that Prozac and Strattera not be used for childhood and adolescent depression, saying that these drugs should be confined to their label indications for obsessive-compulsive disorders and hyperactivity.)

If your child has emotional troubles to cope with, which you suspect are key in triggering her IBS symptoms, what can you do? Homeopathic medicine is one possible treatment.

As we explain in Chapter 9, homeopathy is a natural, over-the-counter therapy that is safe, even for children. While our focus in Chapter 9 is on using homeopathy to reduce IBS symptoms, homeopathy can be very effective in helping with emotional troubles. With the basic information we provide here and in Chapter 9, as well as guidance from a homeopath or from resources that provide more detailed information (see Chapter 21), your goal is to choose a remedy that most closely matches your child's symptoms. You can also choose among potencies.

After you've done your research and determined what remedy and potency to try, give your child one dose and wait to see what happens. If you see immediate improvement, continue to wait and let the remedy do its job. If you don't see any improvement within two days or the initial improvement slows down, give another dose. For severe emotional problems, you can give a dose every hour. For chronic complaints, give one dose three times a day. If you don't see any response to the remedy within a few days, select a different remedy to try.

Alleviating anger

There are many types of anger. If your child displays one of the forms of anger noted here, he may benefit from taking the appropriate homeopathic remedy:

- Chamomile is for finicky anger. The child is fine one moment and angry the next.

- Lachesis is for the anger of jealousy. This child is critical, suspicious, contradictory, and oversensitive.

- Natrum mur is for the child who is very sensitive and gets angry and bursts into tears at any imagined slight.

- Nux vomica is used for great irritability, which leads to headaches and stomach upsets with great sensitivity to noises, bright lights, and smells.

- Staphasagria is for suppressed anger and humiliation that cause headaches.

Altering anxiety

Adults often tease children who appear overly anxious and worried. Of course, that's the worst thing to do. Children can be very sensitive to excitement and upcoming events. For example, children often express a particular type of anxiety that can be called *acute anticipation*.

Following is a list of remedies that may prove useful for specific anxieties:

- Aconite is for chronic fright and fearfulness.

- Calc carb is for children who overwork and overload themselves with tasks and anticipate problems.

- Gelsemium is for acute anticipation or for a child who has never felt well since a particular frightful event.

✔ Lycopodium is for children who will do anything to avoid humiliation and embarrassment or who have not been well since such an event.

✔ Silicea is for children who fear that they will not have enough energy and constantly moan and whine that they are unable to get things done.

Helping hyperactivity

This condition is often misdiagnosed. For example, a "hyperactive" child may just be too bright and active for the adult caregivers in charge. Or she may have food allergies, too much sugar in her diet, a lack of attention and parental discipline, or even mercury poisoning. The following list takes into account a host of other problems that a child with IBS may be dealing with:

✔ Argentum nitricum is used for the hyperactive child with a sweet tooth. The child seems to have a high metabolic rate and is thin, pale, anxious, and can't sit still.

✔ Calc phos is suited to the child who likes to play pranks but is still shy and afraid. Physically, she has swollen tonsils and abdominal gas.

✔ Chamomilla is used to calm the excessively agitated child who cannot sit still for one minute and literally wears himself out to the point of tears.

✔ Kali bromatum is for the child who constantly uses his hands in some form and cannot seem to keep them still.

✔ Lycopodium is used for the child who is exhausted but can't sit still. There is irritability and restlessness, mostly around dinnertime, and lots of gastric distress.

✔ Stramonium is used for a severe case of hyperactivity with violence. There is a characteristic loud and frenetic speech pattern.

Creating confidence

Confidence is a big issue in chronically ill children, and it's important to make sure your child is self-assured and feels supported. The following remedies may be given by the parent, but in difficult cases it may be more useful to work with a homeopathic doctor to determine the correct remedy:

✔ Anacardium is for lack of confidence due to abuse or physical humiliation. The child becomes hard and cold, has no feeling, and may become emotionally cold and violent.

✔ Gelsemium is for poor confidence due to anxious anticipation.

✔ Lycopodium is for poor confidence due to fear of being in public, having been embarrassed in the past.

✔ Natrum mur is for fear of being rejected.

✔ Staphasagria is for poor confidence due to being humiliated. There is deep anger, but the child will do anything to please.

Sensing sadness

Children get sad for many of the same reasons that adults do. The following remedies can treat the effects of a loss in the family due to death of a family member (including the family pet), separation due to illness or divorce, or disappointment:

✔ Aurum is for the loss of a very dear and close relative. When this relationship is lost, the child feels there is nothing to live for.

✔ Ignatia is for acute, sudden, overwhelming, shocking grief; the child can't understand and can't believe what has happened.

✔ Natrum mur is for a child who is emotionally open and whose heart is broken. At that point, she gets stuck, shuts down emotionally, and becomes both guilty and resentful.

✔ Phosphoric acid is for treating a big grief. The child has emotional and physical symptoms of loss of energy, debility, and apathy.

✔ Pulsatilla is for abandonment with grief, sadness, and gentle weeping.

Chapter 16

Keeping Up-To-Date with IBS

*T*his chapter shows how far knowledge about IBS has come in the past decade and how to find out where it's going. Celebrities are jumping on board to bring new awareness to the condition. Research for IBS is accelerating with hopes that new medications will surface. Existing treatments (such as diet and exercise) are proving successful at tackling IBS symptoms. And with all this progress, you have lots of opportunities to continue learning about IBS on your own long after you set this book down.

Raising Awareness of IBS

Every condition needs to have supporters. Foundations, self-help groups, and celebrity fundraisers each have a role to play to offer support to people in need. After people get over the embarrassment of having IBS, they tend to speak openly about their condition and raise awareness. This condition has to battle with dozens of other worthy causes to seek research funding, which means the public has to know it's a problem. In the following sections, we explain how IBS is coming to more and more people's attention.

Marketing medications

Often, awareness of a chronic condition like IBS is raised when someone (usually a drug company) realizes that there's money to be made by talking about it. The positive side is that raising awareness makes it easier for people suffering from the condition to ask for help. The negative side is that the entity that stands to make a profit has a specific agenda and tends to limit the information it provides the public about treatment options.

Expecting cilansetron

A new drug being tested for treatment of IBS-diarrhea is called *cilansetron,* which has the brand name Calmactin. It blocks the activity of serotonin in the gut on the assumption that a person who has IBS-diarrhea has too much serotonin. (This is a big assumption, and we'd like to see the medical community encourage patients to have their serotonin levels checked before agreeing to take a drug that affects them.) Serotonin influences the regulation of pain and motility in the intestinal tract.

Cilansetron had been submitted to the U.S. Food and Drug Administration (FDA) for approval but was rejected in the spring of 2005 because the FDA wanted to see more clinical trials done. The company believes that cilansetron may be beneficial for both men and women, unlike Lotronex, which is beneficial only for women with IBS-diarrhea (see Chapter 8). You can expect to hear more about cilansetron in the near future.

The IBS community received a big shot in the arm with the 2004 launch of an IBS awareness campaign called "Amazing Women." This campaign is part of a larger joint educational campaign supported by the National Women's Health Resource Center (NWHRC) and Novartis Pharmaceuticals Corporation.

While we certainly laud the effort to raise awareness of IBS, we want to point out that this campaign has a specific goal: to market a drug called Zelnorm. Rather than encouraging women to consider how diet, exercise, supplements, or other treatments may help their symptoms, it urges them to talk to their doctors about Zelnorm — a drug that is said to relieve IBS-constipation. Keep in mind that only 25 percent of people with IBS have IBS-constipation; Zelnorm does not treat IBS-diarrhea, which is a much more common problem.

In Chapter 8, we discuss how Zelnorm works and the fact that it isn't effective for a great many people with IBS. And, like many medications, it does have side effects. We aren't saying it isn't useful for anyone; certainly, some people may benefit from this medication. What we're saying is that this medication alone isn't the answer to every person's struggle with IBS. In fact, the vast majority of people with IBS aren't helped by it.

If you have suffered IBS symptoms for a long time, it's normal to feel a certain amount of desperation about finding something that will offer relief. When you see television and magazine ads that seem to speak to you and your symptoms, you may hold out great hope for that drug. We have talked to people who have fought to have access to a certain drug only to find, upon taking it, that their symptoms worsened. We have also heard from people for whom a medication had miraculous results. Always keep in mind that IBS is a very individual illness with symptoms and effective treatments unique to each sufferer.

Brigit had severe IBS-constipation for several years and was willing to try anything. In fact, she believed that she had tried every over-the-counter medication for constipation. When her friend told her that Zelnorm helped her with her IBS-constipation, Brigit asked her doctor for a prescription. Brigit followed the instructions, taking 3 mg in the morning on an empty stomach. Within a few hours, she had a bowel movement. She took another 3 mg at night and awoke with gas and bloating followed by diarrhea. Frankly, the diarrhea was initially a relief after ten days without a bowel movement, but it persisted for a full month and caused her to become lightheaded, drowsy, and dizzy. Her friend didn't have diarrhea when she took Zelnorm, but Brigit figured that everybody was different, and she kept taking the drug. After six weeks, Brigit stopped taking the drug because the diarrhea was so severe and constant that she was afraid to leave the house.

Learning from a self-help group

Two basic types of entities try to educate people about IBS:

- ✔ Foundations and associations supported by drug companies, which promote medications for IBS

- ✔ Self-help groups, some of which may offer books or products to treat the condition

In the previous section, we touch on the types of educational campaigns that are run by foundations and associations supported by drug companies. (In general, the campaigns will steer you toward asking your doctor about a certain medication.) In this section, we turn our attention to self-help groups.

Marjorie lived in a rural area and suffered daily with chronic diarrhea. She found it difficult to leave her home and risk being away from a toilet. Her family bought her a computer with Internet access and taught her how to search for information about her condition. After lots of reading, Marjorie thought that her symptoms sounded like IBS-diarrhea. She signed into an IBS forum and started reading stories from others who had similar symptoms. First, Marjorie felt relief that she was not alone in her suffering. Soon, after posting a couple of messages herself, she gained a better understanding of her illness, enabling her to take control of her IBS. She was able to order some products online and have them delivered to her door. And she also started exchanging e-mails with friends she met in the group.

An online IBS self-help group is the first stop for many people who are newly diagnosed, and even for those who haven't yet received a diagnosis. This type of group is usually a free service that provides support, information, and contact with others who have IBS. In our present healthcare environment, self-help groups fill in the gap caused by the high cost of doctors' visits and the lack of psychological support in the short visit times that most doctors must schedule.

Studies confirm that if you participate in self-help groups, which are really mutual-aid groups, you may benefit in the following ways:

- ✔ You'll know that you are not alone.

- ✔ You'll have a feeling of community with people who have similar problems.

- ✔ If you participate in groups with skilled moderators, you may receive professional advice.

- ✔ You'll experience a sense of belonging and less isolation. This is especially important for people with severe IBS who are confined to their homes due to symptoms (see Chapter 13).

- ✔ You can learn practical information about your condition.

- ✔ You'll acquire coping skills.

- ✔ You may develop an ability to think and act positively about wellness.

- ✔ You'll have support in times of crisis.

- ✔ You gain a sense of empowerment.

- ✔ You may feel more hopeful about your situation.

- ✔ Your self-esteem grows.

- ✔ You may experience a decrease in doctors' visits and hospitalizations.

One drawback of self-help groups is that some participants tend to fall into a complaining mode. The best self-help groups share experiences, hopes, strengths, and victories and try to focus on the positive. One survey of online support groups found that positive comments were seven times more frequent than negative ones, so if you find that a support group you're participating in feels too negative, search for another.

A very positive aspect of online self-help groups is that because participants can remain anonymous, people tend to share their deepest fears about their illness. (Online, you are identified only by your login name and your condition, and that's that.) When they do, they often find out that a hundred other people think the same way. This alone can be tremendously empowering to someone with IBS who is afraid or embarrassed to even talk to a doctor about these problems. Also, when you hear people talking about their symptoms and making jokes about their problems, it tends to lighten your load considerably.

The first online IBS self-help group was formed in 1987 and is said to be the largest Internet community for people with IBS. Members communicate on its bulletin board to share knowledge and experiences with IBS. You can visit this group at www.ibsgroup.org and link to books, studies, medical tests, diagnostic criteria, and medications. The site also hosts an online chat every Wednesday and Sunday evening.

The Canadian Society of Intestinal Research (CSIR) offers information on almost a dozen live support groups at www.badgut.com. (You can also get lots of useful information at this Web site to help answer your IBS questions.) CSIR's focus is on creating a positive, friendly attitude in the groups. And to ensure this attitude, it encourages all participants to make the following statements, which they have generously shared with us, as a commitment to their ongoing support of each other:

- I am in a group of people with a common bond, sharing my concerns, feelings, experiences, strengths, and wisdom.

- Discussions are designed to foster positive attitudes and are directed towards solutions.

- I share my problems but do not dwell on them.

- I do not prescribe, diagnose, judge, or give medical advice.

- I have the right to not use the recommendations of others.

- I respect that personal information shared is confidential.

- Our facilitator will advance discussions but is not there as an expert.

- Most sharing of ideas will come from the group.

- We each have the opportunity for equal talking time or the right to remain silent — we can share as much or as little as we want.

- I actively listen when someone is talking and avoid interrupting and engaging in side conversations.

- I will stick to my own experiences and will avoid generalities.

- The support group meetings supplement, and do not replace, medical care.

- I do not provide nor receive specific medical advice within the group.

- I am not a part of this group for any commercial purpose, nor will I try to sell products or services to group participants at meetings.

- I share equally with the other members of the group the responsibility for making the group run smoothly.

- Having benefited from the help of others, I recognize the need to offer my help to others.

This is one of the most comprehensive guides we have seen for ensuring a successful self-help group. Reading these principles periodically will help members of any self-help group — online or otherwise — focus on the intent of their group.

Direct smooth muscle relaxants

Direct smooth muscle relaxants have not been approved by the FDA and are not currently available for use in the United States. However, they are available in other countries, and a 2002 meta-analysis concluded that smooth muscle relaxants significantly improve the pain and abdominal bloating in IBS patients. The study also concluded that there are few side effects with these drugs, the major one being constipation. If the gut wall muscles slow down significantly, the rush of diarrhea can turn into constipation.

The following is a list of direct smooth muscle relaxants found to be effective that may become available in the U.S. in the near future:

- Cimetropium bromide
- Mebeverine
- Otilonium bromide (octilonium)
- Pinaverium bromide
- Trimebutine

Surfing the 'Net

The Internet is home to more than 100,000 health-related Web sites, everything from university and hospital academic sites to sites run by individuals. In the past, only doctors had access to medical journals and medical articles, but now everyone can access more than 12 million medical papers online. Research shows that complementary and alternative medicine is a hot search topic. And patients are bringing the latest research to their doctors.

More people use the Web to find health information than to shop, check sports scores, or get stock quotes. About half the people who get health information online say it improves the way they take care of themselves, and 60 percent say that information they find online is the same as or better than the information they receive from their doctors.

Infringing on the doctor's turf?

According to the Pew Internet & American Life Survey, one group of individuals is not completely happy about the Internet being the new source of health information: medical doctors. The survey found that consumers are not satisfied with the amount of time their doctors give them in an average appointment and have chosen to look elsewhere for information. But doctors are used to being the gatekeepers of healthcare information and warn consumers about the dire consequences of going it alone.

And we certainly don't encourage you to go it alone either. While you can benefit greatly from doing your own research into IBS and reading everything you can get your hands on, that doesn't mean you should cut your doctor out of your circle of caretakers. Instead, try to use each appointment with your doctor as an opportunity to get her opinions about what you've discovered.

Dr. Ben Gerber and Dr. Arnold Eiser, writing in the *Journal of Medical Internet Research,* propose that the Internet age can actually help improve the patient–physician relationship, because each member of the partnership shares the burden of responsibility for knowledge.

Most doctors have had the experience of a patient bringing information from a Web site to a visit. Naturally, your doctor may react positively if she agrees with the information and the source and negatively if she doesn't. But don't let the fear of a negative reaction discourage you. Most doctors aren't threatened by patients bringing information from other sources to an appointment to discuss.

In fact, many doctors encourage patients to do independent research on their health issues and come to an appointment prepared to ask questions about what they've found. Just don't expect your doctor to agree with everything you're reading. And when she doesn't, be prepared to do some more research before making up your mind about what may or may not work for you.

Knowing your source

It's important to know the source of your IBS information. If you search for IBS information online, make sure you find out who writes the information on a particular Web site and who funds the site. This information should be readily available; if it isn't, e-mail the site's Webmaster and ask for full disclosure.

Be aware that some IBS Web sites are funded by pharmaceutical companies. These sites may restrict their treatment recommendations to the drugs developed by the sponsoring companies. If someone is selling something on a Web site, that doesn't mean the site doesn't contain valuable information about IBS. It simply helps to get full disclosure about who is funding the site and who has written the information, so you can make your own choice about whether to believe the information, follow the advice, or purchase a product.

Surfing for alternatives

If you're looking for information about complementary alternative medicine (CAM), the Internet can be a great resource. For example, you can look up information about supplements (such as those we discuss in Chapter 9) and stress-reducing techniques (such as those we discuss in Chapter 12).

Doctors are generally not taught these modalities in medical school, so chances are you'll find information online that may be new — and possibly very interesting — to your doctor. And if you find that your doctor isn't open to discussing information about CAM, you may want to consider seeking another opinion. You definitely want to give yourself the benefit of working with professionals who have open minds and a willingness to consider all possible means of treating your symptoms.

Reaping the benefits

The benefits of the Internet are many and keep people coming back for more:

- ✔ **Convenience:** You don't have to get dressed up, leave home, be far from a bathroom, or interact with anyone but your computer.

- ✔ **Anonymity:** Nobody else has to know you are looking up the word *sharting*.

- ✔ **Variety of information:** You have the ability to quickly check multiple sources.

- ✔ **Self-empowerment:** You can find out firsthand about any subject.

Seeing Possibilities in Serotonin Research

The biggest news on the IBS front right now seems to be research showing that some people with IBS have an increased concentration of cells that contain serotonin in their intestines. This research supports the production and use of new serotonin-modulating IBS drugs, and it has people with IBS very excited and hopeful. However, the cautions around using a brand new class of drugs (which have a growing list of side effects) are also running high. In the following sections, we present what is known about this research and these drugs so far.

Finding abnormal serotonin levels in the IBS gut

In 2004, the pharmaceutical company Novartis sent out a press release titled "Molecular Defect Found for the First Time in IBS Patients." The subtitle was "New Research Demonstrates that IBS is Not 'All in Your Head.'" (But then, you've known that all along, haven't you?)

A gastrointestinal expert and contributor to the research, Dr. Michael Gershon of Columbia University, said in the press release that "IBS has long been classified as a purely psychosomatic condition. . . . However, IBS is now associated with a very real abnormality in the gut and one that is as biochemical as any other."

This new research, published in the journal *Gastroenterology* in 2004, identified a molecular defect in IBS that does not appear in people without the condition. This research correlates with other findings that have shown that people with post-infectious IBS also have an increased concentration of cells that contain serotonin in their guts. (Note that this study was sponsored through a research grant from Novartis, which markets Zelnorm, a drug that alters serotonin levels in the gut. You can read about Zelnorm in Chapter 8 and earlier in this chapter.)

Realizing that your GI tract has a nervous system

In 1999, Dr. Gershon wrote a book called *The Second Brain* in which he outlined the independent nervous system of the gut, which is driven by serotonin. He emphasized that the discovery of an increased concentration of serotonin in the lining of the GI tract "should revolutionize the treatment of IBS."

Because of the popularity of Prozac, which increases serotonin in the brain, you may think that most of the serotonin in the body is directed at brain activity. That's far from the truth. In *The Second Brain,* Dr. Gershon reports that 95 percent of this neurotransmitter resides in the gut, and only 5 percent affects the brain.

At work in the gut, serotonin binds to specific receptors on nerve cells to make the intestines move. If too much or too little serotonin is bound to receptors, the intestines in someone with IBS are thought to either move too quickly, resulting in diarrhea, or too slowly, causing constipation.

The 2004 research we present in the previous section demonstrates the critical role that normal serotonin signaling plays in regulating GI function and demonstrates that IBS patients have a defect in the way serotonin functions in certain cells lining the GI tract. The researchers say that this defect *may* underlie the way IBS expresses itself with pain, bloating, constipation, and diarrhea.

Supplementing your serotonin

Two supplements may have a positive impact on the serotonin in your gut. One is available at your local drug or health food store. The other, unfortunately, has been pulled from the market. In the following sections, we explain the connection each has with serotonin.

Spicing up serotonin with 5-HTP

Naturopath Dr. Cathy Wong explains that 5-HTP is a precursor to serotonin and may be helpful (in supplement form) in the treatment of IBS. (Her article is available at www.altmedicine.about.com.) 5-HTP is a chemical derived from griffonia seeds and a cousin of *tryptophan,* an amino acid that is also a serotonin precursor. (We discuss tryptophan in the next section.)

Dr. Wong notes that pharmaceutical drugs that increase the action of one particular serotonin receptor (5-HT4) have been clinically shown to improve constipation. However, the precise mechanism involved is not yet known. She also notes that IBS is associated with several conditions that are believed to be related to low serotonin levels, such as depression, anxiety, and sleep disturbances.

Talking turkey (and tryptophan)

We all know the post-Thanksgiving sleepfest that occurs after devouring huge quantities of our faithful gobbler. You may have heard that the sleepiness occurs because turkey contains high amounts of an amino acid called *tryptophan.* Tryptophan is one of the necessary ingredients for making serotonin. It helps the body produce the B-vitamin niacin (B_3), which, in turn, helps the body produce serotonin.

In 1989, tryptophan was a very popular supplement used as a sleep aid and also for treating minor depression and anxiety. Then, a very unfortunate series of events occurred. A Japanese maker of tryptophan introduced a new genetically-engineered component to its process that contaminated the product, leading to some serious side effects and a number of deaths. Tryptophan had previously been used safely for 30 years, but it was pulled from the market as if it were the cause of the problem. At the same time this was happening, Prozac came on the market, and everyone's attention turned to a drug solution for anxiety and depression.

Some naturopaths speculate that if tryptophan were still available over-the-counter, it could be useful as a natural treatment for IBS.

Pros and cons of Modulon

Modulon (trimebutine maleate) is a drug that prohibits serotonin activity. Animal studies have shown that it regulates abnormal intestinal activity but does not affect the bowel if it is behaving normally. This drug is not yet available in the United States but is sold in Canada. (With all the traffic in low cost drugs from Canada, some people with IBS in the United States are already using it.)

Modulon is used for symptoms of IBS pain and also to treat the bowel paralysis that frequently occurs after abdominal surgery. It is not recommended for use by pregnant women or children under age 12.

The list of adverse effects is a long one, and these effects may be aggravated by drinking alcohol. They include dry mouth, foul taste, nausea, diarrhea, dyspepsia, epigastric pain, constipation, drowsiness, dizziness, fatigue, hot/cold sensations, headache, rash (allergic reaction), anxiety, difficulty urinating, menstrual problems, painful enlargement of breasts, and hearing trouble.

Expecting more research

To date, only six or seven studies have been done based on the new research regarding serotonin-seeking drugs (those that modulate serotonin in the gut). Most of the research has been done since 2000. We discuss two of these drugs, Lotronex and Zelnorm, in Chapter 8 and note that neither has been perfected. But because serotonin research provides a possible avenue to find a patented drug to treat IBS, you'll undoubtedly hear much more about it in the near future.

Considering a New Line of Research: The Continuum of Illness

Jini Patel Thompson was diagnosed with Crohn's disease (an inflammatory bowel disease) in 1986 and was immediately given the standard medical treatment. After three years, she was taking 13 pills a day, could hardly eat anything without getting sick, and was chronically weak and exhausted. She mustered up enough energy to read every medical text she could find on Crohn's and realized that her only available options remaining were more rounds of prednisone (which she hated) and surgery.

That's when Jini decided to research other options for her disease, and this bright woman began to investigate what Crohn's disease and all the other gut diseases are really about. Many people ask her what causes gut problems. Here's her answer:

> *I see each of these conditions as points along a continuum, from mild to severe. With IBS at the far left side and Crohn's at the far right. So it would look like this:*

> *IBS—Diverticulitis—Ulcerative Colitis—Crohn's Disease*

The missing link?

We have heard over and over again that IBS, Crohn's, and ulcerative colitis are not related. But is that strictly true? We believe that Jini may be on to something and would like to see research done on this theory.

Like us, Jini has heard many stories of people's gut problems being diagnosed as IBS and then years later somehow transforming into ulcerative colitis and then Crohn's. Jini says many doctors indicate that patients are simply misdiagnosed with IBS in the first place. But if you track symptoms from IBS to Crohn's (see Chapter 2), what you see is a progression of symptoms from functional to physical disease that is localized first but becomes more generalized.

Seeing similarities in causes

There are many causes of gut problems. Just the list of possible causes of IBS, which we address in Chapter 2, is long and varied. Many doctors — and many patients! — have a hard time accepting that fact, because the desire to identify one single cause (and one single cure) is so strong.

Jini lists the following possible causes of IBS, ulcerative colitis, and Crohn's. They're very similar to the causes and triggers of IBS that we discuss in Chapters 2 and 4. Jini says that a personal mix of one or more of these factors can lead to an unhealthy gut and immune system. With her permission, we list them here along with her insightful commentary:

- **Vaccination:** This includes childhood and adult vaccinations, including flu vaccines. Vaccines can cause direct damage to bacterial flora of the gut and long-term immune system damage.

- **Antibiotic use:** Any antibiotic therapy that is not followed by full-spectrum probiotic therapy causes lasting, pervasive damage to the bacterial flora of your gastrointestinal tract (from mouth to anus), which in turn leads to increased infestation of yeast, parasites, viruses, bad bacteria, and other pathogens. These pathogens degrade the mucosal lining and damage the intestinal wall (symptoms include bloating, gas, inflammation, bleeding, and more), which leads to leaky gut syndrome, which then triggers allergic and autoimmune response.

Certain antibiotic drugs can cause pseudomembranous colitis all by themselves (like Novo Clindamycin), and the pharmaceutical information that comes with these products even explicitly warns of this. Yet medical doctors continue to prescribe them and don't follow usage with probiotics. (We discuss probiotics in several chapters of this book, including Chapter 9.)

✔ **Environmental and food-borne toxins:** Processed foods with preservatives, MSG, artificial sweeteners and flavors, nitrites, and other proven toxins and carcinogens; microwaved foods; toxins contained in skincare products, shampoos, cosmetics, furniture, flame retardants in all U.S. clothing, fabrics, and carpets; and airborne pollutants (to name a few sources) — all of these cause cellular and systemic damage and are association with decreased immunity.

✔ **Emotional trauma or abuse:** Don't underestimate the damaging effects of abusive or traumatic emotional experiences on the body, and the gut in particular. For some of you, this may be damage from your past that was never resolved/healed, and/or ongoing emotional patterns or experiences that continue to degrade your health daily.

✔ **Parasites and pathogenic microorganisms:** If your gut ecology is already weakened or imbalanced, travel to a foreign country or ingestion of tainted food or water can be the straw that breaks the camel's back. If your bacterial flora is already imbalanced with a deficit of beneficial bacteria, it's very easy for parasites, yeast, molds, bad bacteria, or fungus to flourish. These pathogens then degrade the health of your intestinal mucosal lining, which can result in ulceration, inflammation, bleeding, and subsequent damage to your systemic health.

Jini says that

Each of these causative factors — including lesser factors like whether or not you were breastfed, your mother's health while you were in utero, hereditary/genetic weaknesses, heavy metal levels in your body, mercury amalgam fillings in your teeth, and pesticide exposure — will contribute in varying degrees and combinations to your particular pathology. Different people are susceptible to different factors and something that strongly adversely affects your friend may only mildly adversely affect you. There is seldom just one factor (pathogen) in isolation that causes IBS or IBD. However, I believe each of us is capable of identifying our own particular pathology, or the causative factors of our own ill health, and then taking the steps that will be particularly healing to each of us.

Focusing on natural healing

You can read more about Jini Patel Thompson's theory in her book *Listen to Your Gut* (Caramal Pub). In it, she warns against trying to find *the* cause of your illness. In her experience with thousands of people who have written to her since she published her book, seeking the one cause and the one treatment can be very frustrating and a waste of time and energy. Instead, she directs people to heal themselves, get in touch with their bodies, and allow them to heal no matter the cause.

Jini recommends a three-pronged treatment for gut problems that addresses disease-causing germs that come in many varieties: yeast, bacteria, viruses, and parasites:

✔ Eliminate these organisms with diet and natural antibacterial and anti-fungal herbs. (However, true amebiasis infection — involving an organism called *Entamoeba histolytica* — often requires allopathic drugs.)

✔ Replace the negative overload with a lot of positive beneficial bacteria and friendly yeast (Saccharomyces boulardii) called probiotics (see Chapter 9).

✔ Heal the mucosal lining and restore/repair the intestinal wall with healing herbs and nutrients.

Again, you can read specifics in her book. One tip we'll share here is that she specifically recommends the brand name Natren for probiotics, and the product she prefers is Healthy Trinity capsules or powder.

We also have learned that it's important to use supplements that contain *human microflora* — the flora that normally inhabits the bowel.

Dr. Nigel Plummer has spent decades studying two of the most beneficial main human microflora: Lactobacillus acidophilus and Bifidobacteria. Dr. Plummer says that because these probiotics are human microflora, they are more compatible with your intestine than nonhuman microflora, such as those found in yogurt. His formulation of Human Microflora Forte (also called HMF Forte) is a product available to health practitioners in North America through Seroyal USA, Inc.

HMF Forte has been tested against the extremely toxic and dangerous bacteria Clostridium difficile. In a group of hospitalized patients on heavy antibiotic therapy, research showed that 67 percent of patients who did not receive HMF Forte developed Clostridium difficile diarrhea. Of those receiving HMF Forte, only 18 percent developed diarrhea, even though Clostridium difficile was present.

Implementing What We Know: IBS Clinics

The future of IBS therapy may lie in discoveries that emerge from new research, such as that we discuss in the previous sections. Or it may lie in simply implementing what we already know. We firmly believe that if clinics were set up today that focused on lifestyle intervention for chronic conditions, we could win the battle against IBS.

As it stands, most of the funding for IBS goes into finding a patented drug for *the cure*. We've seen the same approach taken with other chronic diseases, and it tends to create a tunnel vision approach focused solely on drug intervention.

But, as we explain throughout this book, IBS is a functional disease and has more triggers than you can shake a stick at. Chances are it's not going to be amenable to a single drug treatment. We think the opportunities to relieve IBS symptoms are greater if doctors and patients alike expand their thinking to include changes to diet, exercise, and other lifestyle factors.

That's why, in the following sections, we offer some insight into what IBS clinics could accomplish. We briefly touch on how we can implement what we know about IBS to test for it and treat it. If each major city set up a clinic that focused on accomplishing these tasks, we're convinced that a whole lot of people with IBS would suffer a whole lot less.

Testing for IBS

As we explain in Chapter 7, a wide spectrum of tests is currently used to arrive at a diagnosis of IBS. These tests primarily rule out other conditions with similar symptoms, so your doctor can conclude that IBS must be the culprit.

But we believe that testing for IBS should begin with keeping a food diary (see Chapter 10), and we think an IBS clinic would be an ideal place to walk someone through the process of doing so. Often, what you eat every day can cause bowel sensitivity. Only by tracking what goes into your mouth can you begin to see connections between the foods you eat and the symptoms you experience.

Also, a clinic could certainly offer several noninvasive tests (which we discuss in Chapter 7) to determine whether what you're experiencing is actually a food intolerance or allergy: Hydrogen breath tests to check for lactose intolerance and gluten intolerance; blood antibody tests to check for gluten intolerance; and blood tests to determine food allergies.

Treating IBS

The goal of an IBS clinic would be to provide one-stop shopping for a person with this condition. So in addition to getting guidance on diet, exercise, and stress-reducing techniques, the patient should also be offered treatments such as hypnosis and acupuncture, which we discuss in Chapter 12.

We believe that successful treatment also involves feeling like you're part of a community, so we'd like our ideal IBS clinic to sponsor live support groups. Support groups could be facilitated by clinic staff members or run by members, and some should be open to family members.

Doing your part

It's all within the realm of possibility to create IBS clinics that work. How can you help make this vision a reality? Encourage doctors in your area to get involved. Hand them copies of this book or other research materials that discuss the importance of lifestyle changes in coping with IBS. Be persistent, and if you're a member of a live support group for IBS, ask other members to take up the cause as well. Remember what you've always heard about the squeaky wheel: You deserve to get a little grease (in the form of relief from your symptoms and support for what you're going through), so make as much noise as possible!

Part V
The Part of Tens

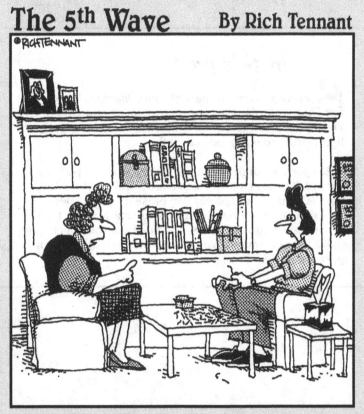

The 5th Wave   By Rich Tennant

"The reason I think stress might be a factor in your IBS is because of research, statistics, and the fact that you've straightened out an entire box of paper clips during our conversation."

In this part . . .

Everybody loves this part of a *For Dummies* book. That's because the chapters are short and sweet, offering great nuggets of information you can easily digest (with no nasty side effects).

In this part, we present ten IBS triggers to be especially wary of. We also give you lists of do's and don'ts to help combat your IBS symptoms. We present ten key medical tests that you and your doctor should know about to get an accurate diagnosis of IBS. And finally, we offer a chapter chock full of resources you can consult to find out even more about IBS.

Chapter 17

Ten IBS Triggers to Avoid

- ▶ Shunning toxic medications and harmful foods
- ▶ Preventing infections and leaky gut
- ▶ Coping with daily and acute stress

*I*n Chapter 4, we discuss all sorts of possible triggers for IBS. One of the toughest parts of having this condition is that you can't rely on your doctor, a book, or your best friend to explain why you have symptoms. The answers aren't that clear-cut because everyone with IBS can have a different set of triggers. That means you have to spend some time paying attention to your body in order to sort through what triggers may be affecting you.

However, certain triggers are more common than others. In this chapter, we present ten of the biggest offenders, along with some pretty powerful ways you can avoid (or at least minimize) them. To find out more information about the topics we discuss here, flip back to Chapter 4.

Avoiding Antibiotics

Some researchers believe that if you are prescribed antibiotics at an early age, your bowels can become irritated because the drugs may harm friendly bacteria, thus causing an overgrowth of abnormal bacteria and yeast.

Just about everyone has taken antibiotics, whether for a serious infection or "just in case." Antibiotics have one purpose — to kill bacteria — and they don't discriminate. So whether you take them for a life-threatening illness or just in case your viral flu turns nasty, antibiotics kill off good and bad bacteria. The bad bacteria you can do without, but losing the good bacteria is a concern.

Good bacteria do a lot of beneficial things for the intestines. One group of bacteria called *anaerobes* (which don't like oxygen) deters yeast. A specific bacteria called *Lactobacillus acidophilus* makes lactic acid, which helps prevent yeast from overgrowing in the intestines. When Lactobacillus bacteria are killed off by antibiotics, nothing deters the yeast, and they take over the neighborhood. (In Chapter 3, we explain why the neighborhood gets nasty when yeast take over.)

Besides making room for yeast to take charge of your intestines, all antibiotics have the potential to cause a severe intestinal disease called *pseudomembranous colitis,* otherwise known as antibiotic-associated colitis. This life-threatening disease is caused when the intestinal flora is destroyed by high doses of IV antibiotics, leaving room for the *Clostridium difficile* bacteria (which normally occurs in low amounts) to grow. Clostridium is resistant to most antibiotics, and its overgrow can have a devastating effect.

Clostridium difficile makes a very powerful toxin that is extremely irritating to the lining of the intestine. In its extreme form, it causes ulceration and bleeding in the intestinal lining, sloughing of tissue, and severe diarrhea. In lesser amounts, we speculate that antibiotic-induced Clostridium overgrowth could be a trigger for IBS.

We advise you to look for alternatives to antibiotics as much as possible, because any amount of antibiotic use has the potential to cause intestinal irritation — or worse. Obviously, we recognize that sometimes you really need antibiotics. If you have a high fever, very stiff neck, prolonged nausea and vomiting, severe abdominal pain that goes on for hours, severe diarrhea with bleeding, fainting, or dehydration, you should seek medical attention. But when your situation is less serious and it's a toss-up whether you need antibiotics or not, look for alternatives.

Sometimes beating off a sore throat can be as simple as holding a clove of garlic in your mouth overnight. Following are a few other natural treatments for mild infections that may keep things from getting worse:

- Barberry
- Echinacea
- Garlic
- Goldenseal
- Oregano oil
- Vitamin C

These treatments can be taken in many forms — as foods, herbal teas, liquid tinctures, or capsules — but they must be taken several times a day for several days to achieve the results you want. For additional tips, read Dr. Carolyn Dean's *Natural Prescriptions for Common Ailments* (Keats Publishing) for advice on handling 100 common ailments.

And when you really have to take antibiotics, make sure you take probiotic supplements or eat organic, plain yogurt that contains Lactobacillus acidophilus and/or Bifidobacteria to build up your good bacteria and crowd out the bad guys. Take the probiotics two hours apart from the antibiotics.

Countering Candida

What's all the fuss about a yeast organism that everyone has anyway? Believe us when we say that this baby can turn on you like a viper! Lazing around in your intestines, yeast is not a problem. Brewer's yeast used in the making of beer — not a problem. Baker's yeast necessary in the bread-making process — not a problem.

But when antibiotics kill off the natural Lactobacillus bacteria in your intestines, or when you eat a high sugar diet, yeast grows wild. It grows out of its boundaries in the large intestine and takes up residence in the small intestine. And just like a viper, it can poke holes in the lining of your small intestine, which can lead to a health problem commonly called *leaky gut syndrome* that we discuss in Chapter 3.

When it grows out of control in the intestines, yeast causes gas and bloating because it produces toxic gases. It can spread to the vagina and cause local burning, itching, and discharge. Moving up to the esophagus and mouth, it causes an oral yeast infection called *thrush*. (Thrush is commonly seen in newborn babies who catch a case of Candida from their mothers — either by traveling through the birth canal that is loaded with yeast or just by picking it up from their mothers' skin when breastfeeding.)

Yeast produces about 180 different toxins that are byproducts of its metabolic functions. Just think of all the urine, feces, sweat, expelled air, and expelled gases that humans produce. Yeast has its own excretions as well, and some of them are mighty nasty. Yeast even produces alcohol that can make you feel and act drunk even though you haven't touched a drop.

What can you do to avoid all these nasty effects?

- ✔ Avoid unnecessary antibiotics.
- ✔ Reduce the amount of sugar, wheat, and dairy you consume.
- ✔ Take a probiotic supplement or eat organic, sugar-free yogurt every day.
- ✔ Read Chapter 3 or visit www.yeastconnection.com for more information.

Reducing Chemical Exposure

In Chapter 4, we discuss chemical food additives, such as MSG and aspartame, and the 60,000 other chemicals in our environment. No, we don't list them all, but we make the point that many chemicals can irritate the bowel.

How much is too much?

Dr. Carolyn Dean wrote part of this chapter while in Rome at a meeting of Codex Alimentarius, the food standard-setting organization of the World Health Organization and Food and Agricultural Organization. Codex member nations had to decide on the level of cadmium that would be allowed in polished rice sold internationally.

Because it is widely known that there is contamination of heavy metals and chemicals in the environment, the question was not whether *any*

cadmium would be allowed, but *how much*. The developed nations asked for a level of .4 mg per kg of food, but several nations that have a high rice diet asked for a lower level — .2 mg per kg. The developed nations won. Some studies show that cadmium is toxic at .4 mg per kg, and others indicate it is safe at that level. There was no consideration of the cumulative health effects on individuals who consume dozens or even hundreds of chemicals in their daily diets.

The National Research Council says that "no toxic information is available for more than 80% of the chemicals in everyday-use products. Less than 20% have been tested for acute effects and less than 10% have been tested for chronic, reproductive or mutagenic effects." What does that mean? It means you'd be wise to limit your exposure to chemicals as much as possible.

Following are some chemical dangers you face in the kitchen:

- ✔ Ammonia is a basic ingredient of most household cleaners. When it's combined with bleach, a toxic brew called *chloramines* is formed.
- ✔ Also included in cleaning products is a poison called formaldehyde.
- ✔ Dish detergents contain naphthalene and phenol.
- ✔ Oven cleaners contain ammonia and lye.
- ✔ Air fresheners don't just cover up odors; they harbor pesticides and oils that coat nasal passages.

Unfortunately, the labeling required for household products does not reflect the danger involved with their use. However, nonchemical substitutes for household cleaners are available, including

- ✔ Vinegar or lemon juice in water, which cleans windows, sinks, and tubs
- ✔ Borax, which is a great laundry detergent
- ✔ Baking soda, an air freshener that people use in the fridge to absorb odors
- ✔ Sea salt, a natural scrubbing agent for ovens and stovetops

✔ Environmentally friendly laundry detergent, which doesn't cause static in your clothes (meaning you don't need to use fabric softener or chemical sheets in your dryer)

✔ Essential oils, such as lavender, which can be used in the dryer to give clothes a fresh scent. Just put a teaspoon on a facecloth and toss it in.

The best way to find nonchemical substitutes for cosmetics, toothpaste, and hair products is to look for ones that are labeled *organic.* That's the only way to be reasonably sure that something does not contain chemicals. You can also use kitchen cosmetics, which can be effective and much cheaper:

✔ Egg white and lemon juice makes a good face mask.

✔ Lemon juice helps fade age spots.

✔ Baking soda is a skin exfoliator.

✔ Avocado makes a rich face mask.

✔ You can use eggs and beer for hair care.

To reduce chemical exposure in the yard, try these nonchemical substitutes for controlling weeds and pests:

✔ Use dish detergent, cola, and beer on your lawn to keep down the weed population.

✔ Plant marigolds and basil to discourage mosquitoes and other bugs but encourage butterflies and dragonflies.

✔ Plant onion, chives, dill, garlic, and mint near plants that you want to protect from pests.

✔ Sprinkle powdered ginger or crushed eggshells to keep away slugs.

✔ Use sprays made from hot peppers or garlic to kill bugs.

✔ Use compost in your garden, which contains helpful bacteria and microorganisms.

✔ Pull weeds before they go to seed.

✔ Identify the pest or weed in your garden before taking drastic measures — it may be protecting your other plants.

Fending Off Family Predisposition

IBS is not passed on through the genes, but like many conditions, it can run in families. If genes aren't to blame, how does the condition get passed down? Here are some possibilities:

✔ Family members tend to eat the same type of diet, and some family members may develop allergies to frequently eaten foods.

✔ The problem may not actually be IBS:

• It may be gluten intolerance (celiac disease), which is inherited. As we explain in Chapter 2, folks with this disease cannot tolerate wheat, the prime source of gluten. Eating wheat results in several symptoms that are identical to IBS.

• It may be lactose intolerance, another cause of symptoms that can be mistaken for IBS. If someone who can't digest milk and milk products eats dairy, it can cause IBS symptoms; when dairy is stopped, so do the symptoms. Lactose intolerance is not a cause or a trigger of IBS; it is a disease unto itself. And it tends to run in families.

As we explain in Chapter 4, another thing that runs in families is the predisposition to illness itself. If parents suffer from chronic illness, their children can actually *learn* how to be ill. So don't go thinking your condition is set in stone until you determine whether it's real or just a bad habit.

What can you do to figure out if bad habits are to blame for your symptoms? Don't eat the same foods every day; get some variety in your life. To start,

✔ Don't eat toast, sandwiches, and dinner rolls every day. And look for wheat substitutes like rye, spelt, millet, rice, and sprouted-grain breads. Buy four loaves of bread, keep them in the freezer, and use a different one every day. That way your body doesn't become overloaded with any one grain.

✔ Don't drink cow's milk every day. Substitutes for cow's milk include almond milk, rice milk, and soy milk.

✔ Reduce your sugar consumption. Substitutes for sugar include fruit and fruit-juice sweetened confections. Also, *stevia* is a noncaloric, natural sweetener available in health food stores in powder and liquid form (see Chapter 10).

The cure for sugar addiction is to avoid it as much as possible for a week or two. After that time, it's very likely that you will no longer crave it. You may even find it much too sweet because your taste buds will have changed.

Eliminating Problem Foods

Food is a huge issue in IBS. The mere act of eating for some folks is torture. That's why it's important to know your food triggers and avoid them at all costs. We discuss food triggers in Chapter 4 and an IBS-friendly approach to finding your triggers in Chapter 10; we strongly suggest looking at those chapters for advice.

Our eating habits haven't always been what they are now. The food on the average dinner table today is light-years away from what people ate 100 years ago. For a farming family 100 years ago, venison, beef, pheasant, turkey, chicken, eggs, vegetables, butter, cream, and fruit were the daily fare. Today's diet is a combination of the menus of a dozen fast-food restaurants. Processed food laced with additives can't compare with fresh, organic home cooking. Intestines do know the difference.

Food allergies

If you have IBS symptoms, you may actually be suffering from a food allergy, even if you don't see outward signs like hives and a rash. As we explain in Chapter 2, the foods that seem to cause the most allergic reactions in the bowel are dairy and wheat.

What can you do if you suspect a specific food may be the culprit? Follow our avoidance and challenge diet, outlined in Chapter 10, to identify your own food allergies. Or ask your doctor about getting blood tests for food allergies.

Food intolerance

Some people discover that what appears to be IBS is actually an intolerance to lactose, gluten, or even fruit. These intolerances are real diseases, and medical tests are available to help diagnose them. The main test is called a *hydrogen breath test,* which we describe in Chapter 7. In a nutshell, when you eat something that your body doesn't digest, it becomes food for intestinal bacteria that produce excess hydrogen, which is measured by exhaling into a machine.

Food sensitivity

Food sensitivities are a bit more difficult to track down than allergies or intolerances. We know that people with IBS are sensitive to fats, spicy foods, and processed foods with a lot of additives. Again, we suggest following the avoidance and challenge diet in Chapter 10 to see what you can tolerate. And if you can't tolerate a particular food, it's best to avoid it entirely.

For example, we've heard cases of people who can't eat salmon without having diarrhea. It's such a fatty fish (rich in omega-3 fatty acids) that some people are just not able to stomach it.

Focusing on Food Habits

Sometimes it's not *what* you eat but *how* you eat that can save you a lot of aggravation and IBS upset. Here are some tips:

- ✔ Eat small meals so your stomach and intestines don't get physically stretched, which can trigger IBS. Small meals also allow your digestive juices to work properly.

- ✔ Chew your food well to help with the digestive process.

- ✔ If you have an important date or meeting, eat only foods that you know are safe for you.

- ✔ Don't eat when you are under severe stress.

- ✔ Don't drink liquids with your meals; doing so pushes food rapidly past its digestive functions.

- ✔ Don't drink carbonated beverages because they can cause gas.

- ✔ Don't drink alcohol.

- ✔ Don't drink caffeine. You may be able to substitute grain coffee for your regular coffee, but test it out first to make sure it doesn't cause symptoms.

- ✔ Don't eat late at night.

Perhaps what you really need to get your IBS under control is a trip to Italy. Dr. Carolyn Dean spent two weeks in Rome and found that her intestines (which are sensitive to wheat and dairy in North America) behaved themselves remarkably well in Rome when she finally indulged in the delicious bread, pizza, pasta, and cheese. The explanation for this reaction — or lack of reaction — is that Italian bread is fresh baked every day, does not contain preservatives, and has far fewer additives than North American varieties. The same can be said for cheeses; they are not pasteurized and processed to the same extent. How can you translate an Italian experience to your own home? Make your own bread from organic flour, and buy Italian cheeses!

Balancing Blood Sugar

We talk about the need to keep your blood sugar in balance in Chapter 4. If it goes too high or too low, the reactions in the body are swift and can affect the intestines. The most noticeable reaction is when your blood sugar falls below a certain level. Low blood sugar can occur when you haven't eaten for many hours or after an episode of high blood sugar (perhaps caused by drinking a couple cans of soda, which contain about 10 teaspoons of sugar each).

How does high blood sugar lead to low blood sugar? Your body wants only about 2 teaspoons of sugar in the blood at any one time. If you consume too much sugar, the alarms are sounded to clear that excess sugar out. If that job is done too well, your blood sugar can fall too far, which sets off another set of alarms (similar to the fight-or-flight response) that floods the body with adrenaline.

Part of a fight-or-flight response is to shut down the bowels, because the last thing you want to do when being chased by a saber-toothed tiger is take a trip to the bathroom. However, the sensitive intestines of someone with IBS can interpret this shutdown as a spasm, which means an IBS attack is on the way.

Fighting Infections

Okay, we're breaking our own rules here. Infection can actually be a *cause* of IBS — which, as we explain in Chapter 2, is very different from a trigger. But we wanted to put this item in this chapter to remind you to avoid gastrointestinal infections at all costs and to make sure that you take probiotics if you have an infection (or if you have to take an antibiotic).

Most researchers think that gut infections that lead to IBS in some people are mostly caused by bacteria, but they could also be caused by viruses, parasites, or yeast. Or you could experience a combination of infections!

Earlier in the chapter, we discuss the problems that an overgrowth of yeast can cause and how to try to avoid it. But viral, bacterial, and parasitic infections come at us from the outside environment, and we should also know both how to prevent them and how to treat them if they occur.

Food poisoning, contamination, or infection

Food poisoning is a huge concern because any source of food can harbor bacteria. Food technologists estimate that between 24 and 81 million cases of food-borne diarrhea occur annually in the United States. (The estimated range is wide because mild cases go unreported and may be mistaken for viral flu.)

The cost of these misadventures in the United States is between $5 billion and $17 billion in medical care and lost productivity. Researchers advise that most cases of food poisoning could be avoided by proper food handling, which includes proper hygiene, packaging, storage, transportation, preparation, and serving — including washing your own hands.

Thousands of bacteria can make our lives miserable with food poisoning, but fewer than 20 actually are the main culprits, including E-coli, shigella, salmonella, campylobacter, and Staph aureus.

And bacteria aren't the only sources of food poisoning; viruses can be passed through body secretions into food. (The classic example is saliva from a misdirected spit or blood from a cut on the hands of a food worker making its way into your salad.) Hepatitis A is a viral infection transmitted in this way.

Parasitic bowel infections are often diagnosed when diarrhea doesn't clear after a week or ten days. At that time, a doctor orders a test for parasites and eggs in the stool and, if the test is positive, prescribes the appropriate drug.

Following are the main symptoms of food poisoning:

- ✔ Diarrhea
- ✔ Fever
- ✔ Headaches
- ✔ Nausea with or without vomiting
- ✔ Stomach cramps

Food poisoning symptoms can show up within minutes or hours of eating food that contains bacterial toxins. However, infection from ingesting live bacteria, viruses, or parasites may take three to five days to appear. The duration of symptoms runs from one to five days. Some people who are infected may not even show any symptoms. (Perhaps people whose intestines are already vulnerable experience the most symptoms.)

The best treatment is to *do nothing*. Eat nothing; just replace your fluids. Especially don't take Imodium to stop the diarrhea, because the diarrhea is trying to flush out the bacteria and toxins from your intestines.

Raw and undercooked foods are the biggest culprits for food poisoning. That means raw meat and fish, but raw fruit and vegetables are also suspect. Here are the best ways to avoid getting (or giving!) food poisoning:

- ✔ Thoroughly wash your hands, utensils, cutting boards, and food processors before and after you prepare food.
- ✔ Use paper towels instead of sponges, which are ideal places for germs to collect.
- ✔ Regularly pour boiling water down your drain, which can harbor super bugs that have grown resistant to antibiotics used in beef and poultry farms.

 ✔ Bacteria make a beeline for foods containing dairy, eggs, meat, poultry, and fish, possibly because they are rich in nutrients. Keep these food refrigerated until it's time to prepare them; don't let them get to room temperature.

 ✔ Store different foods separately. Don't put raw food in with cooked food or leftover food into a container of frozen food.

 ✔ As long as they don't trigger your IBS symptoms, eat acidic foods (like citrus fruits and tomatoes), which are repellent to bacteria and therefore don't harbor their growth.

The best defense against bowel infection is good hygiene. Your mother wasn't kidding when she said you would get a horrible disease if you didn't wash your hands! We don't suggest that you become obsessive about cleanliness, but it's important to know where your hands have been at all times. If they were poking around in something that you wouldn't want to eat, then don't think of picking your teeth or your nose with those dirty fingers.

One other very interesting tip is that washing your hands with cold water may be more effective than hot water because bacteria respond to heat by growing. Yes, washing in scalding hot water kills germs, but it also gives you a second-degree burn!

Travel tips

As we note in Chapter 2, many people suffer intestinal infections when they travel. So it's especially important to protect yourself in this situation.

When traveling, to avoid the local intestinal flora and fauna, take grapefruit seed capsules. These capsules contain a very bitter potion ground out of grapefruit seeds that is toxic to bugs. If you happen to eat a local beastie in your soup or salad, swallowing a couple capsules of grapefruit seed extract, also called *citricidal,* will do a homicidal number on those critters.

Also, avoid drinking the local water and eating anything that may have been washed in the local water. And take probiotic supplements (see Chapter 9) to help build up the good bacteria in the intestines to crowd out yeast and bad bacteria.

Considering the Role of Hormones

Because more than 80 percent of IBS sufferers are women, we have to take a serious look at hormones as a trigger of IBS (see Chapter 5). Obviously, you can't just get rid of your hormones, but if you're female you need to know that your most vulnerable time is around your period. You also need to know that PMS and IBS are two S's that hang together. That's not such a great thing, but knowing it can help you plan your months.

On the bright side, you should know that when your hormones go on holiday around menopause, you will not be so affected by IBS. (And, of course, PMS will be only a bad memory.) While other women are moaning about growing older, you'll be looking on the bright side!

Getting a Grip on Stress

Often, the onset of IBS as a chronic condition can be traced to an emotional upset or trauma, like a death in the family or a divorce. In Chapter 14, we discuss the connection between work-related stress and IBS. In Chapter 5, we point out that physical and sexual abuse are important issues in some cases of IBS, as are a death in the family and the emotional rollercoaster of divorce. Even the stress caused by the humiliating experience of soiling your pants in childhood could lead to a history of bowel problems.

We try to make the point throughout the book that stress is not the predominant *cause* of IBS because we know IBS is not a psychological condition. But you can see how intertwined IBS and stress really are. When you have a sensitive gut and add on stressful events, you can really escalate your symptoms.

In several chapters, especially Chapter 12, we offer tools to help relieve stress, including the stress of having IBS. Self-hypnosis, the Emotional Freedom Techniques, and the relaxation response are all important tools that you can learn easily and adopt into a self-help program.

Chapter 18

Ten Things to Do for IBS

In This Chapter
▶ Being responsible for your body and attitude
▶ Changing your eating and exercise habits
▶ Taking control of stress

*I*f you've read even a couple chapters of this book so far, it's probably obvious to you that we feel diet and lifestyle are the most important aspects of treating IBS. Just consider that IBS really didn't exist 100 years ago. Then ask, "What has happened in our society during the past century that is twisting up our intestines?"

We say it's a combination of bad diet, processed foods, lack of exercise, and massive accumulation of stress with no outlets and few tools to deal with all the above.

We give you lots of tools in this book to help address all these issues. In this chapter, we offer a handy summary.

Taking Charge of Your Body

We can't stress enough that IBS is a medical condition, but it's under *your* guidance and control. The more information you have, the better you will be able to take care of yourself. This is a condition that you experience and you manage; it does not necessarily require ongoing intervention by a doctor. (In the next section, we discuss where your doctor fits into the picture.)

A doctor may not have the time to explain to you the elimination and challenge diet (see Chapter 10), which is key to finding out what's triggering your sensitive gut. A doctor may not know about Emotional Freedom Techniques, the self-administered therapy we discuss in Chapter 12. Neither can a doctor be there with you every day when you choose what foods to eat. Only *you* can make those good food choices and lifestyle decisions.

Working with a Knowledgeable Doctor

While finding a caring doctor is important, you *must* work with a doctor who is knowledgeable about IBS. To rule out inflammatory bowel disease (IBD) and other masquerading conditions, to diagnose IBS, and to identify the possible causes and triggers of your symptoms, you need a doctor who knows what tests to conduct for IBS (which we discuss in Chapter 20) and how to apply them to your case.

We think of a relationship with a doctor as being a partnership. Your doctor has gone to medical school and maybe done specialty training, spending up to a decade learning about the human body. However, you have had a lifetime of experience with your own body. Your doctor needs to listen to your specific symptoms and concerns. Then, together, you can decide what's best.

IBS is not a defined disease with a clear-cut treatment protocol like a wound that needs to be stitched up and bandaged. IBS is a condition that affects every individual differently. Treating it otherwise is a recipe for disaster. Treating it properly with diet, exercise, stress management techniques, and a good attitude is a recipe for success.

Developing a Good Attitude

We all have something that we deal with in life. Whether the issues are physical, emotional, material, or whatever, we all must learn how to cope with life. If you can look at IBS as an opportunity to learn about your body and how to overcome obstacles, you come out on top.

If you have a positive perspective about your illness, you can see it as an adventure, a kind of cosmic test of your patience and endurance. And thinking of it that way — putting your condition in that frame of reference — can go a long way to helping you cope with this adventure. Is your glass half full or half empty? Only you can decide.

One thing we know is true: You are the master of your body. Nobody knows your body better than you do, and if someone says otherwise they are telling a big fib. Paying attention to your body is very important for dealing with IBS. It's also important not to beat yourself up if you have a bad day or even a bad week.

In both our practices, we have seen people with severe health problems who somehow manage to see their problems as challenges. We've all heard stories of people surviving horrendous ordeals and saying that they wouldn't be who they are today if they hadn't gone through all that suffering and pain. These people are the inspiration you need when you are faced with IBS. You have a chronic condition, and many people share the same symptoms and the same agonies that you do. Many of them get through it and become better people.

Listening to Your Body

People with IBS are sensitive folks. You have a sensitive gut that tells you immediately if something is not right. Usually, it's a food that's not right, but that sensitivity also spills over into other aspects of life.

When people say they have a *gut instinct* about this person or that situation, they are relying on the hormonal orchestra in the gut that doubles as our intuition. They go into a room, and it just doesn't feel right. They catch someone's eye and know that person is hiding something. Many women have this gut instinct in a big way. We know when our kids or partners are trying to pull a fast one. We walk into a situation and immediately put our finger on a problem that people are trying very hard to cover up. We feel it in our guts.

If you have IBS, you can put your sensitive gut to good use by paying attention to your gut instinct. How many times have you said to yourself, "I knew I shouldn't have eaten that pastry/chili sauce/ice cream!" From now on, remind yourself that your gut instinct is giving you clues to pay attention to. When it tells you what's good for you to eat and what's bad, you have begun to win the battle with IBS.

Developing a Healing Diet

Call it a top ten list within a top ten list; following are ten good diet habits to follow for eliminating IBS:

 ✔ **Keep a food diary and go on an elimination and challenge diet to learn your triggers (see Chapter 10).**

 ✔ **Drink herbal teas.** Peppermint and chamomile are your best choices.

- ✓ **Eat vegetables.** Avocados, beets, carrots, chestnuts, parsnips, potatoes, squash, sweet potatoes, turnips, and yams are the best because of their soluble fiber content.

- ✓ **Eat fruit sparingly.** Stick to apples and pears and only one or two a day.

- ✓ **Eat whole grains.** Quinoa, rice, corn, and barley are the best because they have the most soluble fiber.

- ✓ **Focus on soluble fiber.** You find it in rice, pasta, sourdough bread, sweet potatoes, potatoes, parsnips, applesauce, banana, and papaya.

- ✓ **Eat kefir and yogurt.** The beneficial bacteria they contain are very valuable for your gut. (However, people with severe lactose intolerance may not be able to tolerate even kefir or yogurt.)

- ✓ **Eat small frequent meals, avoiding large ones.** Stretching the stomach can lead to reflex activity all along the intestinal tract.

- ✓ **Drink plenty of water, especially if you are eating high fiber foods.** For either diarrhea or constipation, you need lots of water.

- ✓ **Eat less spicy food.** For some people, spicy food is a distinct intestinal irritant.

Exercising for Health

As we note earlier in the book, if exercise were available in pill form, the manufacturer would make billions because it has such beneficial effects. The problem with exercise is that you have to do it and do it regularly. It's not like housework, which you can pay someone to do. We all know we should do it, but it's usually the last thing on our "to do" list.

We recommend that you start small. Breathing — yes, simply breathing — can be good exercise. Taking three deep breaths is the way most relaxation programs start, and taking lots of deep breaths is common in most forms of exercise. After you've taken some breaths, consider these simple options:

- ✓ Take a short walk around the block and enjoy yourself.
- ✓ Put on some upbeat music and dance around the house.

When you get your blood moving and your muscles singing, you will begin to feel the benefits within a short time.

We list several forms of exercise in Chapter 11, but it doesn't matter what you do as long as you get moving. Thirty minutes daily does the trick.

Taking Supplements

Dietary supplements come in many shapes and sizes, and sometimes they come with a lot of other binders and fillers that your bowel may not like. With added ingredients like wheat, yeast, lactose, colors, flavors, and even aspartame, they can start causing problems before the supplement can even go to work. Fortunately, many natural supplements are available in your health food store that contain none of the above, and their labels say so.

It's important to read labels and see what's hidden behind the shiny coating. Capsules are usually safer to take because the powder is just stuffed in the capsule; the manufacturer doesn't have to hold it together with something that acts like glue, as happens with a tablet.

Herbs

In Chapter 9, we discuss herbs that may be helpful for controlling your IBS symptoms. Liquid herbal tinctures are even better absorbed than capsules. However, they are usually in a strong alcohol base, which may itself irritate the bowel. But it's easy enough to put your dropperful of tincture in a few ounces of warm water and drink it after a few minutes when the alcohol evaporates.

Another important consideration is to try to use organic or wild crafted herbs so you are sure they are not sprayed with herbicides or pesticides. We know people who get scratchy throats and irritated tongues when they eat sprayed fruit. Imagine how easily that scratchiness and irritation can extend down into the intestines.

Probiotics

Also in Chapter 9, we discuss the benefits of taking *probiotics* — good bacteria. Probiotics help heal the underlying cause of both constipation and diarrhea. Lactobacillus acidophilus is the most important good bacteria in the gut. It is found naturally in some forms of yogurt and is the most common bacteria in the large intestine. It has the special ability to break down sugar into lactic acid, which acts as a protective barrier in the intestinal lining and the vagina against yeast. Lactobacillus not only produces lactic acid, but by using sugar as its food source it is able to snatch sugar out of the greedy grasp of yeast organisms as another way of keeping them under control.

Probiotics are important to take on a daily basis. You can eat yogurt regularly to obtain live cultures of beneficial organisms. Plain, organic yogurt without sugar is the best kind to buy. Because it's organic, it doesn't contain antibiotic or hormone residues; therefore, it is the best yogurt for people with yeast problems. (It's also the best form of yogurt to use as a vaginal douche or to apply externally; a dab or two at night can build up the Lactobacillus you need to create the lactic acid that protects against yeast.)

In a study conducted by Vesna Skul, MD, assistant professor of medicine at Rush Medical College of Rush University and medical director of Rush Center for Women's Medicine in Chicago, women with recurring yeast infections who ate yogurt every day had fewer yeast infections. In other studies, women also had fewer urinary tract infections when eating yogurt daily.

Stonyfield Farm is the brand we recommend because it makes a plain, organic, non-sugar product, and it guarantees six different live bacterial cultures, including Lactobacillus acidophilus. The company's research indicates that probiotics enhance digestion, improve absorption of nutrients, increase the body's natural defenses, and inhibit disease-producing organisms.

If you can't eat dairy but still need probiotics, there are many different varieties of products available. We use brands that contain Lactobacillus acidophilus from Natren and Seroyal. One product you may want to consider is Seroyal HMF Forte. (*HMF* stands for "human microflora.") This product, grown from human Lactobacillus, was created by Dr. Nigel Plummer, who is constantly doing research to prove that HMF is able to actually stick to the human gut wall and replace the good bacteria. Nonhuman microflora may not attach as well or give the same beneficial effects.

Enzymes

Digestive enzymes are found in the body and also on the shelves of pharmacies and health food stores. People with IBS benefit from them because they can help digest your meals. But start with the milder forms of enzymes made from papaya and watch out for ones containing hydrochloric acid that may irritate a sensitive gut.

Incompletely digested foods end up in the intestines as fodder for yeast and bad bacteria. Undigested food can also be absorbed through a leaky gut and cause allergic reactions. See Chapter 3 for more on leaky gut.

De-stressing Your Life

There are many ways to de-stress, but just as with exercise, you have to practice them to get the benefits:

- ✔ **Meditation:** Something as simple as closing your eyes and counting your breaths can sometimes be enough to drop your stress levels. Your heart rate drops, your breathing rate slows down, and the tension in your body eases.

- ✔ **Counting to ten:** This is a time-out tool that you can use whenever you feel your anxiety and tension levels rising. It's also a great tool to use if you think your tension is going to make you blow up at someone.

- ✔ **Emotional Freedom Techniques (EFT):** This is an easy, useful tool that involves tapping on acupuncture points in order to remove energy blocks and emotional blocks. You can read about this technique in Chapter 12.

- ✔ **Laugh therapy:** This therapy is very easy to practice. When you rent movies, get comedies. When you read, stick to the funny stuff. The endorphins produced when you laugh are actually therapeutic.

Starting a Support Group

Obviously, you can join an existing support group if you find one that suits your needs. But if none is available, start your own.

Don't be turned off by the notion of a group of 100 people coming to your house every Tuesday night. Start small. Maybe your first support group will consist of your spouse or partner, your best friend, a coworker, and/or your sister. But as you spread the word, more people with IBS and their support people will join. (Some groups are limited to only people with IBS, and others are more open.) You can also join or start an online IBS support group, which we discuss in Chapters 13 and 16.

Whether live or virtual, everyone needs someone to complain to who will listen. But you have to start with a set of rules. If you just want to be listened to and don't want advice, make that clear from the beginning. Most people are problem-solvers, and if you tell them you have a problem, the human brain goes right to work trying to solve the problem for you. They tell you what doctor to see, what to eat, and what worked for them or their Aunt Minnie. You will be inundated with advice that you may not want. Some of it may strike pay dirt, but often it's distracting if you just want to complain a bit and then move on.

Planning Your Next Move

When you have a condition like IBS, taking charge of it requires planning — lots and lots of planning. You have to plan where you are going and how you are going to get there without having an accident. Gastrointestinal doctors tell stories about patients who have all their travel routes mapped out with all the public washrooms memorized.

It's also important to plan what to eat when you go out. Very often, you have to bring your own healthy snacks so you don't end up eating something that your tummy can't handle. Also, most people learn the hard way not to eat bad foods before an important event.

We're not saying that all this planning ever becomes easy. In fact, it's one of the hardest things to do. When you leave home, you are not really thinking of your next meal. You aren't hungry, and it's just not a priority. However, in a couple of hours, there you are in the middle of a mall or downtown and you are starving and the only restaurants to choose from serve everything fried in gallons of grease.

Sometimes you may kid yourself and think, "I need a treat. I just want to be able to eat what I want." So you plunk down your money and walk away with fish and chips or chicken fingers. But within a few minutes, you are regretting your decision. The only way out of this type of bind is to always carry a healthy snack with you and realize how much better you are going to feel after your snack than after food that tastes like fried cardboard.

Chapter 19

Ten Things to Avoid When You Have IBS

T his chapter is a list of things that don't get along well with IBS. We explain why they cause problems, and we hope we inspire you to avoid them at all costs.

Abstaining from Alcohol

No formal studies have been conducted to prove whether you can drink alcohol if you have IBS. But alcohol has important effects on the gastrointestinal tract, the liver, the brain, and the rest of the body, so we can make a pretty educated guess about what it does to someone with IBS.

Anyone who has been to a high school dance or a college frat party knows what alcohol does to the GI tract. Imbibing too much has the direct consequences of nausea, vomiting, diarrhea, and, in severe cases, GI bleeding. You may be thinking, "But I don't drink that much! One glass of wine shouldn't be a problem." Well, if you have IBS and know you have a sensitive GI tract, any amount of alcohol may be too much for you.

Alcohol is a major distraction for the liver. Under normal conditions, the liver is intent on filtering blood, making hormones, storing glucose for a rainy day, and a thousand other things. But when you drink alcohol, the liver must direct its energy to detoxifying this poison. When it does this (by revving up the enzyme called *alcohol dehydrogenase*), it stops doing many other more important things. By *not* drinking, you save your liver a lot of overtime. Excessive alcohol intake results in the buildup of fats in the liver, creating a fatty liver that destroys normal liver tissue.

And if being kind to your liver isn't enough incentive to avoid alcohol, consider that several medications prescribed for gastrointestinal conditions may react unfavorably with alcoholic drinks:

- Antidepressants used in modest doses for slowing down bowel movements are known to interact with alcohol, causing drowsiness, lack of concentration, and poor judgment.

- Flagyl used for GI infections is a very powerful drug that, on its own, can cause stomach upset and cramps, vomiting, headache, sweating, and flushing. Mixed with alcohol, the symptoms are intense, including relentless nausea, vomiting, and headache.

- Aspirin used for pain causes microscopic bleeding in the stomach. Alcohol mixed with aspirin makes stomach bleeding and stomach irritation much worse.

- Opiates used for pain control can cause diminished alertness and judgment, as well as reduction in brain function, which are made even worse in the presence of alcohol.

- Nonsteroidal anti-inflammatory drugs (NSAIDs) used for pain control can produce stomach irritation and possible liver damage that is worsened with alcohol use.

Crushing Out Cigarettes

Do you remember the first time you tried one of your dad's cigarettes? Chances are you got a woozy head, nausea, and a horrible taste in your mouth — you probably just wanted to throw up. Guess what? The nicotine in tobacco is an *emetic,* a substance that makes you throw up. It does this by irritating the stomach and intestines. That's not what you want if you have IBS.

Some research suggests that smoking may decrease blood flow to the intestines or trigger a response in the immune system. Either one of these effects can result in the aggravation of IBS.

The GI effects of smoking begin with bad breath and continue into the esophagus, where it causes heartburn. The valve between the esophagus and stomach is weakened by smoking, allowing acidic stomach contents to travel up into the esophagus and damage its tissues. The liver is also negatively affected by smoking because, as we mention in the previous section, the liver is charged with filtering out toxins — and cigarette smoke has hundreds of them.

Smoking is also known to cause ulcerations in the GI tract, first in the stomach and then in the duodenum. Smoking reduces the amount of bicarbonate from the pancreas and increases the concentration of stomach acid escaping from the stomach into the duodenum. If smoking can cause ulceration, it can certainly create an irritation of the intestines that can trigger symptoms of IBS.

Reducing Sugar

Some IBS diets insist that sugar is not a trigger for IBS symptoms, but we aren't so sure. There are three main reasons for thinking sugar is not our friend when it comes to IBS:

- **Candida:** Candida is another name for yeast and is one of the bad guys. We talk about yeast overgrowth in Chapters 4 and 17, and we warn that sugar is the best-loved food of yeast. Some people have been known to overeat sugar to such an extent that they produce alcohol from the yeast in their intestines and appear drunk. What they experience is actually called *drunken syndrome* in Japan, and it's a real disease. (Dr. William Crook writes about it in his book *The Yeast Connection,* published by Vintage.)

  We discuss in Chapters 3 and 17 how yeast can create a leaky gut by irritating the GI lining. In some people, that irritation can be enough to cause symptoms of IBS. It also serves as a vehicle for toxins from yeast and abnormal bacteria to get into the bloodstream and cause widespread symptoms.

- **Sorbitol:** Sorbitol is a sugar alcohol that is used in processed food as a so-called natural sweetener. However, for some people with IBS, it can be a gut irritant that leads to diarrhea. Simply chewing a stick of gum with sorbitol can cause symptoms.

- **Fruit sugar:** Fruit sugar, also called *fructose,* sounds safe enough. But especially when it comes in large amounts as high fructose corn syrup, it can have a negative impact on people with IBS. It does all the things that simple table sugar does, but because it hides behind the label "fruit," many people don't know that it can trigger yeast overgrowth. (Fructose is also implicated in the current epidemics of obesity and diabetes.)

Getting Off the Couch

If you think that the advice in this and other chapters is designed just to make you healthier, you're right! We really want to help you stop your nasty lifestyle habits. Obviously, anyone can benefit from a healthy lifestyle, but people with IBS get extra bonuses.

So what, exactly, do we mean by "getting off the couch"? Here's what we want you to do:

- Stop being a couch potato.

- Get up and exercise — start simply (with walking, perhaps) and work up to something more intense (like yoga). See Chapter 11 for lots of ideas.

- Stop eating couch potato foods.

- Exercise your cooking skills in the kitchen and make some home-made food.

- Join a community-supported agriculture (CSA) and eat organic vegetables.

Leaving Large Meals Alone

The more you eat at one sitting, the more likely you are to eat a variety of foods. Sometimes different foods don't mix and match very well in an IBS stomach. As we explain in Chapter 3, different foods compete for the stomach acid, pancreatic enzymes, and bile salts. The whole conglomeration creates gas and fermentation as everything is mixed together, and bacteria make the undigested food their next meal.

Then there is the sheer bulk of the food itself that triggers a lot of unnecessary gut activity. Stretching of the stomach and the various sphincters sends messages of urgency down the entire intestinal tract.

Small frequent meals and snacks seem to be the way to deliver just the right amount of food to the intestines.

Forgetting Fatty Foods

Fried foods soak up too much fat for an IBS stomach to handle. For some people, fatty fish like salmon can even be too much to handle, no matter how it's prepared. And cookies and cakes are usually laden with lard. But the worst fatty food may be ice cream because it has fat, dairy, and sugar all combined in one gooey mess.

Other fats are hidden in packaged and processed foods that claim to be sugar-free. You'll find that fat-free products tend to be loaded with sugar and sugar-free products tend to be loaded with fat. We have to have one or the other to satisfy our junk food addiction.

Some people who have trouble digesting fat must go so far as to stop eating meat, egg yolks, and dairy. We encourage you to look at the elimination and challenge diet in Chapter 10, which can help you determine which foods work for you and which don't.

We're not talking about the dangers of cholesterol when we speak of fat aggravating IBS. Instead, the problem is the way fat stimulates the muscles of the intestines to become more active and the various GI sphincters to open, propelling intestinal contents. It's a very strong reflex, and it's best to give it only minimal stimulation.

Leaving Aspartame Behind

Aspartame is an artificial sweetener found in thousands of diet products. It's produced by combining two neurotransmitters — aspartate and phenylalanine — with wood alcohol (methanol). These elements don't remain together for very long when aspartame hits the small intestine. In the presence of an enzyme called *chymotrypsin,* methanol is broken free of the aspartame molecule.

Actually, methanol can be released from aspartame even before it is ingested. When aspartame products are heated above 86°F, methanol is released. When that product is eaten or drunk, methanol is absorbed directly into the bloodstream.

So, what's wrong with having a little methanol in your system? This chemical, when not in normal foods where it is neutralized, can break down into formic acid and formaldehyde — and it's a serious neurotoxin. Formaldehyde, which is used to preserve dead bodies, is a deadly nerve toxin that accumulates in the body because it's not excreted very quickly. Research indicates that the most methanol you should consume in one day is 7.8 milligrams. However, one liter of diet soda contains about 56 milligrams of methanol.

Methanol causes GI symptoms, as well as headaches, ringing in the ears, dizziness, nausea, weakness, vertigo, chills, memory lapses, numbness and shooting pains in the extremities, behavioral disturbances, and nerve inflammation. However, the most common symptom of methanol poisoning is vision problems, including misty vision, progressive contraction of visual fields, blurring of vision, obscuration of vision, retinal damage, and blindness.

Cutting Back On Medications

Earlier in the book, we tell a story about a woman with IBS who tried a sample of a drug that was designed to treat IBS. Unfortunately, it contained lactose, which completely upset her stomach. Natural dietary supplements often have labels that guarantee they don't contain sugar, wheat, corn, or dairy. However, drug companies don't seem to take into consideration the possibility of food sensitivities when they make their products.

That's one reason to cut back on medications. Another reason is the sheer toxicity of many drugs, which makes them inherently irritating to the intestines. The nonsteroidal anti-inflammatories (NSAIDs), for example, cause so much GI irritation that their major side effect is GI bleeding. Most people are told to take antacids when they have to take NSAIDs. Even aspirin causes small amounts of stomach and intestinal bleeding and is irritating to the gut.

To find out if the medications you are taking cause GI irritation, search your drugs on the Internet for side effects. Or ask your pharmacist for a peek at the CPS drug book and look them up.

If you take a prescription medication, don't stop taking it without discussing it with your doctor. Go to your doctor armed with information on side effects, and talk about reducing the amount you are taking or ask for alternatives. Sometimes stopping medications cold turkey can result in a rebound reaction of more symptoms, whereas slowly reducing them is much easier for the body to tolerate.

Releasing Anger

Throughout this book, we discuss the complex relationship between stress and IBS. The simple take-home point is that stress is bad for IBS, and you need to avoid it at all costs. But how? One way is to work on not letting yourself get worked up when bad things happen. Believe it or not, it *is* possible to avoid getting angry. Here are some suggestions:

- Count to ten when you feel the steam rising — before it drops down into your gut.
- Take several deep breaths for the same reason.
- Try singing the speech you have stored up for your boss, spouse, or child. Even if you don't get to deliver it to the intended recipient, we guarantee singing it will make you laugh and break through the cloud of anger.

If your anger is a consistent problem, try to find out why. Sit with a journal and write out the reasons. Here are some possibilities:

✔ I'm really angry that I'm stuck with a chronic disease.

✔ I'm even more angry that doctors can't help me.

✔ It frustrates me that I have a disease that has no cure.

✔ I'm livid that I have no control over my life; my bowel is in control.

✔ It really bugs me that other people seem to live such a carefree life and I have to dance around my sensitivities.

✔ I'm really mad that I can't eat what I want, go out when I want, and party like most people my age.

These are valid grievances for someone with IBS, and these hot embers of anger may be burning up your guts. Some people torture themselves with being mad about things over which they have little control, and it eats them up inside.

If this is happening to you, write down what's bugging you and get it off your chest and off your gut. In the bright light of day, when these things are written down in black and white, you will slowly be able to resolve some of them.

One exercise to try is to list a sore point and then make a column of pros and cons. For example, if you are really irked that your best friend lives a carefree life and you don't, make a list of what you envy about her life. Then, make a list of ways her life isn't so carefree. Often, this exercise helps you to realize that other people have just as many problems and challenges as you do. It levels the playing field a bit and helps to elevate you out of the victim role that anger seems to create. You can make this pro and con list about anything that's bugging you.

Weeding Out Worry

The advice in the previous section about anger also applies to worry. If you're a worrier, write down reasons why. The list may start with all your concerns and fears about your IBS:

✔ Will I ever be normal?

✔ Will there ever be a cure?

✔ Will I get worse?

✔ What if I have cancer and not IBS?

✔ What if I have Crohn's disease or ulcerative colitis and not IBS?

These are all perfectly acceptable worries to have, but worrying about them won't do one bit of good for your health. Instead, the stress of worrying could make your symptoms even worse.

Psychologists often say that you attract what's uppermost in your mind. So if you spend a lot of time worrying about something, you may be giving your body the impression that you are asking for that thing that you fear — and *voilà,* you have it! No, life is not always that simple. But there is a lot of truth to the adage that you are living what you are thinking:

✔ Think positive thoughts, and you can live a more positive life.

✔ Think negative thoughts, and you can be living under a dark cloud.

In Chapter 12, we present tools to reduce stress, such as the Emotional Freedom Techniques (EFT), meditation, the relaxation response, and deep breathing. They all work equally well on worry.

Chapter 20

Ten Key Medical Tests for IBS

In Chapter 7, we discuss in detail what your doctor needs to do in order to get an accurate diagnosis of IBS. In this chapter, we present the key tests used to rule out conditions that can look like IBS. (Because IBS is not a structural disease, your doctor can't simply run one test and determine whether IBS is present or not.)

The first six tests we discuss are standard procedures done either by your general practitioner or a gastroenterologist. (Keep in mind that barium enemas and upper GI x-rays are not used as often as sigmoidoscopes or colonoscopes these days, but they are still used in areas where scopes are not readily available.) These tests help to differentiate IBS from the inflammatory bowel diseases (Crohn's and ulcerative colitis), and they also make sure there is no evidence of cancer.

The final four tests we present in this chapter help rule out food intolerances, food allergies, and bowel infections. Some of them are not yet used by most doctors, so we explain what they involve and how to contact a lab that conducts them.

Physical and Rectal Exam

Perhaps you find a physical exam to be a comforting reminder that someone is taking care of you. Or perhaps it's a nerve-wracking experience because you're afraid of what your doctor will find.

During a physical exam, your doctor is looking primarily for three things:

✔ Signs of anemia — a pale complexion, a lack of fine blood vessels in the whites of your eyes, or a pale tongue

✔ A white-coated tongue, which is an indication of yeast overgrowth

✔ Signs of vitamin deficiencies caused by malabsorption in gluten enteropathy (celiac disease) or chronic maldigestion

The physical exam is easy, but the rectal exam is not quite as pleasant. However, with enough lubrication and a gentle approach, it should not be too distressing. Your doctor does the rectal exam to find out whether you have hemorrhoids, especially if you have blood in your stool. Just try to relax: Remember that a doctor's finger is much narrower than the stool that passes through the anus.

Occult blood test

After doing a rectal examination and checking for hemorrhoids, lumps, or bumps on your prostate (if you're a man), your doctor will smear a gloved finger on a paper that is impregnated with a chemical that detects the presence of blood cells. If the test result is positive, it's a sign of bleeding in the intestines. This simple test can indicate that there is inflammation in the GI tract, a bleeding polyp, or hemorrhoids.

If the test result is positive, further tests can be done to find the source of the bleeding. These tests include a sigmoidoscopy to check for hemorrhoids, polyps, or tumors in the *sigmoid colon* (the last bit of colon before the rectum and anus). If that test doesn't give you a diagnosis, you will probably also have a colonoscopy. (We discuss both of these scope tests later in the chapter.)

Blood tests

No blood test is available to diagnose IBS, but blood tests are helpful for ruling out other conditions. As part of a regular physical exam, most doctors will perform a series of blood tests:

✔ **Complete blood count (CBC) and differential:** This test measures the amount of hemoglobin and white blood cells in your body. People with celiac disease tend to have anemia, which means they have low hemoglobin counts. If you have protein deficiency or zinc deficiency, you can have a low white cell count.

✔ **Chem screen:** This series of blood chemistry tests uncovers problems with liver and kidney function and electrolytes like sodium and potassium. People with IBS usually have a normal chem screen; if it is abnormal, your doctor will do more tests to find out why.

✔ **CA-125 test:** This test measures the level of a particular blood protein called *CA-125,* which may indicate ovarian cancer. Ovarian cancer has symptoms that can mimic IBS.

Pelvic Exam

If you're a woman, your family doctor may send you to a gynecologist to rule out a pelvic cause for your symptoms. The uterus, ovaries, and fallopian tubes are intermingled with the intestines in such a way that symptoms in one can make you feel like you have symptoms in the other.

A pelvic exam, vaginal swab, and pap test will rule out a vaginal infection and cervical changes that could indicate cancer. When your doctor does the internal exam, she can tell if your uterus is enlarged with fibroids or if there is a sign of enlarged ovaries or ovarian cysts.

Sometimes the pain and pressure from fibroids and ovarian cysts can affect the intestines, even to the point of causing diarrhea and pain. Also, ovarian cancer can sometimes have symptoms of diarrhea and weight loss.

Sigmoidoscopy and Colonoscopy

These are two separate tests, but we discuss them together because the technology is the same.

Sigmoidoscopy and colonoscopy are tests done using what's called an *endoscope* — an instrument that is used to peer into your private parts. (No orifice goes untapped in the hunt for the cause of your symptoms!) An endoscope is a flexible tube with a mini camera at the end. After thorough lubrication, the tube is inserted into your anus. A medium-length tube is used to view the sigmoid region of your colon (the region just above your anus and rectum; see Chapter 3). A much longer tube is used to view the entire colon in colonoscopy.

Your doctor works the controls of the endoscope like a virtual reality game, viewing the action on a screen and moving the camera in on suspect sites. He can even extend a pair of scissors that can snip off samples of tissue. If the doctor finds polyps, which are usually benign outgrowths of the intestinal wall, he can snip them off at their base.

These procedures help rule out the three big C's: cancer, Crohn's disease, and (ulcerative) colitis.

During either type of endoscopy, your doctor is looking for several things: polyps, *diverticuli* (weak, tiny outpouchings of the wall of the intestine that can get filled with debris and become inflamed and infected), ulcerations, and tumors. He is also looking at the lining of the intestines to determine if it looks healthy or not, whether there seems to be equal blood flow to all sections of the colon, and (by using samples from the intestinal debris that remains after thorough purging) whether there is infection or abnormal bowel flora.

To have an endoscopy, you must have a near squeaky clean colon. In order for this procedure to be of benefit, the walls of the intestine must be nearly free from debris. This is accomplished by taking a powerful laxative drink the night before you have your procedure. These procedures are usually sched-uled for first thing in the morning because you aren't allowed to eat before them either.

The endoscopy procedure itself isn't painful, but even the thought of it may make you cringe. Your doctor will likely offer you a bit of relaxing medication. That, combined with a sensitive practitioner, can make the procedure fly by quickly and easily. The sigmoidoscopy lasts only a few minutes, and the colonoscopy is usually done in less than 30 minutes.

At the end of the procedure, your doctor doesn't have to wait for the results. He will probably know immediately whether your colon is healthy or not. However, the specialist doing the procedure may want to send the results to your doctor, who will then give them to you. This formality is not done to frustrate you; your family doctor will give you advice based on the special-ist's advice and will then follow your progress.

Barium Enema

Before endoscopes were invented, x-rays of the intestines coated with barium chalk were all the rage. These days, they are relied on less and less. However, in areas where a specialist who performs endoscopies isn't available, these x-rays can help find polyps, diverticuli, ulcerations, and tumors.

To prepare for a barium enema, you must scrub your colon clean with a strong laxative the night before and arrive for a morning appointment. (You can't eat breakfast.) A well-lubricated tube is inserted through the anus into the rectum, and you are given an enema using a liquid metal called *barium sulphate*. It's white and shiny in your intestines and creates an extreme contrast with your intestines, which show up black or gray on x-ray. Several abdominal x-rays are taken in various positions. If you have ulcers or tumors in the lining of your intestines, they are outlined by the white material and stand out.

You may be given a light sedative to relax you, but you are awake throughout the barium enema procedure. You may feel the pressure of liquid going into your intestines, but you shouldn't feel any pain.

Some people say the time it takes to perform a barium enema from start to finish is around two hours. But it could be more or less depending on how fast your intestines fill up with the barium liquid and how many x-rays need to be taken.

Upper GI Series

As with the barium enema, this test isn't used as frequently as it was before endoscopes were invented. But to specifically rule out Crohn's disease in the small intestine, an *upper GI x-ray with small bowel follow-through* may be used. You swallow a tall glass of chalky barium liquid, and a technician takes many x-rays to look for signs of ulceration that define Crohn's disease.

Hydrogen Breath Test

This simple test is used to detect lactose intolerance. You eat a certain quantity of carbohydrate and then exhale into a machine that measures the amount of hydrogen in your breath. Excess hydrogen is created by bacteria that feed off undigested carbohydrate. If you are deficient in certain enzymes that are supposed to break down that carbohydrate, it will remain undigested and become fodder for millions of ravenous bacteria and yeast in your intestines. These bugs break down the carbs into fatty acids and hydrogen.

In addition, this test is also used to screen for gluten enteropathy (celiac disease) because it's much less invasive than a bowel biopsy — the definitive test for that condition. The presence of a sugar called *D-xylose* in your breath may indicate adult celiac disease. (Most GI specialists, however, feel that a bowel biopsy is still required for diagnosis.)

Tests for Gluten Intolerance (Celiac)

There are several names for gluten intolerance, including gluten enteropathy, celiac disease, and celiac sprue. Whatever you call it, this disease can wreak havoc if it goes undiagnosed (see Chapter 2).

The Celiac Sprue Association has set out three criteria for diagnosing the disease:

✔ A thorough physical examination is conducted, including a series of blood tests, sometimes referred to as the *celiac blood panel*.

✔ A duodenal biopsy is performed with multiple samples from multiple locations in the small intestine.

✔ A gluten-free diet is implemented. When the patient shows a positive response to the diet — symptoms subside and the small intestine returns to its normal, healthy state — the diagnosis of celiac disease is confirmed.

The kicker in this equation is that the gluten-free diet should be initiated only *after* the first two steps. But many people with IBS symptoms eliminate sugar, wheat, and dairy because they are common allergens, and these folks aren't usually sent for celiac testing until much later — if at all.

Some newly diagnosed adult celiacs just rely on the blood testing for their diagnosis. They often have a lifelong history of bowel problems, anemia, and fatigue. When someone points out to them that they may have gluten intolerance (or, more commonly, they make the association themselves from reading about the condition in the mainstream press), a simple blood test is enough for them to make the dietary changes.

However, for young children who are very ill with diarrhea or constipation and failure to thrive, the pediatrician often recommends a small bowel biopsy to really diagnose the condition properly. The reasoning behind this decision is that the diet for celiac disease is so restrictive that it's important to have a definitive diagnosis early on.

Food Antibody Assessment

Food antibody testing is not taught in medical school. It's a specialty test done by labs that investigate nutritional inadequacy. Because IBS is so closely associated with problems with food digestion and absorption, it's important to know that food antibody testing is available.

A simple blood test can identify antigen–antibody reactions to common foods. The test can be used to look for IgA, IgG, and IgM antibodies — three types of antibodies that our immune systems form against allergens. If you are allergic to a food, or even if you have leaky gut (see Chapter 3), undigested food molecules can set up allergy reactions that can be found on this blood test. (Some people who experience lots of symptoms when they eat can have a leaky gut *and* food allergies.)

Food antibody testing is able to give you a list of foods that you form antibodies against. Having this information gives you an opportunity to stop eating these foods for a while so that your body is no longer fighting them.

The most common test uses tiny plastic trays; each tray has a hundred little wells or depressions in it. In each depression is a drop of a food concentrate. A technician puts a drop of your clear blood serum into each depression, and a computer reads the color change that occurs. The test results are highly accurate and can give you answers that would take weeks or even months to find out with other methods (such as the elimination and challenge diet that we talk about in Chapter 10). However, many doctors still feel that the elimination and challenge diet is the gold standard of food allergy and sensitivity diagnosis.

Similar testing is done for other substances to determine if your body is reacting to chemicals in the environment.

For information about labs that conduct these types of tests, see Chapter 21.

Comprehensive Digestive Stool Analysis (CDSA)

The CDSA is a panel of tests that looks for evidence of maldigestion, malabsorption, abnormal intestinal bacteria and ecology, and abnormal intestinal function. This panel tells you the amount of fat in your stool, which implies fat malabsorption; the level of various bacteria in your system, both good and bad; and the amount of yeast in your intestines. This test determines whether you have an overgrowth of yeast or bacteria and, if so, which herbs and/or drugs will kill those organisms.

A simple stool test collected at home is sent to a lab that conducts the CDSA. This test is done in special labs that focus on allergy, GI infection, and nutritional diseases — not in hospital-based labs. Most hospital-based labs don't quantify bacterial or yeast flora; they just check for the presence of organisms.

Because yeast is a normal inhabitant of the GI tract, if it is found in a stool sample, this is recorded as normal. But the specialty labs quantify the amount of organisms present and can tell you if you have too much or even too little of a certain bacteria or yeast.

The doctors that refer people to specialty labs are usually *integrative medicine* doctors (those who incorporate allopathic and traditional medicine) and naturopaths. One of the main labs that does this testing is Great Smokies Diagnostic Lab (see www.gsdl.com).

Chapter 21

Ten (Plus) Additional Sources of Help

In This Chapter

▶ Getting general information and support

▶ Finding resources to improve your lifestyle

▶ Investigating various therapies

Many free resources are available to people who suffer with IBS. In this chapter, we provide Web sites, books, and other resources that can give you more information about your condition and allow you to share everything from recipes to companionship with people who know all about IBS.

While we hope that you find these resources useful, we want to be clear that our goal is to provide information — not endorsements (with a few exceptions). We encourage you to be discerning. A lot of information is available about IBS, especially on the Web. Carefully consider each piece of information that you gather in terms of how it is relevant to your particular IBS symptoms and situation. And keep in mind that the information you get from these sources is not meant to be a substitute for a consultation with an appropriate medical professional.

IBS Organizations and Support Networks

When we did an Internet search for the term "irritable bowel syndrome," we got 927,000 hits. We certainly didn't visit all those sites, and we don't suggest that you do. In this section, we suggest some general IBS-related sites that you may find provide useful information, motivation, and commiseration.

Organizations

Many national and international organizations have Web sites that are full of information about digestive diseases and disorders and include information about IBS. Some sites are devoted to providing information exclusively about IBS. Here are some sites to try:

- ✔ **Canadian Society of Intestinal Research** (www.badgut.com) offers information, live support groups, and online support.

- ✔ **International Foundation for Functional Gastrointestinal Disorders** (www.iffgd.org) is a nonprofit organization dedicated to education and research.

- ✔ **Irritable Bowel Syndrome Association** (U.S. Web site www.ibs association.org; Canadian Web site www.ibsassociation.ca) is a nonprofit organization offering support groups, information, and education.

- ✔ **National Institute of Diabetes & Digestive & Kidney Diseases** (www. niddk.nih.gov) has information about various digestive disorders and diseases, including IBS.

Self-help sites

- ✔ **Help for IBS** (www.helpforibs.com) is a site owned by IBS patient-expert Heather Van Vorous that provides information, education, recipes, and IBS-related products. You can also sign up for online support groups and message boards.

- ✔ **Irritable Bowel Syndrome (IBS) Self Help and Support Group** (www. ibsgroup.org) claims to be the largest online patient advocate and support community for people with IBS.

E-mail lists

By joining a mailing list server, you can receive e-mails from people who are also dealing with IBS. Such lists provide people the opportunity to communicate about their illness and to offer moral support, tips, and remedies to each other.

The Yahoo Web site is host to several e-mail lists that discuss IBS. Each list is owned or moderated by a different group or individual, and each has a different focus. Some are general discussions about IBS, while others are limited to discussions about medicines for IBS. Following are some examples:

- **Irritable Bowel Syndrome** (`http://health.groups.yahoo.com/group/irritable_bowel_syndrome`) is a general list with more than 500 members.

- **IBS Patient Action Group** (`http://health.groups.yahoo.com/group/ibspag`) has more than 250 members and is dedicated to discussion about medication and social issues related to IBS.

Diet Web Sites

As we stress throughout the book, what you eat makes a huge difference in how you feel when you have IBS. Following are two Web sites that relate to the types of diet advice we offer, especially in Chapter 10:

- **The Yeast Connection** (`www.yeastconnection.com`) shows how to eliminate foods that do you no good. Click on the "Yeast-Fighting Program" and then on the "Diet" link.

- **Food Intolerance and Food Allergies** (`www.foodintol.com`) is an Australian Web site dedicated to providing information and education about — what else? — food intolerances and food allergies!

Exercise Resources

As we discuss in Chapter 11, any exercise is beneficial, but certain types of exercise are particularly helpful when you have IBS:

- **T-Tapp** (`www.t-tapp.com`) is a site dedicated to an exercise system designed by Theresa Tapp to improve digestion and elimination, as well as lymphatic flow. Both of your authors use and endorse T-Tapp.

- The **Yoga Journal** is a print publication that is also available online (`www.yogajournal.com`) at a site that contains a lot of free information for yoga beginners.

- **Yoga Basics** (`www.yogabasics.com`) is a great site to explore. It even has yoga you can do to alleviate PMS.

Stress Relief

The connection between IBS and stress is intricate and sometimes frustrating. If you experience stress, you can aggravate your IBS. But just having IBS increases your stress! That cycle is reason enough to check out these resources:

- **The Mind/Body Medical Institute** (www.mbmi.org) is a nonprofit organization dedicated to mind–body medicine and the work of Dr. Herbert Benson, who created the relaxation response (see Chapter 12). The site explains some exercises that can help you reduce stress.
- **EEG Institute** (www.EEGInstitute.com) provides articles, research, and other information about biofeedback and neurofeedback.
- **Learning Meditation** (www.learningmeditation.com) has a pretty self-explanatory name!
- **Delia Quigley** (www.deliaquigley.com) is an associate of ours who has written a book called *Empowering Your Life with Meditation* (Penguin Group), which is available at www.amazon.com.

Information on Other Diseases

A number of diseases and conditions can have symptoms similar to IBS. In the following sections, we list Web sites that provide information about some of them.

Gluten intolerance (celiac disease)

These sites can educate you further about gluten intolerance, which we discuss in Chapter 2 and elsewhere in the book:

- **Canadian Celiac Association** (www.celiac.ca) has general information about celiac disease, as well as recipes, books, and gluten-free product listings.
- **Celiac Disease and Gluten-free Diet Support Center** (www.celiac.com) provides information and resources to people who are gluten intolerant or have other allergies to wheat.
- **Celiac Disease Foundation** (www.celiac.org) works within the health, medical, and pharmaceutical industries to provide information and assistance to people with celiac disease.

✔ **Celiac Sprue Association** (www.csaceliacs.org) is a nonprofit organization that provides information, education, and support to people living with celiac disease.

Inflammatory bowel disease (IBD)

There are two IBDs: Crohn's disease and ulcerative colitis. We explain each in Chapter 2, and you can find out more with these resources:

✔ **Caramal Publishing** (www.caramal.com) is the Web site for Jini Patel Thompson, who was diagnosed with advanced Crohn's disease in 1986 (see Chapter 16). After researching natural and holistic treatments and diets, Jini designed her own treatment plan and has been drug- and surgery-free for over 16 years. The books she has written about her treatment plans are also useful for people with IBS, and they are available for purchase from this site.

✔ **Crohn's & Colitis Foundation of America** (www.ccfa.org) is a nonprofit organization dedicated to finding a cure for, and preventing, Crohn's disease and ulcerative colitis.

✔ **Crohn's Disease Ulcerative Colitis Inflammatory Bowel Disease Pages** (qurlyjoe.bu.edu/cduchome.html) is a Web site created and maintained by a patient with IBD. It provides information, resources, and encouragement to other patients.

✔ **National Institute of Diabetes & Digestive & Kidney Diseases** (www.niddk.nih.gov) has information about various digestive disorders and diseases, including Crohn's and ulcerative colitis.

Lactose intolerance

The Web site www.lactose.co.uk is owned and operated by a scientist whose child has lactose intolerance.

Caring Therapies

The listings in these sections, which relate to therapies we discuss in Chapter 12, can help you take charge of your physical and emotional health.

Emotional Freedom Techniques (EFT)

EFT can help you relieve stress and reduce your IBS symptoms. You can find out more about it at these sites:

- **Gary Craig** (www.emofree.com) is the founder of EFT and hosts a comprehensive Web site with thousands of case studies, free newsletter updates, and practitioner listings. We recommend that you download the EFT Manual available at this site, so you can learn EFT at no cost. EFT training DVDs are also available for purchase.

- **Carol Look** (www.carollook.com) offers EFT resources for food cravings and weight loss, as well as case histories of her work with clients.

- **Christine Wheeler** (www.christinewheeler.com) — who just happens to be a coauthor of this book! — offers EFT tips for dealing with symptoms of IBS.

Hypnotherapy

If hypnosis interests you, check out these two resources:

- **The American Society of Clinical Hypnosis** (www.asch.net) offers educational programs in hypnosis and promotes the use of hypnosis in healthcare and research.

- **The IBS Audio Program 100** (www.ibsaudioprogram.com) offers self-hypnosis tapes that may help you reduce your IBS symptoms.

Transactional Analysis (TA)

TA is a behavioral therapy that we introduce in Chapter 12. These resources provide much more detail than we can fit in this book:

- **The International Transactional Analysis Association** (www.itaa-net.org) offers practitioner listings and resources about TA.

- Books that explain TA include
  - *Beyond Games And Scripts* (Random House) by Eric Berne
  - *Scripts People Live* (Bantam Books) by Claude Steiner
  - *Success Through Transactional Analysis* (Signet) by Jut Meininger

Integrative Medicine

Integrative medicine is a term used by doctors who integrate the best of traditional medicine with the best of allopathic medicine in their practices. The following resources may help as you search for integrative medicine professionals to support you in your quest for health.

Your coauthor Dr. Carolyn Dean offers support to people with IBS as an advisor to www.yeastconnection.com. She also holds health teleconferences, does health consultations, gives health seminars, and has an active Web site at www.carolyndean.com, where you can obtain her many books, link up to her radio shows, and follow her health freedom efforts. With all the above activities, she does not have time to run a private practice!

Environmental medicine

This branch of medicine teaches doctors the cause and effect relationship between the environment and illness. You can find out more from the American Academy of Environmental Medicine Web site at www.aaem.com.

Holistic health

This type of healthcare deals with the whole person and incorporates traditional (natural and alternative) as well as allopathic medical modalities. You can find out more from these sources:

- ✔ **American Holistic Health Association** (http://ahha.org/index.html) is a nonprofit organization dedicated to providing information and resources about holistic health practices. The site includes practitioner listings and links to organizations that support holistic health.

- ✔ **American Holistic Medical Association** (www.holisticmedicine.org) provides a referral directory of holistic physicians and healthcare providers in the United States.

- ✔ **American Holistic Nurses Association** (www.ahna.org) provides a listing of holistic nurse practitioners who practice a variety of holistic healing modalities from acupressure to yoga.

Orthomolecular medicine

This branch of medicine incorporates vitamin and minerals in the *ortho* ("correct") doses. It was originally begun by Dr. Linus Pauling and Dr. Abram Hoffer. You can find out more by visiting Orthomolecular Medicine Online at www.orthomed.org.

Osteopathic medicine

This is a system of comprehensive medical care that includes an emphasis on structural balance of the musculoskeletal system. Osteopathic physicians use joint manipulation, postural reeducation, and physical therapy to normalize the body's structure and promote healing. Find out more at the American Academy of Osteopathy Web site (www.academyofosteopathy.org), which provides a database of osteopathic physicians who are listed with the organization.

Chinese medicine

Chinese medicine is taught in several schools in North America. It is usually a four-year course encompassing herbal medicine and acupuncture. If you want to try acupuncture for your IBS, it's important to see a qualified practitioner who has studied for many years and who has experience with IBS. Check out these resources:

- ✔ **American Academy of Medical Acupuncture** (www.medical acupuncture.org) focuses on integrating acupuncture with Western medical training. The site provides a listing of medical doctors who practice acupuncture.

- ✔ **American Association of Oriental Medicine** (www.aaom.org) focuses on public education about Oriental medicine and acupuncture and features links to research material about acupuncture. The site also provides a listing of acupuncturists in the United States.

Chiropractic

Chiropractic adjustments may help alleviate stress and tension that worsens IBS. Many chiropractors also specialize in nutrition, dietary supplements, acupuncture, and even allergy therapy. To find information or practitioners, try the Web sites for the American Chiropractic Association, www.amerchiro.org.

Clinical Nutrition

A certified clinical nutritionist receives several hundred hours of training, passes stringent examinations, and must maintain ongoing nutritional education to keep her license. As we explain in Chapter 10, the right diet can be very important when you have IBS. A nutritionist may be able to give you the information and support you need. To find information and get help locating a practitioner, try the Web site for the International & American Associations of Clinical Nutritionists, www.iaacn.org.

Herbal, Homeopathic, and Naturopathic Medicine

Naturopathic training also includes training in herbs and homeopathy. However, there are separate schools of herbal medicine and homeopathic medicine that are usually open to the public. People who attend these courses are often regarded as skilled lay healers with a special knack for being able to help others.

Naturopathic medicine

Naturopaths receive four years of postgraduate education in many traditional healing modalities, such as acupuncture, herbal medicine, homeopathy, hydrotherapy, vitamin therapy, and nutrition. To find out more about naturopathy, or to locate practitioners, try these resources:

- ✔ **The American Association of Naturopathic Physicians** (www.naturopathic.org) has a directory for locating licensed naturopathic physicians in the United States.

- ✔ **Bastyr University** (www.bastyr.edu) is a leading academic institution for natural health sciences. The Bastyr Center for Natural Health (www.bastyrcenter.org) in Seattle provides natural health services by appointment.

- ✔ **The Canadian College of Naturopathic Medicine** (www.ccnm.edu) offers a four-year program in naturopathic medicine, and patients can make appointments for treatment in its clinic.

- ✔ **National College of Naturopathic Medicine** (www.ncnm.edu) teaches naturopathic medicine and Chinese medicine in Oregon, and patients can make appointments for treatment in its clinic.

- ✔ **Southwest College of Naturopathic Medicine** (www.scnm.edu) teaches naturopathic medicine and Chinese medicine in Arizona, and patients can make appointments for treatment in its medical center.

Herbal medicine

If herbs (which we discuss in Chapter 9) strike you as the way you want to treat some of your IBS symptoms, here are some resources to help you find a practicing herbalist:

- ✔ **American Botanical Council** (www.herbalgram.org) provides information, education, and news about the herbal medicine field.

- ✔ **Herb Research Foundation** (www.herbs.org) is an extensive site that provides scientific information about the health benefits of herbs.

Homeopathic medicine

Homeopathy (which we also discuss in Chapter 9) is a noninvasive, nontoxic form of medicine that can be very effective for functional conditions. To find out more, try these sites:

- ✔ **American Institute of Homeopathy** (www.homeopathyusa.org) provides information about homeopathy and lets you purchase a directory of licensed homeopaths.

- ✔ **Homeopathic Educational Services** (www.homeopathic.com) has articles and products relating to homeopathy.

Appendix A

Soluble and Insoluble Fiber Chart

∙ ∙

As we note in several chapters, particularly Chapter 10, increasing your intake of fiber (especially soluble fiber) can help alleviate symptoms of both IBS-diarrhea and IBS-constipation. The following chart, excerpted from a chart produced by the U.S. Department of Agriculture, helps you compare sources of soluble and insoluble fiber.

Food	Soluble Fiber (Grams per 100 Grams)	Insoluble Fiber (Grams per 100 Grams)
Bread, wheat, soft	1.26	2.13
Bread, wheat, firm	1.56	4.63
Bread, whole wheat, soft	1.26	4.76
Bread, whole wheat, firm	1.51	5.21
Tortilla, corn	1.11	4.39
Tortilla, flour (wheat)	1.51	0.85
Brown rice, long grain, cooked	0.44	2.89
Oatmeal, regular, cooked	0.42	1.23
Spaghetti, cooked	0.54	1.33
White rice, long grain, cooked	0	0.34
Apple (Red Delicious), raw, ripe w/skin	0.67	1.54
Avocado (California, Haas), raw, ripe	2.03	3.51
Banana, raw, ripe	0.58	1.21
Grapefruit, raw, white, ripe	0.58	0.32
Grapes (Thompson seedless), raw, ripe	0.24	0.36

(continued)

Food	Soluble Fiber (Grams per 100 Grams)	Insoluble Fiber (Grams per 100 Grams)
Mango, raw, ripe	0.69	1.08
Oranges (Navel), raw, ripe	1.37	0.99
Pears, raw, ripe, w/skin	0.92	2.25
Pineapple (smooth Cayenne), raw, ripe	0.04	1.42
Prunes, pitted	4.50	3.63
Raisins, seedless	0.90	2.17
Watermelon, raw, ripe	0.13	0.27
Beans, canned, w/pork and tomato sauce	1.38	4.02
Chick peas, canned, drained	0.41	5.79
Lentils, dry, cooked, drained	0.44	5.42
Pinto beans, canned, drained	0.99	5.66
Red kidney beans, canned, drained	1.36	5.77
Split peas, dry, cooked, drained	0.09	10.56
Beans, green, fresh	1.38	2.93
Broccoli, fresh, cooked	1.85	2.81
Carrots, fresh, cooked	1.58	2.29
Corn, yellow, from cob, farm market	0.25	2.63
Peas, green, frozen	0.94	2.61
Potato, white, baked, w/skin	0.61	1.70
Broccoli, raw	0.44	3.06
Carrots, raw	0.49	2.39
Cucumber, raw, with peel	0.20	0.94
Tomatoes, red, ripe, raw	0.15	1.19
Spinach, raw	0.77	2.43

Appendix B

Glossary

• •

Abdomen: The abdomen extends from below the lungs in the chest to the top of the hips and pubic bone. The contents of the abdominal cavity are the stomach, liver, gallbladder, spleen, pancreas, small intestine, appendix, and large intestine.

Abdominal pain and abdominal spasm: Pain and spasms are a common component of IBS. Intestines stretched by gas or constipation can produce excruciating pain. However, not all abdominal pain is due to IBS.

Allergy: An allergy is a reaction by the immune system against anything foreign, which can be any food or chemical that we ingest or inhale.

Anal fissure: This small tear or cut in the skin of the anus can cause pain and/or bleeding, especially when a bowel movement passes.

Anal fistula: This is a tiny channel or tract that can develop in the presence of inflammation and infection. It is a common symptom in Crohn's disease. Fistulas usually run from inside the rectum to an exit point near the anus.

Anemia: This is the most common abnormal condition of the blood. It means that you don't have enough blood, red blood cells, or hemoglobin in the body.

Anoscopy: This is a test used to examine the anal canal. A lubricated metal or plastic instrument is inserted into the anus to allow the doctor to look for fissures, fistulae, and hemorrhoids in the anal canal.

Anus: This is where it all comes out, the final exit point of intestinal contents. Fecal matter builds up in the rectum before the anal sphincter muscle relaxes, allowing elimination.

Appendix: This 3- or 4-inch long narrow tissue sac is attached to the first part of the large intestine (the *cecum*). Some theorize that its original function was to break down seeds and other hard plant materials.

Ascending colon: This section of the large intestine is located on the right side of the abdomen.

Aspartame: This low-calorie sweetener, also known as NutraSweet, Equal, and Spoonful, is used in a variety of foods and drinks. It is about 200 times sweeter than sugar but has a number of serious side effects.

Barium: When ingested or used in an enema, this chalky liquid shows up on x-rays as a white shadow. It is used to coat the inside of the gastrointestinal tract to find abnormalities.

Bloating: In IBS, bloating occurs in the abdomen. It causes pressure and pain and can expand the waist as gas builds up in the intestines. For fear of passing stool along with gas, some people with IBS don't allow gas to escape through the anus, which may cause a worsening of symptoms.

Borborygmi: The name (pronounced *BOR-boh-RIG-mee*) almost sounds like what it's describing — gurgling and rumbling sounds caused by gas moving through the intestines. It's a much more aesthetic name than *stomach growling*.

Bowel: This is a general term for the small intestine and the large intestine, two hollow tubes that are located in the abdominal cavity.

Bowel incontinence: This term describes the inability to control defecation, which means that feces escapes the rectum and anus.

Bowel movement: This is waste from digested foods that passes through the large intestine and out through the rectum and anus.

CA-125 test: This blood test is designed to detect an elevated level of a protein antigen called *CA-125,* which may indicate ovarian cancer, among other disorders. It may be an important test in the workup for IBS because ovarian cancer has symptoms of abdominal pain and bloating.

Candida albicans: In people who have weakened immune systems or who use antibiotics long-term, this yeast can infect the skin or mucus membranes of the mouth or vagina, or it can cause a serious blood infection. It can also cause another type of yeast infection called *Crook's Candidiasis:*

✔ The overgrowth of yeast in the intestines, which can occur because of antibiotics, birth control pills, cortisone, and a diet high in refined sugar. The yeast changes into a tissue-invasive form and causes intestinal inflammation and leaky gut syndrome, including symptoms of IBS.

✔ Yeast that causes allergy symptoms, such as the burning and itching of various parts of the body: nasal membranes, sinuses, skin, and vagina.

✔ Multiple and sometimes severe reactions in the body to the almost 180 yeast byproducts and waste products.

Carbohydrates: This term designates the sugars and starches in food. *Simple carbohydrates* are sugars found in fruit and table sugar. *Complex carbohydrates* are formed from a large number of sugar molecules joined together and are found in grains, beans, peas, legumes, and vegetables like potatoes, yams, and squash.

Cecum: This is the area of the intestines where the small intestine and large intestine meet.

Celiac disease: See *Gluten intolerance*.

Chronic fatigue syndrome (CFS): CFS is associated with severe, debilitating fatigue and no known cause. A diagnosis is made if the fatigue is present for at least six months and is associated with at least four of these symptoms that resemble a low-grade flu or viral infection: fever, impaired memory or concentration, sore throat, lymph node swelling, muscle pains, joint pains, headaches, poor sleep, and post-exertion exhaustion. Chronic infections such as Epstein Barr virus, toxoplasmosis, and tuberculosis need to be ruled out. Thirty to 60 percent of people with CFS also have symptoms of IBS.

Colitis: This is a general term that means inflammation of the colon. (Note that *ulcerative colitis* is the name of a specific inflammatory bowel disease with physical signs of inflammation and ulceration.)

Colon: This is another name for intestines. Food and water are digested and absorbed, and wastes are eliminated, through this hollow tube that runs from the small intestine to the anus.

Colonoscopy: This test is performed by a doctor to view the rectum and colon. A *colonoscope* — a long, flexible, narrow tube with a light and tiny lens on the end — is used.

Constipation: We don't have to tell you that having constipation means not passing stool as frequently or as easily as you should. IBS-constipation (according to the Rome II Diagnostic Criteria) is defined by having bowel movements three times per week or less. Symptoms of constipation include straining during a bowel movement, as well as having painful bowel movements, gas, bloating, fatigue, and lethargy.

Crohn's disease: This inflammatory bowel disease mostly affects the small intestine with ulcerations, scarring, strictures, and symptoms of diarrhea, abdominal pain, and bleeding. Early cases of Crohn's can be mistaken for IBS.

Descending colon: This part of the large intestine lies on the left side of the abdomen between the transverse colon above and the rectum and anus below.

Diarrhea: The Rome II Diagnostic Criteria define IBS-diarrhea as a stool frequency of greater than three times per day. Associated symptoms include loose (mushy) or watery stools; urgency (having to rush to have a bowel movement); a feeling of having incomplete bowel movements; passing mucus (white material) during a bowel movement; and/or abdominal fullness, bloating, or swelling.

Digestion: The term refers to the ability to break down food in the body into small units that can be used for growth, energy, and repair.

Digestive system: The tissues and organs in the body that help break down and absorb food and liquids create the digestive system, also called the *gastrointestinal tract*. These include the mouth, esophagus, stomach, small intestine, large intestine, rectum, and anus. Ancillary organs that also help with digestion are the tongue, salivary glands in the mouth, pancreas, liver, and gallbladder.

Digital rectal exam: This is a medical procedure in which a doctor inserts a gloved finger through the anus and into the rectum to examine the prostate gland in men and to feel for signs of hemorrhoids, polyps, or tumors.

Diverticulosis: This medical condition, diagnosed with a barium enema x-ray, occurs when small outpouchings (*diverticula*) occur at weak spots in the wall of the large intestine. When the pouches become infected or inflamed, the condition is called *diverticulitis*.

Dysentery: This intestinal infection is often associated with travelers' diarrhea and is accompanied by bloody, frequent bowel movements; abdominal pain; and fever. After such an episode, some individuals may develop IBS.

Dyspepsia: This is an older term for indigestion. Indigestion is not always caused by too much stomach acid; in fact, it's mostly caused by too little stomach acid. The majority of people with IBS (about 75 percent) suffer from indigestion for no known reason.

Endoscopy: This is a diagnostic procedure involving an *endoscope* — a fiber optic tube through which a doctor can see the inside of the gastrointestinal tract. The different types of endoscopy procedures are named for the parts that they visualize: sigmoidoscopy (which views the sigmoid colon), colonoscopy (which views the small and large intestine), and upper endoscopy (which views the stomach).

Eructation: This is a fancy name for gas built up in the stomach and expelled through the mouth (by burping).

Esophagus: This narrow tube, about 9 inches long, forms the first part of the gastrointestinal tract; it joins the mouth to the stomach.

Fecal occult blood test: A small amount of stool is wiped on a specially treated paper, which turns color in the presence of blood.

Fibromyalgia (FMS): FMS is a disorder of the musculoskeletal system associated with pain, fatigue, and insomnia with no known cause. *Fibro* relates to fibrous tissue of muscles, ligaments, and tendons. *Myalgia* means pain. So *fibromyalgia* means pain in the muscles, ligaments, and tendons.

Gallbladder: Shaped like a ball, it hangs beneath the liver, stores bile made in the liver, and releases it to aid in the digestion of fats.

Gas: In the intestines, gas is created from food digestion, from swallowing air, or from the waste products of yeast and bacteria. Gas is released as flatulence or burping.

Gastroenteritis: This term indicates any infection or irritation of the stomach and intestines. The causes of gastroenteritis are many, including food poisoning, bacteria, parasites, and severe emotional stress.

Gastroenterologist: This term (much more classy than *gut doctor*) refers to a doctor whose specialty is disorders and diseases of the gastrointestinal tract.

Gastroesophageal reflux disease (GERD): GERD is a digestive disorder that relaxes the lower esophageal sphincter, which lies between the esophagus and stomach. This weakness of the sphincter allows highly acidic stomach contents to flow back up the esophagus. There is a higher incidence of GERD in people with IBS compared to those without.

Gastrointestinal tract: This term, which means the same thing as *digestive system,* refers to the muscular tube that joins the mouth to the anus. Food passes through it and is digested, absorbed, and eliminated.

Gluten intolerance: This condition, also called *celiac disease,* is often misdiagnosed as IBS because it produces symptoms of diarrhea, bloating, and fatigue. It damages the small intestine, leading to malabsorption of nutrients from food. It is caused by sensitivity to the wheat protein called gluten.

Heartburn: This common gastric disorder, associated with a feeling of burning behind the sternum, may be associated with gastroesophageal reflux disease. There is a higher incidence of heartburn in people who have IBS.

Hemorrhoids: These are swollen, painful, itching, bleeding varicose veins in the blood vessels around the anus and lower rectum. People with IBS-constipation can have a high incidence of hemorrhoids.

Hiatus hernia: In this condition, the opening in the diaphragm is weakened to the point that the stomach slides upward above the diaphragm, causing pain and discomfort that is made worse by bending over or lying flat.

IBD: See *Inflammatory bowel disease.*

IBS: See *Irritable bowel syndrome.*

Inflammatory bowel disease (IBD): An IBD is a disease of the GI tract with signs of ulceration, bleeding, diarrhea, and pain. Ulcerative colitis is an IBD of the large intestine. Crohn's disease is an IBD of the small intestine. Crohn's can also produce ulcers and fistulas in and around the anus and rectum.

Insoluble fiber: This type of dietary fiber comes from plants, is indigestible, and does not dissolve in water. Therefore, it can be an intestinal irritant.

Intestinal flora: This name is given to the living organisms, such as bacteria and yeast, that make up the contents of the intestine.

Intestinal mucosa: The inner lining of the intestines, where food is absorbed in the small intestine and water is absorbed in the large intestine.

Intestines: Also called the *colon* or *bowel,* the intestines are made up of the small intestine (from the stomach to the cecum) and the large intestine (from the cecum to the anus).

Irritable bowel syndrome (IBS): This functional condition affects the gastrointestinal tract with symptoms that include diarrhea and/or constipation, abdominal pain, bloating, and gas.

Kidneys: These organs, located at the back of the abdominal cavity on both sides of the spine, filter wastes from the blood and excrete them in the urine.

Lactobacillus acidophilus: This beneficial bacteria natural to the GI tract, digests excess sugar into lactic acid that protects the bowel against yeast overgrowth. As a supplement, it treats indigestion, diarrhea, and constipation.

Laparotomy: This surgical procedure involves an incision into the abdomen to make a definitive diagnosis of symptoms in the abdominal cavity.

Large intestine: This part of the GI tract runs from the end of the small intestine to the anus.

Laxatives: These medicines are used to induce bowel movements and relieve constipation. If you overuse them, you may become dependent.

Liver: This is the most important organ in the body for detoxifying drugs, chemicals, and foreign materials. It also has hundreds of functions that include making bile, producing hormones, and creating cholesterol.

Lower esophageal sphincter: This muscle, in the form of a ring around the esophagus, separates the stomach and esophagus.

Lower GI series: This term refers to a barium enema x-ray of the large intestine and the lower part of the small intestine.

Malabsorption syndrome: This is a condition in which the small intestine is unable to absorb nutrients from foods. It is evidenced by gas, bloating, stools that contain fat and undigested food, failure to thrive, weight loss, and anemia.

Mucous colitis: This is one of the original names for IBS.

Mucus: A viscous, clear liquid that coats and protects the underlying membranes and tissues is made by cells of the gastrointestinal tract.

Neurotransmitters: These chemicals in the brain and body carry messages to conduct or inhibit nerve activity. Serotonin is a neurotransmitter that conveys messages to make the bowel speed up or slow down.

Occult bleeding: This is blood in the stool that can't be seen but can be found on a special occult blood test. It is an indication of bleeding from aspirin use, ulceration in the bowel from ulcerative colitis, or cancer.

Pain threshold: This is the level of stimulation that causes pain. Some people have a high threshold or high pain tolerance. Researchers say that people with IBS have a low threshold for pain in their intestines and feel it much sooner and more severely than people with a high threshold.

Pancreas: This organ, lying behind the stomach, has two major functions: It produces insulin that regulates blood sugar and produces pancreatic enzymes that digest protein and fat.

Peristalsis: Rhythmic muscular contractions of the entire digestive tract (from esophagus to rectum) force food through areas of absorption in the small intestine and then to be eliminated through the rectum.

Peritoneum: This is a protective lining around the abdominal cavity.

Polyp: This abnormal growth in the large intestinal lining has the shape of a ball on a stalk. It is painless but may cause slight tearing of tiny blood vessels and cause bleeding. Doctors advise that polyps be removed in case they turn cancerous.

Radiation colitis: Colitis or inflammation caused by radiation of the colon for cancer can have symptoms similar to IBS and may be treated with dietary restriction and lifestyle changes.

Rectum: This term refers to the collecting pouch for feces at the lower end of the large intestine connected to the anus. When enough pressure from collected feces builds up in the rectum, this triggers the urge to evacuate.

Rome II Diagnostic Criteria for IBS: IBS diagnosis must be based on at least 12 weeks (in the preceding 12 months) of abdominal discomfort or pain that has two out of three of these features:

✔ Relieved with defecation; and/or

✔ Onset associated with a change in frequency of stool; and/or

✔ Onset associated with a change in form (appearance) of stool.

Serotonin: This neurotransmitter is also found in the brain and platelets, but 95 percent of it is found in the bowel.

Sharting: This slang term describes what happens when a fart is unfortunately accompanied by solid waste matter.

Small intestine: Attached to the stomach at the duodenum and to the large intestine at the ileum with the jejunum in between, the small intestine is crucial in the absorption of nutrients into the bloodstream.

Soluble fiber: This type of dietary fiber dissolves and swells when put into water. Soluble fiber comes from plant sources and is effective in soothing the bowels. Sources include oats, oat bran, dried beans and peas, barley, flax seed, fruits (oranges and apples), vegetables (carrots), and psyllium husk.

Spastic colitis: This term and *spastic colon* were previously used to refer to what we now call IBS.

Sphincter: This circular muscle constricts a tube or closes a natural opening. In a relaxed state, a sphincter opens and allows materials to pass through the opening. When closed, material are blocked from passing.

Stomach: The stomach is an organ in the shape of a pouch with a large upper end and a tapered lower end. It is attached above to the esophagus but separated from it by the diaphragm and attached below to the *duodenum,* the first part of the small intestine. The stomach is responsible for food digestion.

Stricture: This is an abnormal narrowing of a body opening or canal, usually due to a tumor or scar tissue.

Sugar: Refined sugar is produced from beets, sugar cane, or corn. Eating sugar can be detrimental to someone with IBS, causing gas and bloating.

Tumor: This is an abnormal mass of tissue that may be cancerous or benign.

Ulcer: An ulcer is an eroded area of tissue in a mucous membrane.

Ulcerative colitis: This inflammatory bowel disease (IBD) of the large intestine produces tissue damage, ulceration, diarrhea, mucus, and bleeding.

Yeast: See *Candida albicans.*

Index

BUSINESS, CAREERS & PERSONAL FINANCE

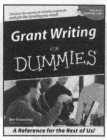

Grant Writing FOR DUMMIES

A Reference for the Rest of Us!

0-7645-5307-0

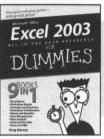

Home Buying FOR DUMMIES

A Reference for the Rest of Us!

0-7645-5331-3 *†

Also available:
- Accounting For Dummies †
  0-7645-5314-3
- Business Plans Kit For Dummies †
  0-7645-5365-8
- Cover Letters For Dummies
  0-7645-5224-4
- Frugal Living For Dummies
  0-7645-5403-4
- Leadership For Dummies
  0-7645-5176-0
- Managing For Dummies
  0-7645-1771-6

- Marketing For Dummies
  0-7645-5600-2
- Personal Finance For Dummies *
  0-7645-2590-5
- Project Management For Dummies
  0-7645-5283-X
- Resumes For Dummies †
  0-7645-5471-9
- Selling For Dummies
  0-7645-5363-1
- Small Business Kit For Dummies *†
  0-7645-5093-4

HOME & BUSINESS COMPUTER BASICS

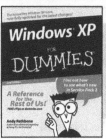

Windows XP FOR DUMMIES

A Reference for the Rest of Us!

0-7645-4074-2

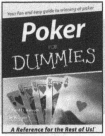

Excel 2003 ALL-IN-ONE DESK REFERENCE FOR DUMMIES

9 BOOKS IN 1

0-7645-3758-X

Also available:
- ACT! 6 For Dummies
  0-7645-2645-6
- iLife '04 All-in-One Desk Reference
  For Dummies
  0-7645-7347-0
- iPAQ For Dummies
  0-7645-6769-1
- Mac OS X Panther Timesaving
  Techniques For Dummies
  0-7645-5812-9
- Macs For Dummies
  0-7645-5656-8

- Microsoft Money 2004 For Dummies
  0-7645-4195-1
- Office 2003 All-in-One Desk Reference
  For Dummies
  0-7645-3883-7
- Outlook 2003 For Dummies
  0-7645-3759-8
- PCs For Dummies
  0-7645-4074-2
- TiVo For Dummies
  0-7645-6923-6
- Upgrading and Fixing PCs For Dummies
  0-7645-1665-5
- Windows XP Timesaving Techniques
  For Dummies
  0-7645-3748-2

FOOD, HOME, GARDEN, HOBBIES, MUSIC & PETS

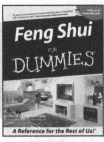

Feng Shui FOR DUMMIES

A Reference for the Rest of Us!

0-7645-5295-3

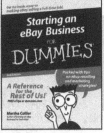

Poker FOR DUMMIES

A Reference for the Rest of Us!

0-7645-5232-5

Also available:
- Bass Guitar For Dummies
  0-7645-2487-9
- Diabetes Cookbook For Dummies
  0-7645-5230-9
- Gardening For Dummies *
  0-7645-5130-2
- Guitar For Dummies
  0-7645-5106-X
- Holiday Decorating For Dummies
  0-7645-2570-0
- Home Improvement All-in-One
  For Dummies
  0-7645-5680-0

- Knitting For Dummies
  0-7645-5395-X
- Piano For Dummies
  0-7645-5105-1
- Puppies For Dummies
  0-7645-5255-4
- Scrapbooking For Dummies
  0-7645-7208-3
- Senior Dogs For Dummies
  0-7645-5818-8
- Singing For Dummies
  0-7645-2475-5
- 30-Minute Meals For Dummies
  0-7645-2589-1

INTERNET & DIGITAL MEDIA

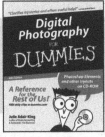

Digital Photography FOR DUMMIES

A Reference for the Rest of Us!

0-7645-1664-7

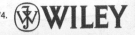

Starting an eBay Business FOR DUMMIES

A Reference for the Rest of Us!

0-7645-6924-4

Also available:
- 2005 Online Shopping Directory
  For Dummies
  0-7645-7495-7
- CD & DVD Recording For Dummies
  0-7645-5956-7
- eBay For Dummies
  0-7645-5654-1
- Fighting Spam For Dummies
  0-7645-5965-6
- Genealogy Online For Dummies
  0-7645-5964-8
- Google For Dummies
  0-7645-4420-9

- Home Recording For Musicians
  For Dummies
  0-7645-1634-5
- The Internet For Dummies
  0-7645-4173-0
- iPod & iTunes For Dummies
  0-7645-7772-7
- Preventing Identity Theft For Dummies
  0-7645-7336-5
- Pro Tools All-in-One Desk Reference
  For Dummies
  0-7645-5714-9
- Roxio Easy Media Creator For Dummies
  0-7645-7131-1

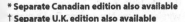 WILEY

FITNESS, PARENTING, RELIGION & SPIRITUALITY

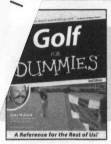

0-7645-5146-9

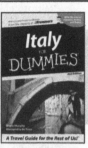

0-7645-5418-2

Also available:
- Adoption For Dummies
  0-7645-5488-3
- Basketball For Dummies
  0-7645-5248-1
- The Bible For Dummies
  0-7645-5296-1
- Buddhism For Dummies
  0-7645-5359-3
- Catholicism For Dummies
  0-7645-5391-7
- Hockey For Dummies
  0-7645-5228-7

- Judaism For Dummies
  0-7645-5299-6
- Martial Arts For Dummies
  0-7645-5358-5
- Pilates For Dummies
  0-7645-5397-6
- Religion For Dummies
  0-7645-5264-3
- Teaching Kids to Read For Dummies
  0-7645-4043-2
- Weight Training For Dummies
  0-7645-5168-X
- Yoga For Dummies
  0-7645-5117-5

TRAVEL

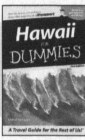

0-7645-5438-7

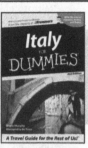

0-7645-5453-0

Also available:
- Alaska For Dummies
  0-7645-1761-9
- Arizona For Dummies
  0-7645-6938-4
- Cancún and the Yucatán For Dummies
  0-7645-2437-2
- Cruise Vacations For Dummies
  0-7645-6941-4
- Europe For Dummies
  0-7645-5456-5
- Ireland For Dummies
  0-7645-5455-7

- Las Vegas For Dummies
  0-7645-5448-4
- London For Dummies
  0-7645-4277-X
- New York City For Dummies
  0-7645-6945-7
- Paris For Dummies
  0-7645-5494-8
- RV Vacations For Dummies
  0-7645-5443-3
- Walt Disney World & Orlando For Dummies
  0-7645-6943-0

GRAPHICS, DESIGN & WEB DEVELOPMENT

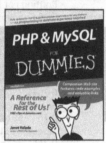

0-7645-4345-8

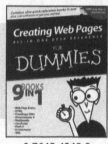

0-7645-5589-8

Also available:
- Adobe Acrobat 6 PDF For Dummies
  0-7645-3760-1
- Building a Web Site For Dummies
  0-7645-7144-3
- Dreamweaver MX 2004 For Dummies
  0-7645-4342-3
- FrontPage 2003 For Dummies
  0-7645-3882-9
- HTML 4 For Dummies
  0-7645-1995-6
- Illustrator cs For Dummies
  0-7645-4084-X

- Macromedia Flash MX 2004 For Dummies
  0-7645-4358-X
- Photoshop 7 All-in-One Desk
  Reference For Dummies
  0-7645-1667-1
- Photoshop cs Timesaving Techniques
  For Dummies
  0-7645-6782-9
- PHP 5 For Dummies
  0-7645-4166-8
- PowerPoint 2003 For Dummies
  0-7645-3908-6
- QuarkXPress 6 For Dummies
  0-7645-2593-X

NETWORKING, SECURITY, PROGRAMMING & DATABASES

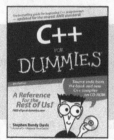

0-7645-6852-3

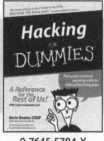

0-7645-5784-X

Also available:
- A+ Certification For Dummies
  0-7645-4187-0
- Access 2003 All-in-One Desk
  Reference For Dummies
  0-7645-3988-4
- Beginning Programming For Dummies
  0-7645-4997-9
- C For Dummies
  0-7645-7068-4
- Firewalls For Dummies
  0-7645-4048-3
- Home Networking For Dummies
  0-7645-42796

- Network Security For Dummies
  0-7645-1679-5
- Networking For Dummies
  0-7645-1677-9
- TCP/IP For Dummies
  0-7645-1760-0
- VBA For Dummies
  0-7645-3989-2
- Wireless All In-One Desk Reference
  For Dummies
  0-7645-7496-5
- Wireless Home Networking For Dummies
  0-7645-3910-8

HEALTH & SELF-HELP

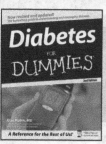

0-7645-6820-5 *†

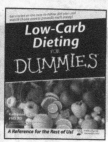

0-7645-2566-2

Also available:
- Alzheimer's For Dummies
  0-7645-3899-3
- Asthma For Dummies
  0-7645-4233-8
- Controlling Cholesterol For Dummies
  0-7645-5440-9
- Depression For Dummies
  0-7645-3900-0
- Dieting For Dummies
  0-7645-4149-8
- Fertility For Dummies
  0-7645-2549-2

- Fibromyalgia For Dummies
  0-7645-5441-7
- Improving Your Memory For Dummies
  0-7645-5435-2
- Pregnancy For Dummies †
  0-7645-4483-7
- Quitting Smoking For Dummies
  0-7645-2629-4
- Relationships For Dummies
  0-7645-5384-4
- Thyroid For Dummies
  0-7645-5385-2

EDUCATION, HISTORY, REFERENCE & TEST PREPARATION

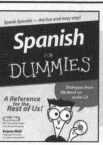

0-7645-5194-9

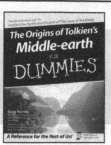

0-7645-4186-2

Also available:
- Algebra For Dummies
  0-7645-5325-9
- British History For Dummies
  0-7645-7021-8
- Calculus For Dummies
  0-7645-2498-4
- English Grammar For Dummies
  0-7645-5322-4
- Forensics For Dummies
  0-7645-5580-4
- The GMAT For Dummies
  0-7645-5251-1
- Inglés Para Dummies
  0-7645-5427-1

- Italian For Dummies
  0-7645-5196-5
- Latin For Dummies
  0-7645-5431-X
- Lewis & Clark For Dummies
  0-7645-2545-X
- Research Papers For Dummies
  0-7645-5426-3
- The SAT I For Dummies
  0-7645-7193-1
- Science Fair Projects For Dummies
  0-7645-5460-3
- U.S. History For Dummies
  0-7645-5249-X

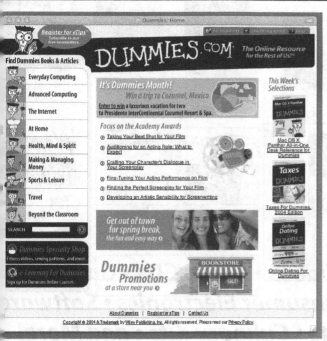

Get smart @ dummies.com®

- **Find a full list of Dummies titles**
- **Look into loads of FREE on-site articles**
- **Sign up for FREE eTips e-mailed to you weekly**
- **See what other products carry the Dummies name**
- **Shop directly from the Dummies bookstore**
- **Enter to win new prizes every month!**

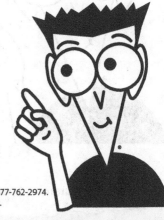

Separate Canadian edition also available
Separate U.K. edition also available

Available wherever books are sold. For more information or to order direct: U.S. customers visit www.dummies.com or call 1-877-762-2974. U.K. customers visit www.wileyeurope.com or call 0800 243407. Canadian customers visit www.wiley.ca or call 1-800-567-4797.

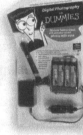
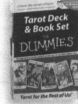
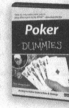
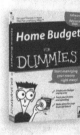
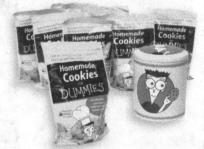
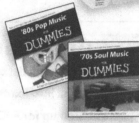
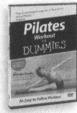
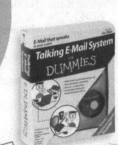
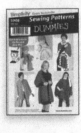
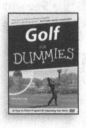
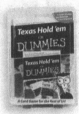
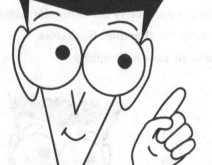